Yoga and Phenomenology on Consciousness

T0387522

SUNY series, Perspectives in Contemplative Studies

Harold D. Roth and Judith Simmer-Brown, editors

Yoga and Phenomenology on Consciousness

GIULIA MOIRAGHI

SUNY
PRESS

Cover credit: *Leaf, flower, and fruit mandala,* Kudle Beach, Gokarna, Karnataka, India 2025. Photograph by Silvana Montini.

Published by State University of New York Press, Albany

© 2025 State University of New York

All rights reserved

Printed in the United States of America

No part of this book may be used or reproduced in any manner whatsoever without written permission. No part of this book may be stored in a retrieval system or transmitted in any form or by any means including electronic, electrostatic, magnetic tape, mechanical, photocopying, recording, or otherwise without the prior permission in writing of the publisher.

Links to third-party websites are provided as a convenience and for informational purposes only. They do not constitute an endorsement or an approval of any of the products, services, or opinions of the organization, companies, or individuals. SUNY Press bears no responsibility for the accuracy, legality, or content of a URL, the external website, or for that of subsequent websites.

EU GPSR Authorised Representative:
Logos Europe, 9 rue Nicolas Poussin, 17000, La Rochelle, France
contact@logoseurope.eu

For information, contact State University of New York Press, Albany, NY
www.sunypress.edu

Library of Congress Cataloging-in-Publication Data

Name: Moiraghi, Giulia, author.
Title: Yoga and phenomenology on consciousness / Giulia Moiraghi.
Description: Albany : State University of New York Press, [2025] | Series: SUNY series, perspectives in contemplative studies | Includes bibliographical references and index.
Identifiers: LCCN 2024057616 | ISBN 9798855803372 (hardcover : alk. paper) | ISBN 9798855803389 (ebook) | ISBN 9798855803396 (pbk. : alk. paper)
Subjects: LCSH: Phenomenology. | Yoga—Psychological aspects.
Classification: LCC B829.5 M636 2025 | DDC 142/.7—dc23/eng/20250115
LC record available at https://lccn.loc.gov/2024057616

To my beloved father,
who showed me the way.
Your dedication to a sincere and lifelong pursuit
will always accompany me.
May the light be with you!

Contents

Acknowledgments		ix
Introduction		1
Chapter 1	What Is Lacking in the Debate on Consciousness?	9
Chapter 2	Epoché and the Horizon Consciousness in Husserl	21
Chapter 3	From Husserl's Consciousness to Heidegger's Being	37
Chapter 4	The Seer and Non-Dual Consciousness	45
Chapter 5	Emptiness and Clear Light Consciousness	65
Chapter 6	Mapping the World Without Independent Essences	85
Chapter 7	The Transformation of Perception in Yoga	99
Chapter 8	A Phenomenological Approach to Practice	123
Chapter 9	Merleau-Ponty and Undoing the Mind-Body Split	143

Acknowledgments

It is because of my students, and because I wanted them to enter the yogic stance in depth, that I developed a phenomenological analysis of the core dimension of the practice. I am immensely grateful to them for having chosen this path and sharing the commitment throughout the years. Thank you for being there.

Without Prof. Bruno Neri, who involved me in the Summer School on Consciousness and Cognition at the University of Pisa, this text would never have seen the light of day: I convey my heartfelt thanks to him for the stimulation and support he provided. Thanks to Prof. Pierluigi Barrotta for trusting me at the beginning of the project. A special thanks goes to Prof. Franco Giorgi, who had the patience to read a draft of the text and encouraged me to clarify a few points. Thanks to Prof. Michel Bitbol for the enlightening conversations we have had in recent years. Thank you to Giacomo de Luca, scholar in philosophy, for having started to explore these matters in depth from the time we met, for the vital exchanges, for the corrections and for his contribution to the enterprise.

I am very grateful to my mother, Maria, who always favored and encouraged my engagement in the practice. With her smiling openness to the world she has set a living example for me.

Finally, an incommensurable thanks to my father, Alfredo, who just passed away due to an illness, for being the first to talk to me about the problem of consciousness when I was very young, for all that he has passed on to me, and for believing in this project even more than I did.

Introduction

This book argues that beneath the content-directed cognitive dimensions of consciousness exists a dimension that is prereflective and embodied. Delving into the world of yoga sheds light on this underlying and overlooked dimension of consciousness.

The methodological key in the approach to yoga is not internal to a specific lineage or tradition, which would lead to a sector-based or cultural line of inquiry but is provided by phenomenology, granted that within this philosophical approach there is no single line of thought but rather a series of developments from a common starting point: the suspension of the "natural attitude" toward reality, in order to experiment with the space of consciousness in which the world gives-itself-out. Yoga, as a psycho-physical practice, though likewise multifaceted and irremediably plural in its expressions, shares this common core: the highlighting of a dimension of consciousness that is prior to any specific content and that is "always already there" when one starts to think about it. In opposition to the current widespread trend of arguing for the nonexistence of yoga as such because of the changing forms it has undergone over time, the author claims that its fundamental invariant feature is a purification process leading to the recognition of the space of the "appearing as such," or the space of consciousness.

The author considers a number of yogic paths aimed at overcoming duality by suspending the discursive conceptual mind, either by going all the way through its dynamic and discovering how it ultimately reveals its empty nature, or by tuning in to the opposite pole: the embodied field of perception. This second strategy has been more carefully looked at because it appears especially useful to explore for Western readers, as they are for the most part unfamiliar with the process of undergoing a deeply embodied experience: an experience in which the body is not merely one more object alongside others, but the fundamental means through which one realizes the underlying *continuum* of subject and world.

From the phenomenological perspective of an experiential fundamentalism, consciousness is not reducible to the physical world but also does not belong to a protopsychic objectlike essence. As the book shows, it is more like a threshold, involving a dynamic between the visible and its horizon; it is an irreducible gap between what is clear and its unclear distant background: the reversibility of touching and being touched.

This book will appeal to both researchers (philosophers, psychologists, cognitive scientists) and to the full spectrum of practitioners of psychophysical disciplines. More specifically it urges researchers to become acquainted with a dimension of consciousness that has been widely neglected in the ongoing neuroscientific debate; similarly, it calls on practitioners from diverse experiential backgrounds to adopt, along with the specific door that opened their personal practice, a "phenomenological stance" that will provide them with a wider and more in-depth understanding of the domain to which they have committed themselves.

Since the publication of *The Embodied Mind* by Varela, Thompson, and Rosch[1] in 1991, an entire strand of research has centered on the similarities between Husserl's phenomenology and Buddhist meditation. This book broadens the topic by taking into account phenomenological insights not only from Husserl but also particularly from his students (Martin Heidegger, Maurice Merleau-Ponty, Francisco Varela, Jan Patočka). On the Eastern side it considers, next to Buddhist meditation, the more comprehensive dimension of yoga, drawing from the *Veda, Upaniṣad*, Nāgārjuna, Patañjali, Padmasambhava, Milarepa, Tzong Khapa, Kālacakra tradition, and Svātmārāma.

Although in contemporary parlance "yoga" has become virtually synonymous with a purely physical activity, even to the point of being set in opposition to "meditation," it is taken here to include the dimension of meditation as a stage along the yogic path, with references not only to Patañjali's yoga *darśana* but also to subsequent *haṭha* yoga traditions, in both the Buddhist and Śaiva matrices.

At the same time, this book offers a detailed discussion of Eastern traditions through a rigorous textual examination, including key original Sanskrit terms, in order to build a comparative analysis allowing Eastern philosophical topics to be translated into Western terminology. The last part of the book offers several applied instructions on how to practice from a phenomenological standpoint.

In our postmodern era, at the end of the great narratives,[2] yoga appears to be one of the few remaining transformative tools capable of shaping everyday life: thus, it needs to be taken into account by philosophical research. With a PhD in philosophy and an engaged and long-term personal yoga practice as favorable starting conditions, the author demonstrates that this connection has been realized on the ground as a knot of intersection between—or even a "short-circuit" of—two lines of investigation; namely, yoga practice and phenomenological exploration. The approach that has been chosen for the investigation is thematic rather than introductory to the various subjects and moments traced along the journey. The aim in fact is to unfold for the reader a synthesis of the path the author has undergone in straddling the two domains and applying certain fundamental features of phenomenology in a direction other than the one to which they originally referred (Husserl's original intention was re-founding of Western science); namely toward the yoga practice itself.

This enterprise has nothing in common with the many instances of the appropriation and assimilation of Indian philosophy by Western authors that date back centuries. Their overall aim was to align Indian concepts with Western ones, despite the often irreconcilable discrepancies between them. In order to promote the reading of Eastern texts and overcome resistance, translators and commentators sometimes tended to emphasize parallels while ignoring differences: there was, for example, a persistent tendency to translate Brahman as God and Ātman as soul.[3] Acknowledging this and other trends toward forced homogenization rightly led, in the late twentieth century, to the emergence of movements exposing those decisions and raising awareness of neocolonialist and Eurocentric tendencies. However, there exists an equally regrettable complementary tendency, which can be described as a form of "learned isolationism." In an effort to preserve the "otherness" of Eastern traditions, these are often kept separate, as if under a bell jar. This move avoids the necessity of integrating Eastern traditions into contemporary philosophical discourse and meaningfully engaging with them. This, too, constitutes a form of violence, albeit more insidious, as it effectively halts dialogue. Under the guise of historicism and ethnography, research on yoga is marginalized and its significance weakened. The Indian philosopher Surendranath Dasgupta, teacher of Mircea Eliade, had already sensed this trend a century ago: "A celebrated Russian Sanskritist once remarked to me that when we had succeeded in making a thing unintelligent, mysterious and dead, then only we say—'Look now it is true and genuine Indian: it looks antique."[4] The excessive fear of encountering the Other by beginning from one's own standpoint, which is indeed essential for a genuine understanding, results in relegating Eastern subjects to a merely taxonomical inquiry that focuses on historico-lexical elements but neglects the vital task of imbuing them with meaning.

By contrast, yogic practices aim at a kind of universalism, seeking to reach everyone, regardless of religious or geographical background.[5] To honor that calling, this book deploys phenomenology as a tool in the service of yoga; it is a tool that aims to be universal in its revelatory capacity. The two domains, by renouncing any form of rigidity or preeminence, engage in a close dialogue and mutually transform each other. This, in the belief that the search for an original yoga alongside the assertion of a true phenomenology, is a recurring superstition of which we should be wary.

The author has lectured on some of these topics for the last five or so years at the interdisciplinary Summer School on Consciousness and Cognition and at the Master Program on Neuroscience, Mindfulness and Contemplative Practices of the University of Pisa and has been asked to write a book on these subjects so that students around the world could be provided with a text. That is how this project began. As the writing process evolved, the work became more of a monograph with an unprecedented thesis, without losing its original didactic intention and interdisciplinary nature. It is worth noting that the book fits within the framework sought by the University of Pisa when hosting the First Symposium "The Mindscience of Reality" in 2017 (with His Holiness the Dalai Lama as guest of honor), which led to the first institutional agreement between the University of Pisa and the Sera Jey Monastic University for Advanced Buddhist Studies & Practice.

Chapter-by-Chapter Description

Chapter 1 introduces some fundamental terminology in the debate on consciousness as it appears in analytical philosophy and cognitive science, highlighting how that debate does not yet cover the problem of consciousness to its full extent because it ignores the question of a "horizon" or "background" consciousness. The author argues that taking a closer look at the experiential dimensions opened through a phenomenological approach to yoga might reveal the paradox in the study of consciousness that confronts current scientific research. Toward the end of the chapter the author explores the relationship between this overlooked dimension of consciousness and the question of embodiment.

After having explained some basic aspects of Husserlian phenomenology, chapter 2 argues that Husserl, especially in his later works, was interested in a dimension that exceeds intentionality. Husserl sketches a transcendental domain that is described in Gestalt terms as the domain of a distant consciousness. This dimension of consciousness does not concern a specific content but the relationship between that content and its unclear horizon; in other words, it involves a dynamic taking place between something clear and its undetermined background.

Chapter 3 seeks to bridge Husserl's insights into the rarely tackled theme of the background consciousness with Heidegger's philosophy. More specifically, Heidegger's notion of Being, which is generally considered a completely different outcome of the phenomenological inquiry in respect to Husserl's premises, is connected to Husserl's interest in the transcendental domain of the horizon consciousness. The author argues that Heidegger, through the exploration of the attitude of "letting be," also provides the reader with some practical advice on how to recognize a dimension of consciousness that is unhooked from the psychological "I."

A time and place shift takes place in chapter 4: the focus of the inquiry turns eastward. More specifically, the author suggests that the aforementioned dimension of consciousness is at the center of Eastern yogic traditions. The author argues that the goal of yogic practices is a process of purification leading to a higher state of consciousness that is disconnected from the empirical "I." The concept of purification is explored from its Vedic origins to its popular thematization in Patañjali's *Yogasūtra*. The author then uses a comparative analysis to show how the concepts of epoché and purification from phenomenology are useful in understanding what is at the heart of yoga.

Chapter 5 deals with the unobjectifying demands concerning the theme of consciousness in Buddhist yogic milieux and their kinship with a phenomenological approach that avoids reification. It considers the meaning of emptiness and dependent origination in the thought of Mahāyāna Buddhist philosopher Nāgārjuna, in dialogue with Heidegger. Drawing on Tibetan yogic teachings (Padmasambhava, Milarepa, Tzong Khapa, and the Kālacakra tradition), the author argues that the notions of emptiness and clear light consciousness refer to the dimension of consciousness to which phenomenology has been pointing from the start.

The previously explored denial of the concept of "inherent existence" is connected at the beginning of chapter 6 to relational interpretations of quantum physics, reflecting the interdisciplinary perspective that characterizes the book as a whole. The value of a pragmatic approach to science, according to which the scientific result has no inherent nature but is a tool to efficiently orient in the world, is traced back on one side to Heidegger's analysis of scientific idealities and on the other to Varela's concept of enaction and structural coupling. The debate on consciousness introduced in the first chapter is recalled in relation to Varela's contribution in terms of neurophenomenology.

Chapter 7 suggests adopting the phenomenological distinction between the body-as-object and the lived-body in order to overcome many of the misunderstandings around the notion of body in Eastern traditions. After having explored the subtle yogic physiology, as it appears, for example, in the *Haṭhayogapradīpikā,* it is argued that it has strong value in terms of deconstruction in that it is capable of undermining previous crystalized habits. At the end of the chapter, the dominant view—according to which bodily postures heavily characterize only modern yoga—is questioned.

In chapter 8, the meaning of the *āsana* is taken to reside particularly in its capacity to undermine the identification with the empirical "I." It is argued that from a phenomenological perspective, the required physical effort experienced in the *āsana* has the role of inhibiting and dismantling previous trends and habits, whereas the ensuing phase of release is the perfect cultural space to access the dimension of the appearing, a dimension that Patočka has defined as an a-subjective consciousness. Two moments are thus traced within a phenomenologically inspired practice: a moment where "doing" prevails, and a moment where "letting be" takes over.

The final chapter is an in-depth exploration of Merleau-Ponty's insights into the theme of body and perception. Through a close reading of Merleau-Ponty's use of language, the author identifies several hints in order to reframe the question of the physical to advance the understanding of consciousness. Practical cues and detailed instructions are provided so that the reader can start testing on the ground what may have previously been intuited solely on the intellectual level. Future outcomes of the inquiry are outlined at the end of the chapter.

The reader will note that key terms in German and Sanskrit have been included between square brackets within the text. This has been done for the sake of transparency, since much too often scholarship on both phenomenology and Eastern traditions lacks sufficient references to the original terms and thus risks becoming an arbitrary instrument of questionable usefulness. Certain key terms (like *Tapas* in Sanskrit and *Leib* in German) are used instead of English terms once they have been carefully defined so that even the reader new to phenomenology, to yoga, or to both, will know what they mean.

Chapter 1

What Is Lacking in the Debate on Consciousness?

A Paradox in the Study of Consciousness

The current debate on consciousness in the philosophy of mind and cognitive science generally assumes that a conscious state can be recognized by the presence of information in the cognitive system available for verbal report and behavioral control, within an overall sense of selfhood. This volume interrogates this dominant axiom that binds consciousness with cognitive functions,[1] with information availability in terms of representational contents, and with the sense of I-ness. There are in fact many cases of yogic or meditative states that are not paired with content availability and verbal report and in which the identification with the "I" subsides; in the West, these are called "non-ordinary states of consciousness." It is these very states that are considered in Eastern traditions the most significant and representative occurrences of a conscious experience. By contrast, what we consider our default state of consciousness—that of a normally alienated egocentric individual mastering ordinary cognitive abilities—in the East is generally considered a detrimental state and in no way represents the benchmark of how a conscious state should unfold.

The paradox in the study of consciousness that we are currently facing is that the incidental conscious state of a well-educated twenty-first-century Westerner is described as the intrinsic conscious modality of the human being as such. In other words, a highly contingent dimension of consciousness, linked to a specific time set and to specific worldly practices, is surreptitiously setting the standard for what is considered worthy of devotion in terms of study.

Making the effort to zoom out of our cultural and geographic constraints to see the bigger picture concerning the theme of consciousness will certainly make a difference not only in theoretical research but also in connected applications like the domains of artificial intelligence and robotics. Furthermore, considering the modification of our concept of consciousness according to values and worldviews that differ from the dominant paradigm will also have crucial impacts on the ethical debates over issues like the end of life and vegetative states.

William James himself, the founder of the debate on consciousness in the English-speaking world, in *Varieties of Religious Experience* claims that, next to the "ordinary state of consciousness [. . .] there lie potential forms of consciousness entirely different" and that "no account of the universe in its totality can be final which leaves these forms of consciousness disregarded," concluding that "at any rate, they forbid a premature closing of our accounts with reality."[2]

Objecting that nonrepresentational dimensions of consciousness[3] would by definition fall outside the domain of denotative language and thus be impossible to identify is a weak argument. The Aha! moments each of us lives through—whether they be connected to love or death, to a particular natural scene or a work of art—are all beyond the domain of what is describable through the *logos*, but few would venture to state that such dimensions do not exist or are not worthy of examination. What is so important about yogic states compared to these occurrences is that they offer the possibility of tuning in to an underlying, prereflective dimension of consciousness not by chance but in a programmatic way. In other words, if one can enter the condition of realizing the a-subjective continuum of consciousness in the face of a natural scene, this fortunate moment might not be enough to shake the usual identification with a unified pole of cognitive material because that identification has stabilized and crystalized over time. By contrast, yogic practices offer a specific deconditioning training to realize this preordained dimension of consciousness: the dimension of appearing as such.

At the same time, this volume urges taking a very close look at the school of phenomenology. The phenomenological lineage is a notably unique example within Western philosophical panoramas of an inquiry centered on exploring this overlooked continuum of consciousness. For this reason, familiarizing oneself with the phenomenological stance means becoming empowered with a tool to access yogic dimensions.

A Brief Overview of a Few Concepts in the Debate on Consciousness

Before devoting further introductory remarks to the enterprise attempted here, it is worth dedicating a few paragraphs to support what has been claimed to this point. This will be done through a brief overview of a couple of concepts that are central to analytical and neuroscientific inquiry and that have had a powerful influence on the ongoing discussion about the mind.

Philosopher David Chalmers claims that "wherever there is conscious experience, there is some corresponding information in the cognitive system that is available in the control of behavior, and available for verbal report. Conversely, it seems that whenever information is available for report and for global control, there is corresponding conscious experience."[4] In cognitive scientist Bernard Baars's global workspace theory,[5] consciousness concerns information accessibility in terms of representation,[6] with prereflective layers of consciousness simply ignored. In a more recent article, Baars envisages the space for a "consciousness without content" that he calls "silent consciousness" and calls for a "principled method to study the psychophysics of momentary silent consciousness," which is still to be worked out.[7] Stanislas Dehaene refines Baars's assumptions in what he calls a global "neuronal" workspace model according to which, again, what consciousness stands for is the broadcasting of global information across the brain available for computation, report, and self-monitoring.[8] Higher-order theories[9] according to which experience can be conscious only because of another state of a higher order about that same experience, are still representationalist theories.[10]

Daniel Dennett, for his part, ends up considering in his multiple draft model (in which the idea of a special unified center in the brain is discarded) only the potential reportability of a specific mental content.[11] Dennett reaches the point of saying that any theory separating "consciousness" from "function" should also be discarded: "We argue that all theories of consciousness that are not based on functions and access are not scientific theories."[12]

Continuing this brief review, reference should be made to a recent article in which neuroscientist Thomas Metzinger takes into account the experience of "phenomenality" as encountered in a number of meditation reports.[13] This is an encouraging enterprise in that it programmatically seeks to create the initial foundations of a study of "pure consciousness" in its own right that, according to Metzinger, is usually neglected in neuroscientific inquiry. However, Metzinger starts off by defining this experience as a "minimal phenomenal experience" in that it would entail a low-complexity and nonagentive variety of knowing.[14] Defining the luminous consciousness typical of yogic states as a "minimal phenomenal experience" sounds quite odd, for in contemplative practices it is instead considered the maximal experience a human being can come across. Metzinger acknowledges a possible functional correlation of the minimal phenomenal experience with "tonic alertness," a functional property of the cingulo-opercular (CO) network[15] after having established six constraints that emerged from a number of case studies.[16] Metzinger does not hide his theoretical strategy of re-including "pure consciousness" in a representationalist model of the mind and turning the specifically "content-less" phenomenal state reported in first-person accounts of pure consciousness into an alleged "abstract form of intentional content."[17] But it is especially the ambivalence toward the question of the body within "minimal phenomenal experience"(both excluded in terms of the "absence of low-level embodiment" and "interoception" and reclaimed as a "maximally abstract form of embodiment"[18]) that does not receive a clear thematization and thus calls for a deeper understanding of the relationship between body and consciousness.

Nearly half a century ago, philosopher Thomas Nagel chose the mental experiment of imagining "what it is like" for a bat to be a bat[19] and thus acknowledged the existence of a fundamental dimension of consciousness not linked to a given representational content; Joseph Levine pointed in a similar direction when speaking of *qualia* or "qualitative sensory experiences"[20] and acknowledging the existence of an "explanatory gap" between the brain's neural processes and the experiences related to them. This explanatory gap is what Chalmers later defined as the "hard problem of consciousness." In fact, while the "easy problems of consciousness" concern "an explanation of cognitive abilities and functions"[21] that entail only a correlation between a function and an underlying physical-neural mechanism, the hard problem of consciousness lies in investigating why "the performance of these functions [is] accompanied by experience."[22] However, as noted above, Chalmers considers conscious experience as happening only in combination with cognitive faculties, by virtue of what he calls the principle of "structural coherence" or "correspondence" between "the various functional phenomena that are associated with consciousness," understood as "those information contents that are accessible to central [cognitive] systems,"[23] and the experiential dimension.

Philosopher Ned Block brought the well-known distinction between "phenomenal consciousness" and "access consciousness" into the discussion, with the first involving experiential dimensions and the second referring to "cognitive, intentional or functional"[24] properties within the general "executive system." However, instead of clearing up the confusion that surrounds the concept of consciousness, which he defines as "hybrid" or "mongrel" in that it connotes "a number of different concepts," Block retains significant ambiguity regarding the concept of "phenomenal consciousness," which is oddly connected both to sensations and perceptions (the "what it is like" experience) and to "thoughts, desires and emotions."[25] Furthermore, Block takes phenomenal consciousness to be "distinct from any cognitive, intentional, or functional property"[26] but at the same time "often representational."[27] For this reason, we will not employ the term "phenomenal consciousness" when referring to the experiential conscious domain here at stake.

This continuum of consciousness, this wide field of awareness, is so unbound from cognitive functions that, according to Eastern yogic perspectives, it also remains unbroken during dreamless sleep. And this is the point at which Eastern and Western views on consciousness diverge without return. In fact, the philosopher John Searle has stated that consciousness begins when one wakes in the morning and continues "throughout the period that one is awake until one falls into a dreamless sleep, into a coma, or dies or is otherwise, as they say, unconscious."[28] Searle's words have recently been echoed by psychiatrist Giulio Tononi, who claims that "everybody knows what consciousness is: it is what vanishes every night when we fall into dreamless sleep and reappears when we wake up or when we dream. It is also all we are and all we have: lose consciousness and, as far as you are concerned, your own self and the entire world dissolve into nothingness."[29] However, it is well known that in different Eastern philosophies in the Vedanta, Buddhist, and Śaiva traditions, dreamless sleep is actually considered a fuller state of consciousness than those experienced during ordinary wakefulness and dreaming. It is very similar, according to the *Māṇḍūkya Upaniṣad*,[30] and other sources, to the states of consciousness found in meditation and called "Prajñā." The fact that once awake one forgets about that particular experiential state does not imply that consciousness was absent but should rather be taken as a sign of the fact that memory was not triggered in the usual way in that condition. Though detailed memory is lacking, there is still a trace of the quality of what is experienced during sleep[31] that justifies the common expression "I slept well last night."

What Tononi points out[32] is that dreamless (i.e., non-REM) sleep happens as a result of a loss of ordinary connectivity and integration among cortical areas. Recent studies have shown how a similarly altered brain connectivity that reverses the flow of neural connectivity from the anterior to the posterior regions of the cortex[33] also takes place during slow nasal breathing stimulation.[34] This artificial process partly simulates what happens to the olfactory bulb (and to the connected brain cortex) during the slow *prāṇāyāma* breathing of yoga. In other words, the pattern of neural connectivity that emerges during sleep appears to have something important in common with the one present during the *prāṇāyāma* state.

In fact, if neural connectivity, which is also called the "connectome," is according to Sebastian Seung[35] what makes us "who we are," yogic conscious states are likely related to a dramatic modification of this connectivity. Yoga and contemplative practices are precisely all about suspending "who we are": holding in abeyance the belief in what we think we are enables us to access a level of consciousness different from the ordinary one, a dimension in which one forgets about the "I."

It should be noted that in ancient Indian inquiry the nose was considered the receptor of the *prāṇa,* the vital energy within the body that modulates the different states of consciousness accessed by the mind-body complex. In the *Bṛhadāraṇyaka Upaniṣad* it is said that the nose, meant to be a perceptive organ, is the receptor of vital energy: "*prāṇo vai grahaḥ.*"[36] Is there any reason why the ongoing debate on consciousness should not consider in fine detail the inner experiences that yogis carried out in previous millennia on the subject of consciousness, which Westerners have only seriously been debating for little more than a century? The connections between the olfactory bulb and the states of consciousness that contemporary neuroscience is discovering appear to have been anticipated by a couple thousand years in the first-person explorations of the yogis, in terms of inner empiricism.[37] The renowned suspension [*nirodhaḥ*] of the fluctuations [*vṛtti*] of the mind-space [*citta*] invoked by Patañjali when defining yoga[38] could be taken as an extended metaphor to describe what is now identified as a dis-facilitation of ordinary neural integration. If Tononi's integrated information theory (IIT) considers cognitive functions to be the result of a reduction in uncertainty and thus an increase in information, could it not perhaps conversely show that certain states of consciousness, such as yogic states, are related to a functional change in the human connectome and to an increase in uncertainty?[39]

These working hypotheses might very well be discarded or ruled out in the following steps when tested with appropriate rigor, but they can only be examined—in both senses of the term—from an interdisciplinary standpoint. It is for this reason that it is worth researchers making the effort to enter yogic traditions in depth; the journey will certainly bring unprecedented hints and perspectives to the ongoing inquiry into consciousness.

Therefore, instead of rushing to discover the missing "extra ingredient," next to physical properties that would account for consciousness, we should take a step back to become clear with what is actually at stake when we are referring to consciousness. Before launching into metaphysical issues and taxonomies involving materialist,[40] nonreductionist,[41] monist, or dualist views of the world between which to choose—that is, before trying to envisage the place of consciousness in nature—the very concept of consciousness needs to be worked out from a more comprehensive point of view. Prior to establishing whether consciousness is a fundamental property of reality that takes its place next to physical properties (along with the Cartesian reminiscence of the *res cogitans* and *res extensa*) or if it is reducible to them, we need to return to the unseen assumptions that stand under what people generally mean by consciousness.

Philosopher Evan Thompson, after having distinguished consciousness viewed as "perceptual or cognitive awareness, that is, the kind of awareness that targets a specific object" from consciousness as "the total field of awareness,"[42] points in the direction of reframing the question of the "physical" in order to advance the understanding of consciousness: "We need to work our way to a new understanding of what it means for something to be physical, in which 'physical' no longer means essentially nonmental or nonexperiential."[43] For this reason, entering yogic traditions will help us to understand the problem of the body and its nonunivocal status.

The Overlooked Dimension of Consciousness and Embodiment

In this book, yoga is explored with the aim of offering different insights into the theme of consciousness and addressing some of the key questions that ongoing research has left unanswered. The key to carrying out this exploration will be phenomenological because phenomenology from the outset has concentrated on bringing to the surface this usually unseen dimension of consciousness. Edmund Husserl calls it "transcendental consciousness," Martin Heidegger refers to it as the "forgotten dimension of Being," and Maurice Merleau-Ponty intends it as that intertwining of subject and world that very much influenced Francisco Varela's idea of a structural coupling.

The central claim here is not that phenomenology, as initially conceived by Edmund Husserl, has striking similarities with yogic or meditative practices (which are of course present along with some differences). This has already been attempted in a few pioneering essays; the authors proposing these connections have the merit of highlighting certain fundamental shared features but nevertheless end up reaffirming the notion that Husserl's commitment to reflection and intentionality does not leave enough space for a far-reaching comparison with the deeper dimensions of absorption explored, for instance, in Patañjali's yoga.[44] Other authors have been particularly focused on reclaiming a conceptual and discursive status for Indian philosophies and, to achieve that goal, bend them toward the rational approach of phenomenology.[45]

Instead, this volume shows that by understanding certain phenomenological features, one can not only describe in detail and away from esoteric drift what is actually going on within yoga practice but also, and consequently, orient the practitioner coming from a Western cultural background toward the goal of accessing this overlooked dimension of consciousness. This enterprise is attempted, on the one hand, by concentrating on what in Husserl overwhelms the vexed question of intentionality and on the other by taking into account phenomenological insights not only from Husserl but also and especially from his students: those who have taken up his phenomenology and developed it in deeply personal and specific directions.

This book emerged not as a result of a scholarly inquiry, at least in the first instance, but as an inevitable outcome of just such a personal experience: the author had to come to terms with a phenomenological mindset and a committed, lifelong yoga practice. For this reason, there is no intention of entering into the historiographical debate on phenomenology or on the different yogic practices taken into account. That would take us back to the specializing tendencies dominating the academic world that fragment knowledge and that were denounced by Husserl in the *Crisis of the European Sciences*.[46] In a context in which Eastern studies are still almost exclusively the preserve of Sanskritists and Indologists[47] and thus have no chance of dialoguing with ongoing research on consciousness, which in turn exempts itself from considering conceptual problems coming from a non-European matrix, this work overcomes the persistent Hegelian insistence[48] on the inferiority of non-Western philosophies, still mainly considered sector-specific and cultural fields of interest. "The exclusion of India from the history of philosophy,"[49] as Wilhelm Halbfass put it, always appears more anachronistic in a period like the current age, when an overwhelming increase in the popularity of and interest in yoga in the Western world is clear to everyone.

The insights that emerge from this enterprise will lead to unprecedented yoga practice methods, phenomenological yoga practices that are capable of disclosing a dimension of consciousness that is the total field of awareness or the condition of possibility of any single experience. Before any specific content can fill our mind, and even prior to the awareness of being a specific, individual self, there is an undeniable evidence[50]: the evidence that the lights are on or that there is a "no-thing-ness" [*Nichten*], a null, an emptiness, which comes before any single entity and is a kind of receptacle that ultimately coincides with Being itself, as Heidegger puts it.[51] The question of to whom this evidence is given would not be appropriate in reference to a dimension of consciousness that has no owner, that overcomes not only the borders of the "I" understood as selfhood but also overflows the very boundary we have learned since childhood to posit between what we call "subject" and what we call "object."

The fact that this dimension of pure consciousness has been taken for granted, if not ignored or denied by some authors in the West is no proof of its lack of existence but more likely results from the fact that it is not an object, as suggested in the *Bṛhadāraṇyaka Upaniṣad* when referring to the dimension of the Seer: this Ātman is "never seen, but is the Seer [*Draṣṭṛ*]; It is never heard, but is the Hearer; It is never thought, but is the Thinker; It is never known, but is the Knower."[52] In our everyday natural attitude, we are always and only searching for objects and have "unlearned to desire anything other than *objects*,"[53] so it is little wonder that contemporary research sometimes confuses consciousness with objectifiable processes in the brain. Fortunately, both phenomenology and yoga teach us to desire something else, to place our interest on what Jan Patočka calls the "appearing as such."[54] This fundamental and preordained dimension of consciousness can be recognized and hinted at through a phenomenological-yogic stance because it appeals to the lived body. In fact, no matter how surprising it may sound, the door to entering this dimension of consciousness, which is both unobjectifiable and unaccountable through merely denotative language, is neither disembodied nor dematerialized. On the contrary, the gateway to it stems from the very depth that we share with the world, from that "intertwining" that Merleau-Ponty calls "la *Chair*." It is our embodiment that enables us to tune in to it: "The thickness of the body, far from rivaling that of the world, is on the contrary the sole means I have to go unto the heart of the things, by making myself a world and by making them flesh."[55] Merleau-Ponty also points out that "this ultimate consciousness is not an eternal subject perceiving itself in absolute transparency . . . it is the consciousness of the present. In the present and in perception, my being and my consciousness are at one."[56]

In the last few decades, several studies have centered on the idea that the notion of mind should include its somatic embedment and the interactions with the environment, leading to concepts such as "embodied cognition"[57] or the "extended mind."[58] However, what is explored more specifically in this book is the fact that living our body according to specific corporeal and breathing techniques can disclose normally unnoticed dimensions of consciousness. This approach is taken in the firm belief that a "return to the body" will become more than a mere motto or manifesto from the moment it is grounded in something more than the simple assessment of the presence of a body, irrespective of its placement in space and time and of its relation to the breath. The embodiment taking place within a practitioner,[59] in which moments of intentional effort followed by release are experienced according to a specific dynamic, is radically different from what happens within a body that is nailed to the chair. Many of the exponents who have fostered and encouraged a return to the sensory realm (starting with the great phenomenologists of the last century) actually kept themselves from coming to terms with a more radical involvement with the potentialities of a lived-through body: this is nothing less than bizarre[60] and calls for contemporary research to put aside any underlying prejudice about what would be compromised with corporeal shallowness and to plunge into this fundamental mode of existence: our incarnated Being.

Chapter 2

Epoché and the Horizon Consciousness in Husserl

Husserl and the East

Edmund Husserl's first love was the hard sciences: he obtained his PhD with the work *Contributions to the Calculus of Variations* and published *Philosophy of Arithmetic* in 1881 and *Logical Investigations* in 1901. With a background as a mathematician, he placed the principle of absolute justification and apodicticity[1] at the base of his enterprise. Husserl's initial goal was gnoseological: he wanted to re-found Western science on a more solid basis and to reach a universal justified starting point. However, he realized along the way that a phenomenological approach to reality brought about a "complete personal transformation"[2] and ended up speaking about "the greatest existential conversion"[3] that takes place within the phenomenologist. In Husserl's view, this existential enterprise could eventually involve the whole of humanity: "the possibility of radically changing all human existence through this epoché which reaches into its philosophical depth."[4] What could the reason be for this shift in language and tone?[5] Was Husserl influenced by Eastern traditions in developing his phenomenology?

Husserl left an enthusiastic review of the Neumann edition of the Buddhist *Suttapitaka*, claiming that the Buddhist method is "of the highest dignity for spiritual purification and pacification, a method thought through and carried out with an internal consistency, an energy and a nobility of mind which are almost unmatched" and concluding that "Buddhism can be paralleled only with the highest formations of the philosophical and religious spirit of our European culture."[6] However, Husserl later returned to espousing the traditional superiority that Western philosophy had always claimed in relation to Eastern forms of knowledge, which he considered mere "empirical anthropological" types,[7] arguing that Europeans capable of rightly understanding themselves would thus never "Indianize."[8] Had Husserl's "examination of other systems indeed been sufficient, both as to quantity as well as to quality and method"[9] to reach such conclusions? According to Husserl scholar Karl Schumann, it had not. So, is the present volume's attempt to apply certain phenomenological insights to yoga and contemplative practices flawed from the start? Quite the contrary. Precisely because Husserl's knowledge of Indian philosophy was limited, in both the phases of encomiastic praises and in those of his distancing, the convergences between the insights on consciousness coming from Eastern traditions and those stemming from phenomenology come from the things themselves; that is, from their internal reason, rather than from biographical contingencies or an ideological veneer.

The claim of this work is not that phenomenology is a type of meditative practice, but rather that there are strong points of convergence between phenomenology and yoga that are capable of justifying the hypothesis explored here: that certain fundamental assets of phenomenology can help to understand what is going on within yoga from a nondoctrinal stance.

It should however be said that when the frequent objection is made that meditation should come clear on its aim and establish whether it is a question of exploring the world in a nonjudgmental way or a question of attending to one's own experiences,[10] what seems to be ignored is that these two aspects are not in opposition. Rather, they come together so that it is not a matter of "ambiguities": in both yogic states and phenomenology these two moments are deeply intermingled—two sides of the same coin, as it were—because of the fundamental correlation between world and consciousness, as I make clear below. In yoga and contemplative practices, the process of suspension can become much more radical than in phenomenology, ultimately entailing a phase in which even "perceptual judgements" are neutralized; in phenomenology, at least as it was initially intended by Edmund Husserl, it is mostly "evaluative judgments" that are asked to be set aside.

Husserl's initial goal required that all pregiven sciences and more generally all assumptions and prejudices [*Vorüberzeugungen, Vorurteile*] undergo an overturning [*Umsturz*].[11] He was interested in "a science of the universal how of the pregivenness of the world, i.e., of what makes it a universal ground for any sort of objectivity."[12] To put it bluntly, Husserl had the feeling that science had followed its objects of study so far that it had lost its connection with the firsthand experience from which they stemmed. Normally, we move into a world about which we have already been told and take for granted. It is somehow already established that the world is out there and made of certain things: trees, tables, computers, people, and so on. This is somehow settled and decided once and for all. Phenomenology asks us to suspend this kind of imprinting and, for a moment, take the world just as it appears in the space of consciousness without having decided whether or not it actually exists out there. A suspension of the ordinary attitude of encountering the world takes place in the form of a neutralization of any judgment about the existence or nonexistence of any object.[13] In other words, the world is taken just as it appears and within the limits in which it appears, without adding anything to this appearing: this is the hard part.

Husserl's attempt to obtain a positive start and a sphere of "first knowledge" unthreatened by doubt entails turning the gaze to an experience of the world in which nothing is taken for granted.[14] In order to gain access to this new type of experience, one must subtract oneself from the naïve beliefs [*Glauben*][15] about the world: "Our purpose is to discover a new scientific domain, one that is to be gained by the method of parenthesizing."[16]

Ordinary Perception vs. Phenomenological Perception

Husserl notes that within ordinary perception [*Wahrnehmung*], there is nothing "pure and adequate,"[17] for an anticipation of a further perceptive confirmation always takes place: "It is essentially impossible for even the spatial shape of the physical thing to be given otherwise than in mere one-sided adumbrations [*Abschattungen*]."[18]

Perception, as normally intended, takes the form of an always better "approximation"[19] to a presupposed external and "transcendent" object that is never given in evidence: "the pure thing seen, what is visible 'of' the thing, is first of all a surface, and in the changing course of seeing I see it now from this 'side,' now from that, continuously perceiving it from ever differing sides. . . . This implies that while the surface is immediately given, I mean more than it offers."[20] From Husserl's point of view, what is called perception consists in an anticipation of a future attunement [*Einstimmigkeit*],[21] including all the corrections needed in view of this ideal approximation [*Aproximationsideal*].[22] Transcendent things end up being nothing more than constituted unities of possible attuned perceptions [*konstituierte Einheiten möglicher einstimmiger Wahrnehmung*].[23] A belief thus happens surreptitiously within ordinary perception and without this belief,[24] perception stops being a perception as normally meant.

As a mental exercise, Husserl suggests that we imagine not positing the existence of any external entity corresponding to the corrections made by approximation. Husserl is not questioning the empirical existence of the world, as a skeptic would,[25] but wants to find out how the experience of the world is given to us when we do not posit any transcendent reality; "transcendent" refers here to an external substance independent from the subject. Husserl wants to discover what is left when the "presumptive" belief in the existence of a world out there is placed out of validity [*ausser geltung setzen*].[26] This means differentiating between the habitual "seeing what" of visual judgment and "seeing as," which sticks to mere appearance; it is about letting go of interest toward objects, be they material entities or concepts intended as theoretical objects (fundamental for our survival in evolutionary terms), and shifting the interest toward the space of consciousness in which these alleged objects are given; the space of attention, which is usually unseen as such, for it is considered simply a means to obtain objects: "But while I am perceiving I can also look, by way of purely "seeing," at the perception, at it itself as it is there, and ignore its relation to the ego, or at least abstract from it. Then the perception which is thereby grasped and delimited in "seeing," is an absolutely given, pure phenomenon in the phenomenological sense, renouncing anything transcendent."[27] In the natural attitude, one tends to single out portions of reality—transcendent objects—within interpretive patterns and strategies fit for survival that entail labeling and classification. In phenomenology, precisely the interest in the objects correlated to the perception taking place is bracketed in favor of an interest in the way things appear and are given firsthand within the space of consciousness; that is, the intentional objects. Husserl exerted an influence on the research of Gestalt psychologists because they were all interested[28] in how things appear (literally, "are positioned [*gestalt*] in front" of the eyes[29]), when our logicizing tendencies are inhibited.

Through a direct examination of experience, Husserl seeks to reach the evidence of perception [*Evidenz der Wahrnehmung*]:[30] "Perceived 'things' are not inferred entities."[31] For example, when one says that "the sun is hot," one is making a statement that entails positing the existence of a transcendent object out there about which heat is being predicated. By realizing that perceiving is different from ascertaining and that in perception no opinions should be created and no conclusions drawn, Husserl defines the "principle of all principles" that will guide the phenomenological method: "that every originary presentive intuition [*Anschauung*] is a legitimizing source of cognition, that everything originarily (so to speak, in its 'personal' actuality) offered to us in 'intuition' is to be accepted simply as what it is presented as being, but also only within the limits in which it is presented there."[32]

Let us take the example of the house from Husserl's repertoire and elaborate on it freely.[33] Imagine someone who has long wanted to buy a house. After years living in rented accommodations, she finally finds herself in the financial position to buy a house with a garden. Consider this person, walking up and down the road waiting for the real estate agent to arrive while looking at the gardens visible from the street, trying to guess which house is the one she will soon see and possibly buy. In this condition, the person is completely caught up by her interest in the house as a transcendent object. The object-house, however, is not a fundamental datum of perception but a "projection of transcendence,"[34] a posited and conceptually fabricated entity that takes up certain meanings within a given community. The person is not perceiving the phenomenon "house" but the entire conceptual apparatus built on it. Only if, as Husserl says, the interest in the house is put out of play—an interest that ultimately equals a directedness toward possession [*Habe gerichtet*][35]—a conversion of both gaze and attitude can take place. The person would only now be able to see a new object of perception, which is not the house but her own "directedness to the house"; that is, how the house is given within the space of consciousness, regardless of whether or not the house X, as we normally intend it, exists out there.[36] Being directed to the house given in perception or volition is the "intentional act" and, according to Husserl, the fundamental datum of experience with which we are confronted once all posited empirical factors have been removed.

It's Not All about Intentionality

At this point, it must be stressed that the analysis of the concept of intentionality developed by Husserl based on Franz Brentano's earlier efforts is usually considered the core of phenomenology as taught in classes on the history of philosophy. Brentano, a psychologist whose major work, *Psychology from an Empirical Standpoint*, was published in 1874 had taken up the scholastic term "intentionality" and reexamined and refined it in psychological terms, concluding, broadly speaking, that consciousness is always directed toward an object and always has a specific content. Husserl began investigating the different acts of consciousness (perceptions, imaginations, memories, and so on), the intentional acts[37] with their constituting elements of the "noesis" (the intentional act as it is given in consciousness), and the "noema" (the content itself of this act), on the basis of Brentano's teachings. It is also true that Husserl dedicates many pages to analyzing cognitive faculties and their specific contents, as some authors coming from a philosophical analytical context contend.[38] However, what is usually not stressed when presenting phenomenology is the fact that Husserl, starting from these elements, comes to envision a dimension of consciousness that overflows the boundaries of intentionality. As will become clear below, what allows Husserl to discover the realm of the transcendental—the very heart of his contribution to philosophy—is the recognition that, surrounding the object-directed field of consciousness, a nonobject-directed space of "mute-validities" arises, a "constantly flowing undetermined horizon."[39] This space, which Husserl at times calls the "background" or "horizon consciousness," is empty of content. The present volume centers on the understanding of this content-free horizon and will lead to rediscovering a dimension of consciousness that is now overlooked. According to the phenomenologist Jan Patočka, the horizon "is not an intention that might be filled";[40] indeed, Husserl is considered by his Czech disciples as the thinker of the horizons of experience,[41] the author who placed the accent on the difference between object-consciousness and horizon-consciousness.[42]

The first move required on the part of the phenomenologist is breaking the tendency to take the world as an end, in the words of Husserl's pupil Eugen Fink,[43] which is achieved by the introduction of a tool that interrupts the attraction toward the mundane interests in which people are caught up in everyday life. The free act of suspending judgment [*freie Tat der Urteilsenthaltung*],[44] which amounts to placing out of validity all the beliefs regarding transcendent existence or nonexistence and consequently of possession, is defined by Husserl as the "phenomenological epoché [ἐποχή],"[45] resorting to the ancient Greek term ἐποχή,[46] which literally means "suspension."

In referring to the "epoché," Husserl speaks of a form of abstention [*Enthaltung*] that breaks with the former way of life and brings about transformation:

> A . . . universal *epoché* is possible, namely, one which puts out of action, with one blow, the total performance running through the whole of natural world-life and through the whole network (whether concealed or open) of validities—precisely that total performance which, as the coherent "natural attitude," makes up "simple straightforward" ongoing life. Through the abstention which inhibits this whole hitherto unbroken way of life a complete transformation of all of life is attained, a thoroughly new way of life.[47]

Husserl argues that his epoché is different than the skeptical version:[48] "I am not negating this 'world' as though I were a sophist; I am not doubting its factual being as though I were a skeptic;

rather I am exercising the 'phenomenological' epoché which also completely shuts me off from any judgment about spatiotemporal factual being."[49]

The epoché "denies to all thematic objects . . . interest in their validity. And obviously in this consists the phenomenological switching-off [*Ausschaltung*]."[50] Husserl refers to the same concept with the expression "method of parenthesizing" [*Methode der Einklammerung*]:[51] "we apply to the object a bracketing, so to say, that shuts it off, an index that says here I want to inhibit every validity, every interest in being [or not being] and in value; I want to attend only to the object as an intentional element of its act, of the act that confers on it validity."[52] This method of bracketing is the method of the phenomenological reduction;[53] it is a reduction in the sense that the transcendence of mundane objects is put out of play, with every "pre-understanding" [*Vormeinung und Mitmeinungen*][54] set aside and not the slightest position or opinion taken about it [*Stellungnahme*].[55]

Husserl reassures us by adding that this bracketing does not imply becoming blind toward the object [*Objektblind*]; on the contrary, it entails remaining a "seer of everything" [*für alles bleibe ich sehend*].[56] But everything is seen as bearing its sense and validity within consciousness: "Strictly speaking, we have not lost anything but rather have gained the whole of absolute being which, rightly understood, contains within itself, constitutes within itself, all worldly transcendencies."[57] "Losing everything means winning everything" and is the necessary way to come to live a real, ultimate life [*letztwahres Leben zuleben*].[58]

Everything is seen as it is given, precisely in as much as it is bracketed [*als eingeklammert gesehen*], and the very self exists both as simple seer and as pure practitioner knowing itself [*als zugleich schlicht Sehender und als reine Selbst erkenntnis Übender*].[59] Husserl makes the point that "I am not the one who dreams and that is dumped into the dream; on the contrary, I am the observer of dreaming and of what is being dreamt, of the fantasizing and of what is fantasized."[60]

Husserl argues that though consciousness itself [*Bewußtsein selbst*][61] tends to remain unseen and hidden [*verborgen*][62] in the ordinary stance, one can bring it to light through the "new" way of observation [*Betrachtungsweise*], the "unnatural stance" [*unnatürliche Einstellung*] from which to consider oneself and the world.[63] This transcendental vision [*transzendentaler Schau*] of the observer trained in the phenomenological method fosters philosophical amazement [*philosophische Staunen*].[64] Husserl compares it to the situation of a blind person who needs to learn to see from scratch: "At the beginning we are in a similar position to that of someone blind since birth who has cataracts removed and must, from that moment, truly begin to learn to see."[65]

Husserl insists that one should suspend [*behalten*][66] everything that is implied and co-posited with the world of experience [*jede Mitsetzung der Erfahrungswelt*] and every statement about its Being or not-Being [*Sein und Nichtsein*]. In order to access the transcendental subjectivity [*transzendentale Subjektivität*], every interest in the existence of the world must be inhibited [*inhibieren wir jedes Interesse am Weltsein*],[67] together with every practical interest [*praktische Interesse*] concerned with value [*Wertinteresse*].[68] This is how the phenomenological method [*phänomenologische Methode*] discloses a new kingdom of experience [*Erfahrungsreich*] alongside the ordinary one.[69] Husserl sometimes speaks of different levels and degrees of epoché: the "phenomenological epoché" is a kind of first stage of the second and more radical moment of the "transcendental epoché," which he also calls the "transcendental reduction" [*transzendentalen Reduktion*].[70] The terms "epoché" and "reduction" are used virtually synonymously in many instances.[71] The first stage of the suspension, the phenomenological epoché, concerns the objectivities of the world. Their transcendence is bracketed in order to gain access to the subjective acts in which the object is given; that is, to acts of consciousness as such, be they perceptions, recollections, or anticipations. The second stage, the transcendental epoché, entails a bracketing of the acts of consciousness in order to reach pure consciousness itself: that which is left when "the whole world with all physical things, living beings, and humans, ourselves included"[72] is parenthesized.

Echoing the Cartesian "hyperbolic doubt,"[73] Husserl supposes that even if the world did not exist [*Weltnichtigkeit*], together with the "I" as human being,[74] there would not be "nothing" in the sense of a null. Something would remain; namely, this very perception of the world [*Weltwahrnehmen*] in terms of the experiencing itself [*Erfahren*].[75] The hypothesis of an annihilation of this universe [*Zunichtemachen dieses Weltalls*] entails the disappearance of the empiricist psyche [*empirische Seele*][76] but not of its "pure" component, pure subjectivity [*reine Subjektivität*],[77] because consciousness is not a "piece of the world."[78] To access this dimension, which Husserl calls the "transcendental experience [*transzendentale Erfahrung*],"[79] mundane ordinary "transcendent" experience must be placed out of validity or "out of play."[80]

The Overcoming of the Empirical "I"

Husserl's intent is to overcome the egoistic and psychological dimension of the "I," its empirical-objective coating [*empirisch-objektive Gewand*],[81] in favor of a transcendental experience that he sometimes calls the "transcendental I" [*transzendentale Ich*][82] that has no owner in terms of belonging. According to Husserl, it is not easy to un-conceal the dimension of this disinterested spectator [*uninteressierter Zuschauer/Selbstschauer*],[83] who takes a distance from the empirical "I," endures within the space of experience, and becomes the knower of itself [*Selbsterkenner*].[84] In the ordinary stance, this dimension is veiled [*verhüllung*].[85] It is through breaking the habit of losing oneself in mundane objectifying tendencies that one can access this transcendental purity [*Traszendentalen Reinheit*].[86] When speaking of the hardship [*Schwierigkeiten*] of the task of training in phenomenology, Husserl says that the phenomenologist must exercise a systematic ἐποχή [*systematische* ἐποχή] through which every mundane component can be transcendentally spiritualized [*transzendental vergeistigt*].[87]

Husserl argues in favor of the existence of a "field of pure consciousness" that "is not a component part of Nature"[88] and therefore remains untouched by the suspending procedure: "Consciousness has, in itself, a being of its own which in its own absolute essence, is not touched by the phenomenological exclusion. It therefore remains as the 'phenomenological residuum' [*phänomenologische Residuum*] as a region of being which is of essential necessity quite unique and which can indeed become the field of a science of a novel kind: phenomenology."[89] Within this frame, the epoché is the "operation necessary to make 'pure' consciousness, and subsequently the whole phenomenological region, accessible to us."[90]

It is important to stress that this pure subjectivity, which Husserl often calls the "reduced ego," is not a piece of the world and should be understood as no less than an "a-subjective" dimension, as noted by Jan Patočka.[91] Husserl is excluding both a transcendent view, in which consciousness is a thing among others, and a radical immanent idealism, in which the existence of something other than the subject is excluded: "Just as the reduced Ego is not a piece of the world, so, conversely, neither the world nor any worldly Object is a piece of my Ego, to be found in my conscious life as a really inherent part of it, as a complex of data of sensation or a complex of acts."[92] And this is what the term "transcendental" actually means in the phenomenological sense: what appears has its origin in something other than subjective conscious experience, but its meaning is determined and comes into being precisely because of this conscious "stage" or platform. There is something that resists the arbitrary coating of the subject and determines the experience to unfold in one specific way more than in another. There is a core that, for example, directs the efforts of a scientist working in a lab, testing theories and revising the initial hypothesis to make it more convergent to the experimental results.[93]

What is this field of pure or transcendental[94] consciousness? How can we get a feel for what Husserl is referring to?

Figure-Background Dynamic and Horizon Consciousness

According to Husserl, we must turn our attention [*Wendung der Aufmerksamkeit*] from the object in which we usually place our interest during any act of perception to the spatial background [*räumlichen Hintergrund*][95] from which it stands out and that usually remains unnoticed [*unbeachtete*]: "Speaking of a 'twisting' [*Wendung*] of attention is significant; . . . that to which it is turned was already present in the field of consciousness as a background object, without being noticed; that is, without its being the thematic object of an act. . . . The same thing to which I now specifically pay attention was already in my perceptive field; it was already there; I had only not paid attention to it."[96] If we think of optical illusions and paradoxes such as Rubin's vase, we realize that when we spot the vase, we lose the shape of the two profiles. Conversely, if we try to single out the outlines of the two profiles, we can no longer clearly distinguish the vase. In order for one of the two shapes to be seen, the other one must be on a level of strong indetermination, as a mere background. For something to be singled out, what is at the bottom must remain latent.

There is a latency that allows something else to come forth. Husserl also argues that something perfectly clear [*vollkommen Klare*] upon closer examination reveals its inner horizon of a relative lack of clarity [*inneren Horizont der relativen Unklarheit*]; together with the possibility of becoming clearer and clear, it harbors a relative distance [*relative Ferne*].[97]

Husserl's point is deeply radical; he is not merely claiming that any visual object stands out on a background, as illustrated in the previous gestalt images. He goes much further, saying that any shape means more than what it is. This meaning more is the invisible part of the image that we posit, even though we do not see it. Take the image on the above left (figure 2.4): what we actually see is a dark grey square shape flanked by two lighter grey rhomboid shapes. However, we usually infer from what is visible the invisible sides of this hypothetical cube, the sides that are only adumbrated by the visible sides but remain undetermined. Meaning more than we actually see, we come to see a cube as illustrated

Figure 2.1. (left) Rubin's Vase. *Source:* Public domain.[98]
Figure 2.2. (center) Rabbit-Duck. *Source:* Public domain.[99]
Figure 2.3. (right) Young and old lady Gestalt. *Source:* Public domain.[100]

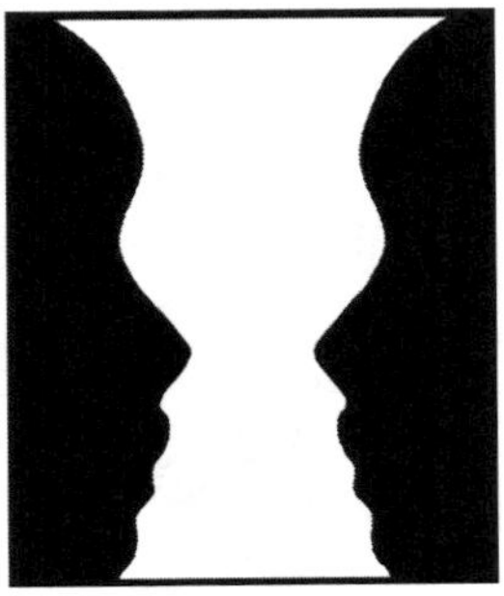

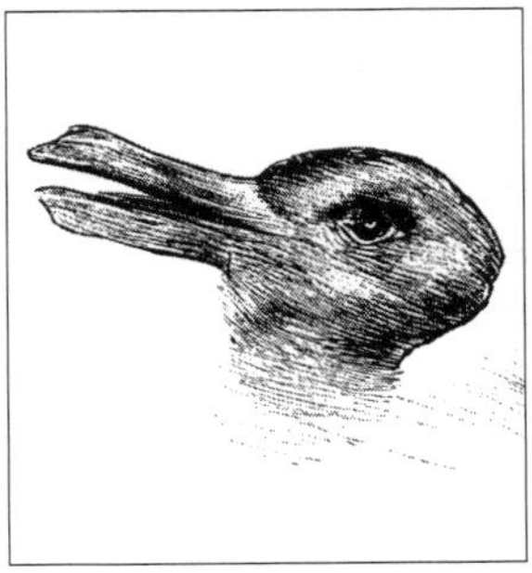

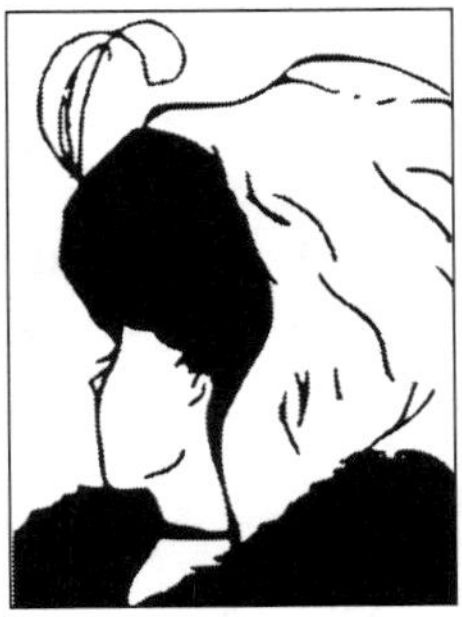

Figure 2.4. (left) 3D cube. *Source:* Public domain.
Figure 2.5. (right) Transparent 3D cube. *Source:* Public domain.

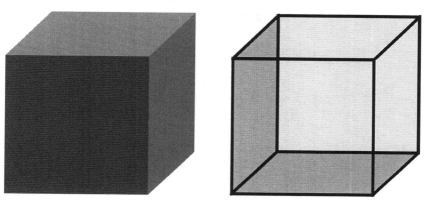

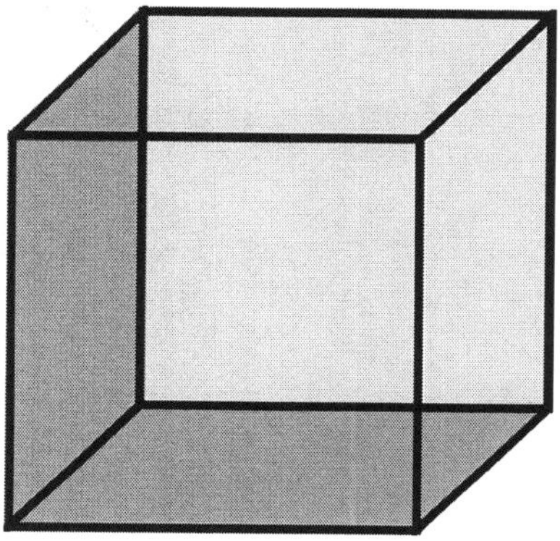

in the image to the right (figure 2.5). In this case, the horizon or background consciousness is the awareness of the existence of undetermined and latent sides of the visible. In the *Ideas Pertaining to a Pure Phenomenology and to a Phenomenological Philosophy,* Husserl anticipates this theme through the concept of "passive synthesis," saying for example that "the objectivity that must be constituted through this act is 'passively' there in consciousness in a confused state."[101] Furthermore, in the *Cartesian Meditations,* Husserl speaks of a "passive genesis": "In any case, anything built by activity necessarily presupposes, as the lowest level, a passivity that gives something beforehand; and, when we trace anything built actively, we run into constitution by passive generation."[102] The question of the passive synthesis[103] recurs in Husserl's inquiry, but it is in the 1923–1924 *Lectures* on the theme of the phenomenological reduction, published as *Erste Philosophie* [*First Philosophy*], that this question is tackled on the basis of a close investigation of the theme of the "background consciousness" [*Hintergrundbewußtsein*] or "horizon consciousness" [*Bewußtseinshorizont*],[104] the deepening of which may be crucial for understanding what Eastern philosophies aim at when they speak of consciousness: "What is clear [*Klare*] always brings with its empty horizon of lack of clarity and lack of distinction [*Unklarheit und Undeutlichkeit*]."[105] Husserl delves into greater detail regarding this horizon consciousness when he claims that "everything perceived has, so to say, in itself its background; each one is only given by showing a visible anterior side with invisible inner and back sides."[106] He argues that we "never have something perceived without a horizon consciousness; however, we seize and limit the perceived [element]."[107] This horizon consciousness is a "consciousness empty of view" [*anschauungsleere Bewußtsein*],[108] in the sense that it is empty of meaning: there is no "being-directed" in it. It can be understood as the condition of possibility of experience itself [*Möglichkeit der Erfahrung*].[109] The empty horizon [*Leerhorizont*] of consciousness actually encompasses the entire world [*umspannt eigentlich die ganze Welt*]. As Husserl says, it is "an infinite horizon of possible experience [*einen unendlichen Horizont möglicher Erfahrung*];"[110] it does not coincide with experience because it is the condition of possibility of experience as such. It is an endless kingdom of the still unknown [*unendliche Reich des noch Unbekannten*], but at the same time latently foreshadowed [*vorgedeutet*].[111] After all validities and objectivities are rendered powerless [*Geltungen in eins außer Kraft zu setzen*], the constant awareness of the horizon [*beständige Horizontbewußtsein*] that accompanies every actual present in life [*das jede aktuelle Lebensgegenwart begleitet*] can emerge.[112]

Becoming aware of the consciousness of the horizon implies a capacity to linger over what is not graspable through concepts but that can nonetheless be sensed as the bottom of the overall unity of the endless life connections.[113] Furthermore, by tuning to the horizon of the present moment [*gegenwärtigen Horizonte*],[114] an overview of oneself [*Selbstüberschauung*] can arise.

In *The Idea of Phenomenology* (1907), the early Husserl goes in this same direction when offering cues like the following:

> Thus, as little interpretation as possible, but as pure an intuition as possible (*intuitio sine comprehensione*); in fact, we will hark back to the speech of the mystics when they describe the intellectual seeing which is supposed not to be a discursive knowledge. And the whole trick consists in this, to give free rein to the seeing eye and to bracket the references that go beyond the "seeing" . . . along with the entities that are supposedly given and thought along with the "seeing," and finally, to bracket what is read into them through the accompanying reflections.[115]

Discussing this horizon consciousness, Husserl also refers to it in terms of a faraway or distant consciousness [*Fernbewußtsein*][116] that grows in the continuous stream of the present moment, and this specification is fundamental to begin envisioning this consciousness as something that crosses the boundaries of the empirical subject and points to an ulteriority that Husserl calls the transcendental.[117] This dimension belongs to Being as such, a notion introduced in contemporary philosophical inquiry by Husserl's most promising student, Martin Heidegger.

Chapter 3

From Husserl's Consciousness to Heidegger's Being

The Oblivion of Being

Martin Heidegger is often charged with having led Husserl's starting points to a completely different philosophical outcome and to an alleged kind of mysticism, and it is true that Heidegger's notion of releasement [*Gelassenheit*] recalls Meister Eckart's one in many respects.[1] However, it is equally true, that Heidegger's insights are the natural evolution of Husserl's, though they are hardly in dialogue with one another because Heidegger upends the philosophical terminology and invents his own unedited lexicon. This move by Heidegger had a precise intention: he wanted to break with the objectifying tendencies hidden in Husserl's language that in Heidegger's view undercut Husserl's enterprise from the inside without his even noticing. There are indeed some instances in which Husserl warns of the constant risk of confusion that awaits those who exercise the method of reduction,[2] likely referring to the mistake of taking the phenomenological analysis as an object itself and of hypostatizing its components. But Husserl does not directly impute this risk to the language on which he draws, a technical terminology inherited from the tradition of natural studies in psycho-physiology. Husserl's lexicon was imported from the scientific sphere, and he at times gives the impression of seeking to apply also to the phenomena of phenomenology the method that natural sciences usually impress on their objects of study, restricting them and extracting them from the totality of being.

However, when Husserl states that "we must return to the 'things themselves' " [*zurück zur sachen selbst*] in reference to phenomena, he is not discussing new reified and crystallized things but the fundamental dynamics of experience: "We can absolutely not rest content with 'mere words,' i.e., with a merely symbolic understanding of words. . . . Meanings inspired only by remote, confused, inauthentic intuitions—if by any intuitions at all—are not enough: we must go back to the 'things themselves' [*Wir wollen auf die Sachen selbst zurück gehen*]."[3] In addition, the evidence to which phenomenology appeals is very different from the kind referred to in logic,[4] for instance, because it is a form of what is purely lived-through within a subjective act:[5] "Every truth derived from pure self-evidence is a genuine truth and is a norm."[6] Subjective does not mean arbitrary; the criterion of validity of this evidence is intersubjectivity. Phenomenological descriptions are not personal but do have an intersubjective validation.

Phenomena represent a relational space; they embody the coming into view of the world in the space of awareness. In order to account for this revolutionary shift in the discussion that phenomenology brings to the philosophical debate, Heidegger decides to reinvent the lexicon and adopts a completely different terminology, which has given the impression of a clean break with Husserl's project. However, if a link is established between Heidegger's notion of Being and Husserl's notion of consciousness,[7] one realizes that the turn that Heidegger imprints on Husserl's phenomenology is not that radical, just like the turn that developed in Heidegger's own thought.[8]

Heidegger's famous distinction between the facts of the world and their underlying being or, in his terminology, the ontological difference between the entities of the world [*seiendes*] and Being [*Sein*] as such[9] recalls, in this view, Husserl's distinction between the objectivities (entities) and their undetermined or partially concealed background, the horizon consciousness. Just as Husserl suggests discovering [*entdecken*][10] the residual [*übrig*][11] experience of the world [*Welterfahren*][12] that remains after everything else has been inhibited [*inhibieren*],[13] Heidegger speaks of the task of overcoming the oblivion of Being [*Seinsvergessenheit*][14] that he regards the West as having undergone at least since Descartes, when the world became entirely representation,[15] and the entity (the represented-object) became the center of all interest: all to the detriment of the dimension of Being, which grew more and more concealed, unseen, and forgotten. The dimension of Being that is not to be identified with God or with a "foundation of the world,"[16] might be unhidden, for Heidegger, by removing the layers of concealment and covering that prevent it from revealing itself and shining forth.

Heidegger argues that prior to the ordinary and apparently obvious concept of truth as concordance or conformity,[17] according to which truth corresponds to the concordance between the thing and the concept (along with Thomas Aquinas's "*Veritas est adaequatio rei et intellectus*"), there is another one: truth as "unconcealedness" [*Unverborgenheit*]. Heidegger regards the ancient Greeks as having a word for it: ἀλήθεια [*a-letheia*] meaning revealing, disclosure, literally un-concealedness (with λήθε meaning veiling and concealment and a privative ἀ as a prefix).[18] Despite having a word that harbored the authentic meaning of truth, the Greeks in Heidegger's view were not able to think all the way through the essence of this term and, after initial insights by pre-Socratics like Anaximander, later Greek thought laid the foundations for the derivative concept of truth as conformity, which in modern times became the only conceivable one.

According to Heidegger, the ancient notion of *a-letheia* must be restored to counteract the oblivion of Being. In this term, coming into presence happens as an unveiling, and thus a peculiar link is established between what is unveiled and what is veiled, between presence and absence: "That which shows itself [*sich zeigt*] and at the same time withdraws [*sich entzieht*] is the essential trait of what we call the mystery [*das Geheimnis*]."[19] In opposition to the widespread modern ideal of reaching the fully graspable and displayable, the notion of *a-letheia* treasured the inextricable connection between what is clear and the unclear horizon from which it stems.

Letting Be and Disclosure

My claim is that the dynamic of veiling and unveiling at the core of Being and truth outlined by Heidegger had been foreseen by

Husserl in terms of a dynamic between figure and background and considered by the founder of phenomenology the structure of consciousness itself.

And just as a specific time is needed for both shapes of a *Gestalt* to show up, with only one often emerging for a long period, the process of unveiling takes time and attention on the part of the one who is contemplating.

This unconcealedness is sometimes rendered by Heidegger through the notion of "disclosure" [*Erschlossenheit*], which conveys the sense of how the world comes into being with a peculiar kind of independence with respect to human agency. Heidegger also hints at this disclosure with the notion of "clearing" or "lighting" [*Lichtung*], like a clearing in the woods. The clearing is not an entity but the precondition for any fact to emerge. A clearing is needed in which anything at all can appear, just as a preordained dimension of consciousness must be implied for any mental content to be given:

> In the midst of being as a whole an open place occurs. There is a clearing, a lighting. Thought of in reference to what is, to beings, this clearing is in a greater degree than are beings. This open center is therefore not surrounded by what is; rather, the lighting center itself encircles all that is, like the Nothing which we scarcely know. That which is can only be, as a being, if it stands within and stands out within what is lighted in this clearing. Only this clearing grants and guarantees to us humans a passage to those beings that we ourselves are not, and access to the being that we ourselves are.[20]

In the essay "Gelassenheit," published in 1959, Heidegger introduces the notions of "openness" [*das Offene*] and "the region" [*die Gegnet*][21] to which everything can return and rest [*ruhen*].[22] The capacity that is needed to realize this open horizon is not being able to represent [*vor zustellen*] what offers itself in order to subject it [*unterstellen*] and thus assure it [*gesichern*] to what is already known;[23] rather, what is required to realize it is a welcoming attitude of releasement: "Letting be [*Gelassenheit*] is not only the way, but the movement [itself along the way]."[24] For Heidegger, this letting be is awakened [*erwacht*][25] when we allow ourselves to be released to what is not a "want" [*wollen*].[26] This letting [*lassen*] hides "a higher sense of action [*Tun*] than the one that crosses all worldly actions and the bustling about of humanity. . . . Because letting happen doesn't belong to the kingdom of will [*Willens*]."[27]

In a dialogue between a scientist, a scholar, and a teacher,[28] Heidegger highlights that the passage [*der übergang*] from want [*wollen*] to letting be is the most difficult.[29] Heidegger envisions a new way of thinking in respect to traditional representational thinking. According to this new paradigm, instead of being pinned under the firm grasp of concepts [*Be-griffen*], manifestation is looked after. It is all about an elevated act [*Tun*][30] in which we have nothing to do and nothing to represent. Instead, we must attend and safeguard: "nothing should we do, but wait,"[31] and "waiting means to release oneself into the openness"[32] where everything is gathered together in relation to every other.

Phenomenon and Phanes

Heidegger suggests an attitude toward the world of a quiet resting in receptivity and acceptance,[33] which is the fundamental trait of yoga and meditative practices. It is a matter of coming together and abiding in the wide quietness.[34] Though Heidegger makes no direct reference to it, there was an ancient Greek deity who presided over the unconcealment of reality: Phanes ("light"). The word *phenomenon* comes from the Greek *phainomai* (φαίνομαι)[35] which means "to appear," "to show oneself," "to be given," "to come into view," and it intends nothing beyond itself. *Phainomai* (from the root "*phaos*," φῶς) in turn has its origin in the term *phanes*, which in Greek means "light" and is the medium of all manifestations.

Phanes is a primordial deity; he is the "first-born," the protogonos who comes before all the others. Roberto Calasso notes that Zeus had to swallow Phanes to absorb his power and take his place as the new king of the universe.[36] Phanes was the god of procreation and was also called Erikapaios, the "giver of life." Phanes emerged at the dawn of the universe as a golden embryo that gave rise to everything and is represented in sculptures inside a sort of cosmic egg. Phanes is also lord of the animals when he is represented with three or more animal heads and a snake coiled around him. Phanes (figure 3.1), who is sometimes depicted as a young, beautiful hermaphrodite (thereby surpassing the duality of gender) with golden wings, emerges from fire, with flames as headwear. In some instances, the blazing fire makes him a manifestation of Eros or desire. He becomes manifest to the cosmos precisely because of the luminous splendor that his fire radiates. Thus, from the early days of the West, Phanes has driven the process of manifestation of reality. The world comes forward in its shining manifestation thanks to a divine power, but to allow Phanes to reveal himself, a welcoming and vigilant stance must be embraced, and Heidegger's phenomenology is a reminder of the importance of learning to "let be."

Figure 3.1. Relief of Phanes of Loggia Cornaro. *Source:* Bia123gio, Wikimedia Commons. CC BY-SA 4.0.

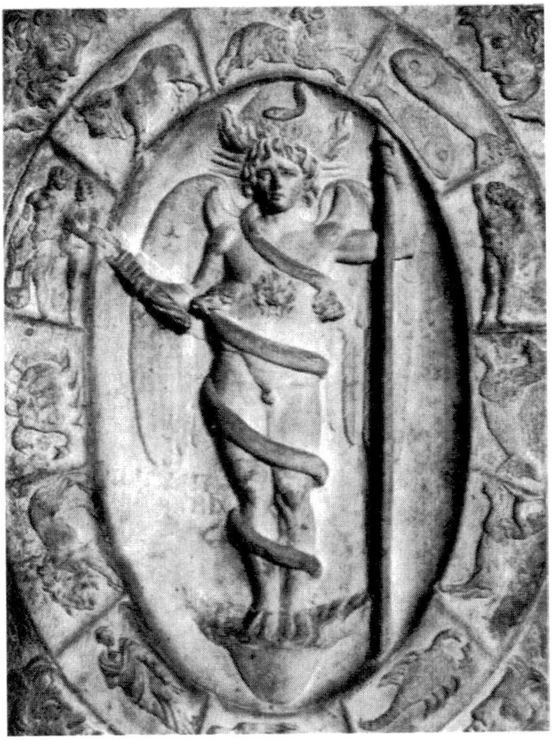

The current debate on consciousness should try to follow phenomenological inquiries and insights not for the sake of mastering Continental philosophy but to obtain a glimpse of this luminous space of appearing that comes beforehand and opens up at its own initiative. Having followed Husserl's analysis has enabled us to recognize the necessity of doing something, of suspending and inhibiting the pregiven objects of the world. Only when particular objectivities are bracketed in favor of what we can call the bigger picture can the existence of the wider horizon of all-encompassing consciousness be sensed. Husserl brings us to the edge of this new realm that he calls the mothers of knowledge: "when we no longer move on the old familiar ground of the world but rather stand, through our transcendental reduction, only at the gate of entrance to the realm, never before entered, of the 'mothers of knowledge.'"[37] Turning to Heidegger helps us make the second step of addressing to the realm of Being. This is phrased in very similar terms as presented in the Upanishadic literature, where it is said that the practitioner, after having chosen a clean place and settled in purity, should "dedicate to the study of Being [*sat*], become an advocate of Being, meditate on Being and offer himself to Being."[38]

Being Equals Appearing

When invoking releasement and the capacity of allowing to be, Heidegger explicitly unfolds the kind of attitude that is required to access this all-pervading dimension of consciousness in the background. It is about dropping master-hood and ceding control over reality and discovering that once our urge to intervene has burned away, we are not left as impoverished as we might have feared. Rather, we are filled with wonder, as the scholar muses in the dialogue: "Then wonder can open what is locked?" The scientist's response is powerful in its simplicity: "By way of waiting."[39]

In other words, once the natural tetic attitude and validity of a specific object have been put out of play through the suspensive effort of Husserl's reduction,[40] an unveiling moment might occur, as hinted at by Heidegger's phenomenology. The first moment requires action (in the sense of suspending), while the second moment requires "letting happen" in the sense of entering a welcoming stance in which a wider, more luminous horizon becomes accessible.

The great revolution of phenomenology is claiming that "being means appearing"[41] and that "what is" is the "phenomenon."[42] It is a "Copernican reversal"[43] because the being of things is not placed beyond them, as had been true of earlier metaphysical philosophy. In phenomenology what appears is not mischievous or doubtable in favor of a true hidden essence considered reliable. What appears is also not a mere representative that stands for something else, like the noumenon in Kantian terms: "And this is not to say that the things once more exist in themselves and 'send their representatives into consciousness.' This sort of thing cannot occur to us within the sphere of phenomenological reduction. Instead, the things are and are given in appearance and in virtue of the appearance itself."[44]

However, we have seen that this appearance is not fully displayable and harbors within itself the veils and layers of concealment that allow it to appear. The phenomenological key to approaching reality is essentially nonesoteric and nonmetaphysical. In other words, no ideal world, independent of the one we are allowed to know, is posited. No hierarchy is established between a higher world and a lower one, if for no other reason than no theory of the world is offered. Every preexisting theory is systematically bracketed and set aside in order to come closer to what is happening in the space of consciousness.

Chapter 4

The Seer and Non-Dual Consciousness

Knowledge and Liberation

Having laid out a few key building blocks of the phenomenological enterprise, we now set out toward the East in an effort to find out what happens when this frame of reference is applied to yoga. Unlike Western traditions, there is no intellectual value in knowing, per se, in the Eastern view: knowing is never an end but a means toward a different course of action[1] and, ultimately, a means to liberation. Understanding or removing ignorance [*avidyā*] has a soteriological function; it leads to "salvation" [*mokṣa*]. The starting point in embarking on the path of understanding is the acknowledgment of the condition of suffering into which one has been thrown. That suffering depends on the ignorance in which one is immersed, which is literally the inability to see what's in front of oneself, mistaking one's own projections [*adhyāsa*] for what is really there. It is out of the decision to free oneself from suffering that one sets off on the quest for knowledge and removes the layers of ignorance that dull the sight.

Evidence of this can be found across different traditions, though the most celebrated example is in the Four Noble Truths[2] of Buddhism. Around 526 BCE, in the Gazelle Park of Sarnath (Benares), Siddhartha Gautama taught the existence of "suffering," the fact that this suffering has an "origin," and that it can "cease" when that origin has been removed. The fourth truth points to the path that leads out of ignorance and thus to the "cessation of suffering."

The same concept appears in Patañjali's *Yogasūtra*: "for the one who discerns, everything is suffering [*duḥkham eva sarvaṁ vivekinaḥ*]"[3] and in later *haṭha* yoga traditions: "*haṭha-yoga* is a refuge for the ones who are afflicted from every kind of suffering."[4] In the *Śvetāśvatara Upaniṣad,* it is said that through yoga the embodied being becomes free of pain [*vitaśokaḥ*][5] and that "one has neither disease nor old age nor death, having won a body made of the fire of yoga [*yogāgni*]."[6] In ancient Greek philosophy, a similar approach appears in Plato's metaphor of the cave: turning toward the path of knowledge and education is compared to rescuing oneself from the condition of being a slave forced to watch only the shadows of the world.[7]

And what is the interest in turning to Eastern traditions and practices when exploring consciousness? Are phenomenological analyses not sufficient? Husserl makes a fundamental contribution with his epoché and the necessity of sticking to the phenomenon in terms of what shows itself, moment after moment, in the space of consciousness, while Heidegger highlights the kind of receptive attitude required to allow the dimension of the background consciousness to unfold. But something else fundamental is missing in the analysis of the phenomenologists: a practice within which to train the abovementioned phases. Contemporary phenomenologists complain about the lack of practical techniques or even hints in phenomenological philosophy: "Although phenomenology should have been pure method, it became theory instead."[8] Michel Bitbol admits that "the lack of methodological instructions is undoubtedly phenomenology's greatest weakness and biggest lack."[9]

Turning to yoga and contemplative practices and applying a phenomenological key to them[10] gives us a few thousand years of refined practice in which to train our phenomenological insights. Whereas Western culture has only become deeply interested in consciousness in the last few centuries, in India yogic techniques have been inner laboratories in which to explore different layers and dimensions of consciousness for millennia.

States of Consciousness in the Vedanta

The Vedas, literally meaning "vision," are a collection of texts made up of hymns and invocations with which the Aryan people sought to establish communication with the realm of the invisible; they are the most ancient set of scriptures other than those in Mesopotamian cuneiform writings and Egyptian hieroglyphs. The *Rigveda* is the oldest of the Vedic scriptures (c. 15th–13th century BCE), and the *Bṛhadāraṇyaka Upaniṣad* is the oldest of the Upanishads, a heterogenous corpus of philosophical texts that inquire into and elaborate on the concepts and themes exposed in the Vedas that date from the ninth and eighth centuries BCE. If in Western culture historiographical interests and the question of dating has been of major concern ever since, in India a lack of concern for issues of the precise dating and attribution of the texts delivered by tradition must be acknowledged: dating can span a range not just of several years but of centuries. Indian philosophers, commentators, and scholars were interested in internalizing and transmitting the deep meaning and content of traditional texts. For their purposes, the original author and date were usually of little or no importance.[11]

It is in this context that one finds an anticipation of what today could be called a classification of different states of conscious experience. In the *Māṇḍūkya Upaniṣad*, four (more precisely, "three plus one") states of consciousness [prajñā][12] are outlined in detail and connected to three letters (and the following silence) that together make up the sound A-U-M [*Om*]. This is the primordial sound, carrier of the vital energy from which all other sounds stem: "The syllable AUM, the imperishable Brahman, is the whole universe. All that is past, present and future is, indeed, AUM/Om. And whatever else there is, beyond the threefold division of time—that also is truly AUM."[13]

The first conscious state taken into account, Vaiśvanāra, the letter A, is the waking state [*jāgarita*] defined as the state "with consciousness turned outwards [*bahiṣprajñā*];"[14] that is, with consciousness directed toward external objects. The second one considered is the state of consciousness turned inward [*antaḥprajñā*]. This is the dream state of Taijasa, the letter U, in which consciousness is directed toward internal objects [*pravivikta*].[15] The next state marks a vast difference from current debates on consciousness, as anticipated in the introduction. In fact, what is taken into account as the third state of consciousness is precisely "deep sleep" or dreamless-sleep, prajñā,[16] here intended in the strictest sense, the letter "M." A state that many contemporary neuroscientists consider exempt from consciousness[17] was taken two thousand years ago not only as a state in which consciousness is maintained but also as the state of "a sheer mass of consciousness" [*prajñānaghana*]. Within this state of deep sleep [*suṣupti*], "becoming one" takes place [*ekibhūtaḥ*]. The text also offers some important information about how this conscious state is given. It is not a purely intellectual or dry experience of unity. Rather, this state of unification brings with it ample amounts of joy; it is essentially blissful [*ananda*].[18] And this is not all: there is a fourth state to consider. Turīya, or Caturtha, literally the fourth, is beyond language and duality. It is the silence without measure that follows the syllable Om. This state is not definable and for this reason is only hinted at through the gradual Vedic process of negation expressed through the "neti neti"—"neither this, nor that"—that is so effective in its power that nothing is said to be higher:[19] "not with consciousness turned inward, not with consciousness turned outward, not with consciousness turned both ways," "not conscious, not unconscious," "not a mass of consciousness [*na prajñānaghana*]," "unseen, inviolable, unseizable, signless, unthinkable, unnamable," "peaceful, beneficial [*śiva*]," "without duality [*advaita*]."[20]

The commentator Gauḍapāda, master of the famed Śaṅkarācārya and considered one of the first exponents of the Advaita Vedānta lineage,[21] cautions that the third and fourth states are similar in that both entail a nonperception of duality [*dvaitasyāgrahaṇaṁ*][22] and point toward a nondual dimension, although in the fourth, Turīya, there is a fuller realization of that nonduality [*advaita*]. This is because the dimension of prajñā accessed through the third state is still conditioned (like the first two stages) by external contingencies such as the fact of sleeping, whereas the fourth dimension is not conditioned at all: "Prajñā, however, is conditioned by cause [*kāraṇa*]. But in Turīya those two [cause and effect] don't exist."[23] In the *Yoga Tarvali*, a text attributed to Śaṅkarācārya, a "mindless pose" [*amanaska*] is mentioned.[24] This condition is referred to in terms of "conscious-sleep," yoga *nidrā*, and it is blissfully experienced by the one who is established in the fourth state, the Turīya.[25]

When referring to this conscious dimension beyond language and duality found in the Turīya (and partly in the prajñā), the

Upanishads (and not only the *Māṇḍūkya*) resort to notions like Brahman, Ātman, Prajñā (in the broad sense), and Om. These are different words that point in the same direction to the space [*ākāsa*] of Being-Consciousness-Bliss [*sat-citta-ananda*],[26] though each has a slightly different nuance. In philosophical terms, one could say that Brahman has a more ontological and universal hue, whereas Ātman a more ontic and existential one, although in the *Chāndogya Upaniṣad* the Brahman is said to be both the space outside the person and the one inside: the space inside the heart.[27] Prajñā, often translated as "wisdom," refers to the dimension of Being and consciousness in general and specifically indicates the third state of deep sleep.

The translatability of these terms, one into the other, becomes evident by way of just a brief listing of the renowned sayings of the Advaita Vedānta, the Mahavakyas: "All of this [universe] is Brahman;"[28] "It is one, without a second;"[29] and "I am that."[30] There are the four most famous sayings: "You are that,"[31] "this Ātman [self] is Brahman,"[32] "I am Brahman,"[33] and "Brahman is Consciousness."[34]

The task of the practitioner according to the Vedanta consists in noticing that the subjective experience of being a separate independent and mortal entity typical of the state of ordinary wakefulness is a delusive and deceptive projection stemming from ignorance [*avidyā*]. In phenomenological terms, this state of ordinary wakefulness can be understood as the "natural attitude" that characterizes the tendency to single out within the continuum of experience only objects, including one's own body and self. In Vedanta, this level of consciousness must be overcome to realize one's essential and fundamental identity with the Brahman, the wider self. In phenomenology, the natural objectifying tendency of the ordinary attitude must be overcome to access the transcendental or background consciousness that, like the Brahman, is not a piece of the world and has no owner. This wider self, often called the seer [*draṣṭṛ*], coincides with the condition of the possibility of any experience; that is, with a concept of consciousness that overflows the boundaries of the empirical subject.

Husserl highlights the fact that having access to the realm of the transcendental requires bracketing the constitutive objects of the natural attitude; in the *Māṇḍūkya Upaniṣad*, to access the third and fourth state, one must overcome both the ordinary waking state in which interest is directed toward external objects, and the dream state, in which interest is still directed toward objects, though they are internal. In the *Maitry Upaniṣad*, it is also said that the mind directed toward external objects is to be restrained and placed under control through the yoking action [of yoga], by the wise one [*tathānyatrāpyuktaṁ yadā vai bahirvidvānmano*].[35] The "one who sees" [*vidvan*] must remain stable without forming concepts and by setting aside any mental projection [*niḥsankalpa*].[36] This mental cleanliness is to be interpreted as the most essential form of purification: in the *Muṇḍaka Upaniṣad*, yoga appears as a practice of purification [*saṁnyāsayogādyatayaḥ śuddhasattvaḥ*].[37] In the *Śvetāśvatara Upaniṣad*, it is stated that the dimension of consciousness [Ātman] is realized within oneself by means of *satya* [being-truth] and *tapas*,[38] the purifying heat. It is precisely the dimension of *tapas* that is connected in the pages below to the phenomenological stance, which is why it merits a closer look.

The Meaning of Purification

Usually translated as "austerity," "discipline," or "penance," *tapas* is one of the most frequently recurring concepts in the texts (it is central to the Veda and the *Rigveda* in particular and continually comes up in the *Upaniṣad*).[39] However, it is the most rarely thematized in subsequent literature. "Austerity," "penance," and "asceticism," the first translations put forward by missionaries and other religious people, whose interpretations tend to reduce Brahman to "God" and Ātman to "soul" in a highly Christianizing way, have made this a thorny issue from the outset. After all, given the visible spirituality of India—the land of *sādhaka*, ascetics, and devotees ready to undergo the most outlandish mortifications—did the act of converting *tapas* into such a familiar concept not free oneself from the trouble of thoughtfully and painstakingly defining it? This seems to have been the thinking of many Indologists; in addition, the spread in the West of a kind of Hinduism expunged of any tantric component promoted by figures like Vivekananda and Mohandas Gandhi was no help.

However, the occurrences in the *Rigveda*, the most ancient text, do not justify any translation other than "heat" or "warmth," whereas a meaning closer to "discipline"[40] arises later on. This transformation of the meaning of *tapas* is largely due to its frequent linking with the term *śrama* in the texts, which relates more specifically to "effort."[41] The connected meanings in the sense of "penance" and "mortification" that have developed are therefore a distorting evolution[42] of an original core that essentially meant "heat" and "energy." The root *tap-*, a cognate of the Latin *tepor-*, can be found in a number of compound nouns and means "giving out" or "releasing heat" and "being hot";[43] it thus refers to both the power of heat and the burning required to generate it. From an etymological perspective, *tapas* shares a root with the English "tepid." It essentially means "heat," "ardor," "fervor,"[44] but it also denotes warmth, thus making the connection with tepid clearer; the term only later came to mean asceticism in its original sense of "exercise."

The true Lord of *tapas* [Tapaspati] is the fire Agni, born from the heat of *tapas*.[45] Of all the deities invoked in the Vedas, Agni is called upon most often, sometimes under the names of the "Ancient One" or the "Red One"; the *Rigveda* opens with an encomium to Agni.[46] This is not surprising when one considers that fire has always been humanity's first line of defense against the wildness of nature, an ally against ferocious beasts and the bastion that holds back encroaching darkness. Not only does it clear a path through the jungle and open up communication between the earth and the heavens, but it is also the key transformational tool in moving from a diet of raw foods, common to animals, to one based around cooked foods. Its ability to control primordial matter can also be seen in the production of earthenware and in metalworking, an art typically steeped in magical or alchemical values. Agni, which in the Vedic texts is often referred to as *tapasvin*—he who is possessed or marked by *tapas*—in more recent Hindu iconography is often depicted with three heads.[47] Riding a ram (also a fire sign in the Western zodiac) and holding a ladle or spoon for offerings, Agni wields the *vajra*, the lightning bolt that represents the destructive flame capable of consuming enemies, and has burning teeth and a burning head (figure 4.1).

Figure 4.1. Agni riding a ram. *Source:* Wikimedia Commons. Public domain.

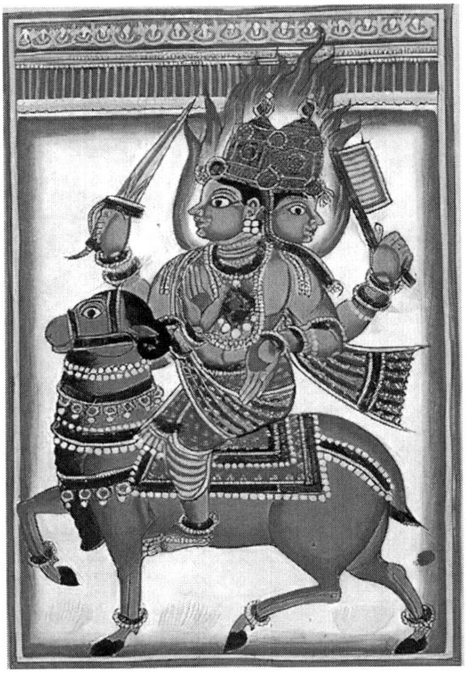

Tapas, through the power of Agni, consumes the flesh during cremation ceremonies but is also a weapon: the offensive heat that can turn enemies to ashes, be they demons, *Raksas*, or *Asura*, primordial fallen deities in later literature. "Do you, Agni, injure with heat [√*tap*] the unfriendly among us; do you injure with heat [√*tap*] the ritual purpose of the grudging outsider who would do us harm: do you, the very pious, injure the impious with heat [√*tap*]."[48] As Walter O. Kaelber emphasizes, Agni is asked to "pierce the raksasas with most hot (flames)."[49] Because it is able to neutralize enemies, it takes over the power of purifying evil.[50]

The Two Faces of *Tapas*

But there is another side to *tapas* in which generation is central. In order to develop into a creative force, *tapas* must first be used as a destructive force, as we can infer by the fact that in Vedic mythology creation could only take place following the destruction of the demons Vala and Vrta, who prevented creation from unfolding.[51] In the Vedic literature, the creative and generative capacity of *tapas* is represented by the sun, Sūrya,[52] which "produces heat more than any other."[53] Furthermore, there is a clear link between *tapas* and sexual heat. Not only is *kāma*, desire, homologized with the *tapas*-possessing fires,[54] but it rises from *tapas* as a result of intercourse.[55] Aside from the image of the *Tapta-gharma*, the ritual cauldron that when heated up symbolizes orgasm, the Vedas contain the metaphor of kindling that links the churning of two sticks with erotic intercourse, through which the creation of *tapas* leads to birth.[56]

This facet of *tapas*, meaning "tepid heat," no longer carries us toward the flame that burns and incinerates but instead takes us under the wing of a hen, into the warmth of brooding.[57] Prajāpati, the primal deity of the Vedic pantheon and identifiable with the universe itself, who would become the Brahman in the later Upanishadic tradition, in certain passages dealing with creation, is about to incubate the worlds.[58] He is sometimes depicted as a golden embryo, *hiraṇyagarbhāya*, born from heat [*tapaso jatam*], the famous *brahmāṇḍa* or cosmic egg, representing both the macrocosm and the microcosm (figure 4.2). Indicating this process of brooding we find another derivative of *tapas*,[59] "*abhi- √tap*," meaning "to irradiate with heat":[60] the warmth irradiated by *tapas* brings the eggs to hatching. In addition to the burning aspect, the warm dimension of egg hatching is also treasured in *tapas*: it is a warmth that includes protection, attention, and care. When brooding, no aggressive heating effect or pressure should be applied; rather, space and ease is needed so that the birthing process can develop autonomously. It is a question of providing the space, time, and ease to allow what has been prepared to occur.

Therefore, in *tapas*, alongside a component strongly linked to doing or inhibiting, there is a dimension in which "allowing to happen" and "letting be" are central. To open a clearing and a space of careful listening, the layers and remnants of the past must be burned. This dynamic between doing and letting happen, which we have seen at play in phenomenology in terms of the phase of the reduction and the ensuing surfacing of the transcendental consciousness (or, in Heideggerian terms, the revealing moment

Figure 4.2. Brahmāṇḍa. *Source:* Photo by the author.

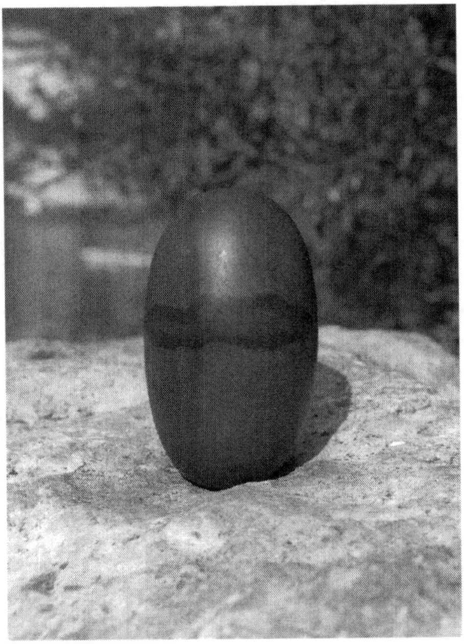

of Being), can be exemplified in very basic terms and within reach of an everyday language by describing a familiar setting and task such as tending the fire, in which everyone has engaged.

There is much to do when lighting a fire. The area where the fire will burn must be prepared by sweeping the ashes from the fireplace. Dry logs, neither too big nor too small, have to be gathered. Finer twigs and brushwood that burn more easily and pages of old newspapers to ball up are needed. At this point, the best—and most difficult—part is still to come. These elements cannot be tossed randomly into the fireplace: a detailed structure must be observed. First comes the paper, followed by a layer of twigs with plenty of space, allowing the fire to breathe. Finally, without suffocating this delicate nucleus, smaller logs in the shape of a pyramid are placed in the fireplace. Everything is now ready for the triggering act: one of the central balled-up pieces of newspaper is lit with a long match. Then comes the crucial phase of the whole procedure, in which it is no longer so much a question of doing something but rather of allowing the process to happen.

Of course, once the flame has reached the twigs and struggles to spread to the first logs, one can certainly still try to do something, such as blowing on the nascent fire or lightly stirring the logs with a stoker. However, one must be careful, because the temptation to overdo it always lies in wait: by dint of blowing or stoking the fire too vigorously, one might extinguish it. At that point, the greatest discouragement would be having to start all over again. If the task is not to be given up on by resorting to electrical heat, one needs to focus on the subtle step of simply letting the fire happen, although that does not mean, once the early stages have been successfully navigated, abandoning the fire to its fate. In this case, the fire would most likely be destined for a short life. One has to tend the fire: without necessarily doing anything visible, this means being able to pause for a while on its "happening." Sitting back and simply "passively" watching the fire will not suffice. It is rather a question of taking into account the givenness of the event, with the light and warmth that emanates from it. Only when careful attention is paid to the crackling of the fire, intervening intuitively with a few well-timed prods (that stoke rather than extinguish the flame) becomes possible.

In tending the fire, there is a constant flow between doing and allowing to happen. Neither can prevail: becoming excessively active or overly rapt and lazy will lead to the fire's inevitable extinction. It is all about dwelling within this rhythm between doing and letting be, not only as to lighting a fire but also as to understanding the essence of *tapas* that is at the very heart of yoga, because yoga, as the *Maitry Upaniṣad* relates, is the very radiance of the fire and the sun [*tejaścaivāgnisūryayoḥ*].[61] As writer and scholar Roberto Calasso recalls, "The most important step in the task of setting up the fires is the attempt to transfer the fires from the outside world to the remotest depth of the sacrificer's body. The whole doctrine of yoga rests on this operation."[62]

Yoga

The origins of the term "yoga" are ancient as the Vedas, where the root *-yuj* refers to the process of linking something to its counterpart: to "tie together," to "connect," to "create bonds."[63] The root -yug occurs in the *Rigveda* as the "yoking"[64] of animals (horses) to the chariot before battle. It appears in compound form in the term "*Ṛta-yukti*,"[65] which means "union with the cosmic order" or "to be yoked with the cosmic order," in the sense of "moving in the correct way," with *Ṛta* a prelude of the later cosmic law of *Dharma*. In the *Śvetāśvatara Upaniṣad*, the metaphor of yoking animals is placed in direct contact with the control of the unquiet mind: "The wise one, heedful, should control the mind as a chariot yoked to bad horses."[66] The same text contains a reference to yoga as action or exercise [*karāṇi yoge*],[67] and the location in which it should be carried out is described in detail.[68] In the *Kaṭha Upanishad*, the state of yoga is defined as a stable concentration of the senses [*sthirāmindriyadhāraṇām*]:[69] the supreme goal is stilling the five perceptions, along with the mind, when the intelligence is not dispersed [*buddhiś ca na viceṣṭati*].[70] In the *Maitry Upaniṣad*, the union with the "infinite One" [*eko'nanta*][71] is realized through the procedure and method of yoga [*tatprayogakalpaḥ*],[72] which entails a oneness of the breath, the mind, and the senses [*ekatvaṃ prāṇamanasorindriyāṇāṃ*].[73] On the other hand, Patañjali's classical *yoga darśana*, emphasizes in yoga the complementary dimension of discrimination [*viveka*],[74] discernment, the capacity of separating what the discursive objectifying mind tends to conflate together [*saṃyoga*].[75]

Often misunderstood as a religion, yoga is actually a "means," a method in the sense of a practice, a way, and at the time an "end" and a worldview [*darśana*] in the philosophical sense. This psycho-physical discipline includes, throughout the Indian subcontinent, countless variations, each different from the next, some forms being systematic and highly educated and others being popular and unsystematic. In fact, beyond being one of the six *darśana* or philosophies of Hinduism, yoga is a cross-sectoral approach present in different spiritual and religious Eastern traditions such as Buddhism,[76] Tantrism, and Śivaism. The Buddhist text *Questions of Milinda* [*Milinda Pañha*], for instance, refers to the fact that the yoga practitioner [*yogāvacara*], by holding the mind with attention, cuts through afflictions with wisdom, just as a barley harvester takes a bundle with the left hand and cuts through it with a sickle in the right hand.[77]

Returning to the relationship between fire and purification, the shift from the outer to the inner fire may be interpreted as passing from the ritualized, formalistic dimension of the Vedic world[78] toward a deeper dimension, where sacrifice seeks to represent the return to unity and is no longer carried out by commission but is instead internalized by those embarking on a path of reintegration like the *muni*, or proto-yogin. However, this transformation is anticipated in certain Vedic passages: "He with the long loose locks supports Agni, and moisture, heaven and earth: He is all sky to look upon: he with long hair is called this light."[79] According to Calasso, this figure is the "first defector (refugee), not because he rejects the complex system of interaction on which ritual is based, but because he seeks to absorb it, within himself, in the inaccessible space of the mind."[80] One of the first steps in the process of internalizing *tapas* is taken in the *Atharva Veda*, when Agni is placed inside the body as an ascending vital air.[81] Historian Mircea Eliade notes that heat is also produced "by disciplining or arresting the respiration; this allows the assimilation of yogic techniques to orthodox Brahminic methods, just as it allows the yogin to be assimilated to the *tapasvin*."[82] It is in the epic poem *Bhagavad Gītā* that the inner sacrifice is elevated and considered superior to the ritual one: "Some yogis perform sacrifice to the gods alone. . . . Others offer as sacrifice the outgoing breath in the incoming, and the incoming in the outgoing, restraining the courses of the outgoing and the incoming breaths."[83]

The transition from the oblation of clarified butter to the fire (the *agnihotra* carried out morning and evening) to the "daily sacrifice in respiration," *prānāgnihotra*,[84] is considered by Calasso to be "the first case of the complete internalization of an event, an invisible ceremony that takes place in an individual's 'breath,' " in which "there is no longer any fire, there is no longer any milk to pour on it, the words of the texts are no longer to be heard. But all this still exists: in silence, in the activity of the mind."[85]

Patañjali's Yoga

The internalization of *tapas* is the heart of Patañjali's *kriyā* yoga, which is often referred to by the more general expression *rāja* yoga and renowned for having set out an eight-step path leading to liberation [*kaivalya*]. In an intertwining of history and mythology, Patañjali, who according to the vulgate was "he who fell from heaven as an offering" in what we assume was the early centuries of the current era, systematized the multifaceted and varied tradition of yoga in a unified vision, which later was the base of the yoga *darśana*.[86] It is worth listing Patañjali's eight stages of the path [*aṣṭāṅga-yoga*],[87] if only to have an account of how meditation (the seventh limb) is related to the others: (1) prescriptions toward others [*Yama*],[88] (2) prescriptions toward oneself [*Nyama*],[89] (3) posture [*Āsana*],[90] (4) breath control [*Prāṇāyāma*], (5) withdrawal from external objects [*Pratyāhāra*],[91] (6) concentration [*Dhāraṇā*], (7) meditation [*Dhyāna*],[92] and (8) absorption [*Samādhi*].

Patañjali, allegedly a doctor and grammarian, has gone down as the author of the *Yogasūtra*, even if his chronological placement is deeply controversial and his very historical existence has been called into question and is still surrounded by a halo of mystery. His *Yogasūtra* are widely considered the Bible of yoga, although they are not without chosen sides and omissions of yogic elements that would be attributed to Tantra in later centuries, when the shift from an oral to a written tradition of these practices took place. Furthermore, recent studies show the influences of Buddhist traditions[93] like Yogācāra[94] and Madhyamaka[95] on Patañjali's *Yogasūtra*. The term "cloud of dharma" [*dharma megha*] in Yogācāra literature (like the Mahāyāna *Laṅkāvatāra-sūtra* or the *Daśabhūmika sūtra*) as the ultimate *bhūmi* appears also in Patañjali as the kind of *samādhi* stemming from the highest degree of discriminative wisdom,[96] which further confirms the fact that Patañjali appears to have reworked concepts from different traditions and translated them into his own terms.

An attempt is made here to show how Patañjali's teachings center on the concept of purification and what follows it and that the core notion around which everything revolves is precisely *tapas*, not least because of Patañjali's choice to define his method [*sādhana*][97] in terms of *kriyāyoga*, the yoga of purifying action.[98] Patañjali defines *tapas* as the tool through which impurities are destroyed [*aśuddhi-kṣayāt tapasaḥ*][99] and through which perfection [*siddhiḥ*] of the body and senses [*kāyendriya*] is brought about. He thus returns to the original meaning of *tapas*, a flame that incinerates, purifies, and opens up a clearing in which something new can be born. In the key aphorisms of his collection of 195 sutras, Patañjali appears to be exploring, using different terms and images, this central concept of purification, which entails two moments: one neutralizing and one revealing. There is a cyclic development within the sutras: at the beginning of the second section [*pāda*]__which is dedicated to the method or exercise [*sādhana*]___he uses different words to characterize the same idea that he introduces at the beginning of the first section, which is dedicated to absorption [*samādhi*], and that he picks up again at the beginning of the third section, dedicated to the powers [*vibhūti*]. In addition, within each section there is a recurrence of the central concepts, which appear in a number of variations of the same theme.

After introducing the notion of *kriyāyoga*, Patañjali defines it as capable of weakening [*tanū-karaṇa]* the afflictions [*kleśa*][100] and bringing about *samādhi*.[101]

Yoga is not only a path of transformation [*pariṇāma*] but also a soteriological path to liberation or isolation [*kaivalya*][102] from afflictions. These afflictions are ignorance [*avidyā*],[103] ego [*asmitā*], craving (attachment to the mental object) [*rāga*], aversion (avoidance of the mental object) [*dveṣa*], and clinging to life (attachment to life as an object) [*abhiniveśāḥ*];[104] they are subtle and "are to be destroyed when [the mind] dissolves back into its original matrix [*pratiprasava*]."[105] In the traditional classical commentary on the sutras, Vyāsa compares these afflictions to seeds that literally need be burnt: "When these impediments have been reduced to the condition of scorched seeds, they become absorbed in (their cause, in the shape of) the yogin's mind whose [ordinary] functioning has come to an end."[106] Through the purifying ardent action of yogic practice, these seeds of mental objects are neutralized along with their potential seminal power, just as enemies are turned to ashes by the burning flame of *tapas*.[107] In the third section, Patañjali returns to this concept by saying that the seeds—inertial drives [*saṃskāra*] directed to external objects—need to be suppressed or restrained [*nirodha*],[108] just as Husserl insists on assigning a "zero index" to any transcendent object through the suspending action of the epoché.[109] The attainment of the higher states of *samādhi* requires restraining the dispersed mind from the many transcendent objects [*sarvārthataikāgratayoḥ*][110] and directing it to a single, pointed concentration [*ekāgratā*][111] that evolves into meditation and eventually into *samādhi* in the strictest sense.

The Stilling of the Mental Vortices

The famed second aphorism of the first section, "*yogaś citta-vṛtti-nirodhaḥ*"[112] is the core of Patañjali's yoga, a manifesto of his entire enterprise: "Yoga is the inhibition (restraint, stilling, neutralization) [*nirodhaḥ*] of the fluctuations [*vṛtti*] of the mind-stuff [*citta*]."[113] Drawing on the phenomenological framework to interpret this statement, one can say that within the natural attitude the space of the mind-stuff[114] is crossed by countless mental events, connected with one another by continuous associations that can be compared to fluctuations, swirls, ripples, or vortices. This is how cognition works; it is all about the establishment of connections between different objects playing a role in life and singled out in the continuum of experience. From the perspective of both biological and cultural evolutionism, the dispersed mind, focusing on a number of different things at the same time, is fit for survival when, for example, random connections lead to a useful solution to a problem one is facing. Making endless associations between the objects of mental events is the grasping mind's natural way of working. These fluctuations can take the form of correct knowledge and valid proof or false knowledge and error; they can take the form of fantasy and conceptual anticipation or of recalling past memories.[115] Patañjali lists three types of correct knowledge [*pramāṇa*]:[116] the first [*pratyakṣa*], commonly translated as "direct perception," should be intended as an ordinary perception in which linguistic and categorial aspects are threaded with an appropriative self-centered framework rather than as a phenomenological perception as has been outlined until this point. Indeed, purified forms of perception or meditation (compatible with the requests of phenomenology) are encountered when approaching more advanced stages of absorption.[117]

The stream of the mind space that some Western writers have tried to describe in detail in the stream-of-consciousness genre can take the form of the analytical procedure of intellectual knowledge, the one of a disturbing inner chatter, or the form of a random association that brings the solution to a problem on which the mind has been stuck; it might be accompanied by the expression "I've got it!" Therefore, according to Patañjali, fluctuations may be detrimental [*kliṣṭa*] or nondetrimental [*akliṣṭāḥ*],[118] but they are in any case to be controlled and inhibited [*nirodhaḥ*] if one wants to enter the yogic state. For this reason, the yogic stance is an un-natural stance. Eliade summarizes this point: "The worldly man is 'possessed' by his own life; the yogin refuses to 'let himself live.'"[119] Both phenomenology and yoga are essentially un-natural attitudes toward the world, or, one might say, anthropotechnics,[120] in the sense that they do not come as a consequence of the process of growing up; on the contrary, they require a distancing from the habitual way of observing the world. They both need a strong commitment and firm discipline. In *First Philosophy*, Husserl states, "Hence in fact, it is all about a completely unnatural stance [*unnatürliche Einstellung*] and of a completely unnatural observation of the self and the world;"[121] in the *Crisis*, he emphasizes this point by speaking of "a total change of the natural attitude, such that we no longer live, as heretofore, as human beings within natural existence."[122]

In yoga, the ordinary pattern of the mind needs to be inhibited, parenthesized, or put out of action, *nirodha*, in terms that are similar to the phenomenological epoché. When the *vṛtti-s* are inhibited with their specific reifying and hypostatizing tendencies, one can realize the underlying horizon, the flowing continuum of consciousness, which in phenomenological terms is called the "transcendental consciousness." In the third aphorism of the *Yogasūtra*, this background consciousness, the realization of which represents the goal of the practitioner, is referred to in terms of the seer, the condition of possibility of any experience: "The seer is merely the power of seeing [*draṣṭā dṛśi mātraḥ*]."[123] Only when the swirls and ripples are stilled through yogic practice does the seer come to dwell in its own form.[124] The term *draṣṭṛ* comes from the root *dṛś*, which means "to see," and practicing the phenomenological stance entails, for Husserl, remaining a "seer of everything" [*für alles bleibe ich sehend*].[125] In this condition of concordance and equality [*samāmpatti*],[126] the mind becomes like a transparent gem [*maṇi*] and, unlike with the natural attitude in which the object is taken as something independent from the subject, it realizes the fundamental correlation between the knower [*grahītṛ*], the knowing [*grahaṇa*], and the known [*grāhya*].[127] In Husserlian terms, this could be framed as the structure of intentionality, in which what is known is called *noema* and the act through which it is known is called *noesis*. Both are related not only to one another but also to the space of consciousness. Patañjali continues by saying that otherwise [*itaratra*], if the fluctuations are not inhibited, consciousness conforms [*sārūpyam*] to these objectifying fluctuating mental events and identifies with them, thus calling on, in phenomenological terms, the ordinary condition of the natural attitude.[128] When the identification with the objectifying tendencies takes place, an unfortunate *saṁyoga* happens, Patañjali warns:[129] that is, an undue conflagration between the seer [*draṣṭṛ*], consciousness, and the seen [*dṛśya*] (e.g., the mind or the eye).

The Seer and the Seen

In the *Drgdriśyaviveka,* a text with no certain attribution but traditionally traced back to Śaṅkarācārya, the most famous exponent of the Advaita Vedānta tradition,[130] it is said that "the form is perceived and the eye is its perceiver. It (eye) is perceived and the mind is its perceiver. The mind with its modifications is perceived and the Witness (the Self) is verily the perceiver. But It (the Witness) is not perceived (by any other)."[131] What in the *Drgdriśyaviveka* is called the "Witness" corresponds to what Husserl calls the "observer." In both cases, an attempt is made to single out the space of consciousness in which any act can take place, be it a perception, a dream,[132] or a fantasy. The undue conjunction, or confusion [*saṁyoga*] between seer and seen is avoided through the capacity of discriminating [*vivēka*].[133] For this reason, the path of yoga entails both a yoking process and a separating action: dividing the world of mental objects, *praḳrti,* from the dimension of consciousness, *puruṣa.*

With the first aphorisms, Patañjali thus summarizes what yoga consists in and briefly sketches the two phases that we have come to learn through phenomenology: a moment in which "doing" something prevails, in terms of burning, the phase of neutralizing the natural objectifying tendency, attained through the "nirodha" and corresponding to the epoché, and a moment of "letting be" and a tepid incubation, the ensuing revealing phase of the seer, that can be another way to indicate the surfacing of the transcendental consciousness, a consciousness that realizes the essential interrelatedness and interdependence of experience.

In the aphorisms that follow, Patañjali explains that the fluctuations are inhibited by means [*upāya*] of "reiteration" [*abhyāsa*] and "non-attachment" [*vairāgya*].[134] The first term refers to the importance of practicing on a regular basis, to the necessity of a reiterated exercise. Husserl argues in similar terms: "The 'transcendental' epoché is meant, of course, as a habitual attitude which we resolve to take up once and for all. Thus it is by no means a temporary act, which remains incidental and isolated in its various repetitions."[135] Similarly, when it comes to yoga, it is not enough to capture the general idea regarding the inhibition of the fluctuations of the mind; a theoretical insight will not suffice. This understanding needs to be grounded in a constantly renewed practice. Referring to "what makes so extraordinarily hard the acquisition of the proper essence of phenomenology,"[136] Husserl admits that "these are hard demands," but "nothing less is required":[137] he concludes that the task of the phenomenologist is "by no means an easy one."[138] Patañjali also claims that this reiterated practice [*abhyāsa*] requires effort [*yatnaḥ*][139] but goes even further in his demands for engagement by the practitioner by stating that the "practice becomes firmly established when it has been cultivated uninterruptedly and with devotion [*satkāra*] [literally the attitude of the one who "makes/attends' to the Being"], over a prolonged period of time."[140]

The second term singled out by Patañjali, *vairāgya*, indicates the nonattachment or dispassion of the one who is without craving [*vitṛṣṇasya*] for external objects.[141] This connects with the phenomenological idea of desiring something other than objects and thus avoiding reducing consciousness itself to an object. This is what happens in contemporary debate when one or more cognitive faculties are regarded as standing for consciousness: "The conjunction [*saṁyoga*] between the seer [*draṣṭṛ*] and that which is seen [*dṛśya*] is the cause [of suffering] to be avoided [*heya*]."[142] Patañjali appears to have offered an advance warning against the now-recurring temptation of taking certain neural patterns that are correlated to attention or another determinant feature for consciousness itself. Even if a biological mechanism correlates to the ability to see in the broad sense, we should not mistake it for the seer, because it is something that can be "seen" [*dṛśya*] through, for example, an imaging technique such as functional magnetic resonance imaging. The seen—the neural corelates of consciousness (NCCs)—are not to be conflated with the seer that can never be seen because it is not an object but the condition of possibility of the visible. Herein lies the purifying nature of Patañjali's enterprise. Husserl also considers his own effort a "pure inquiry,"[143] a form of "purification,"[144] and of "transcendental purification"[145] with which "the spirit returns from its naive external orientation to itself"[146] through "pure intuition"[147] to an "ontology of the experiential world purely as such."[148] *Ideas for a Pure Phenomenology* is the beginning of the title of Husserl's major work, and the various forms of *rein*, the German term for "pure," recurs hundreds of times within his texts. Against the constant reifying and hypostatizing tendencies hidden in language and discursive thought that lead us to take the dimension of the seer (the transcendental consciousness) as the new real thing with which to replace the old concepts, Patañjali argues that the dimension in which the seer is realized, the absorption of *samādhi* in which the mind does not cling to any transcendent object but becomes steady, pain-free [*viśokā*], and luminous [*jyotiṣmatī*][149] is a state that intrinsically lacks a self-sufficient and independent nature. Just as the transcendental consciousness does not exist independently but appears through a *Gestalt* dynamic (as the undetermined background of anything determined that surfaces), Patañjali's *samādhi* is devoid of its own form [*svarūpa-śūnyam*].[150] Patañjali reaches this point when discussing the last three limbs of his eight-step path that lead to the insightful state of prajñā, another term with which to refer to the dimension of the seer. More precisely, through the union of concentration, meditation, and absorption [*saṁyama*] comes prajñā,[151] which is defined by Patañjali as a state in which the cosmic order [*ṛta*] is borne [*bhāra*].[152]

Fixing the mind on one place is called concentration [*dhāraṇā*],[153] and extending this action over time is called meditation [*dhyāna*]. Eventually, a stage is reached in which, through the shining forth [*nirbhāsaṃ*] of content alone [*arthamātra*], the mind is devoid of its own form [*svarūpa-śūnyam*]; this is called absorption [*samādhi*].[154] The stage of enlightenment is thus closely related to the dimension of emptiness [*śūnyatā*]: it is not graspable because it is empty of own substance and nature.

Chapter 5

Emptiness and Clear Light Consciousness

Emptiness in Nāgārjuna

At this point, it is inevitable to refer to the one who is famed for being a *śūnyavādin*; that is, for having gone about telling the *śūnyatā* and for having devoted no less than seventy stanzas to emptiness: the Buddhist philosopher Nāgārjuna.[1] This inevitability is not a matter of any historical influences of the ideas of Nāgārjuna on the *Yogasūtra*, which likely exist but might also be called into question in the context of Eastern philology, in which dating is an issue that is never settled. Delving into the tenets of Nāgārjuna's Madhyamaka will help avoid the common metaphysical substantialist and dualist approach to yoga[2] and contribute to clarifying how the nonrealist and interdependent key of interpretation with which phenomenology has equipped us is particularly suitable to understand deeply what is at stake not only in Patañjali's yoga, but also in the *haṭha* yoga traditions of the Buddhist and Śaiva matrices. In addition, the clarifications of notions coming from the Vedanta such as Ātman and Brahman will take advantage of Nāgārjuna's contribution.[3] In fact, in the *Maitry Upaniṣad*, it is said that when the Ātman is thoroughly penetrated—that is, when the Ātman is realized through Ātman [*ātmanātmānam*]—the Ātman becomes devoid of Ātman or non-ātman [*nir-ātmā*].[4] This and several other Upanishadic passages[5] clearly justify a nonsubstantializing and nondualist interpretation of such notions, a phenomenological interpretation that envisages a third way between idealism and realism and recognizes world and subject as the provisional and ever-changing outputs of a circular movement of co-determination.

Nāgārjuna, who lived in India around the second century CE, is the most influential Mahāyāna Buddhist philosopher. He wrote the fundamental work *Mūla-madyamaka-kārikā* [*Fundamental Root Verses on the Middle Way*] and established the Madyamaka doctrine, in which the notion of emptiness is central on the basis of the teachings contained in the *Prajñāpāramitāsūtra*. These can be summarized by the famous lesson that the Buddha offers to his disciple Śāriputra in the *Hṛdaya Sūtra* [*Heart-Sūtra*]: "Śāriputra, form is not different from emptiness, and emptiness is not different from form. Form itself is emptiness, and emptiness itself is form."[6] As a dialectical philosopher, his tight argument is analytical and often resorts to the *prasaṅga* argument, which is the Buddhist form of the *reductio ad absurdum*. The target of his criticism is the realist tendency of substantializing things; that is, the metaphysics of reification and hypostatization [*prapañca*].[7] Nāgārjuna seeks to show that the notion of intrinsic or inherent existence [*svābhva*] is incoherent and to replace it with the one of emptiness [*śūnyatā*].[8] The doctrine of the "an-ātman" [*anatta* in Pali], of the noninherent existence of the Ātman (which in Buddhism comes to indicate more specifically the personal self[9] and not so much the transcendental consciousness to which the term pointed in the Advaita Vedānta),[10] is a general Buddhist tenet; what is emphasized in Mahāyāna (the second turning of the *dharma* wheel),[11] especially through the intermediation of Nāgārjuna's philosophy, is the idea of extending this emptiness of intrinsic existence to other things.[12] Nāgārjuna argues in favor of the famed doctrine of "dependent arising" [*pratītya-samutpāda*]: "the dependent existence of things is said to be emptiness, for what is dependently existent is lacking substance."[13] Thus, "emptiness" does not mean "inexistence" but a lack of intrinsic nature, in the sense of "own": "for whom there is emptiness, there are all things. For whom there is no emptiness there is nothing whatsoever."[14] What is refuted is the idea that something exists independently from everything else, as is found in the Western scholastic concept of substance, bearing the cause of itself in itself and not in something else: "Something that is not dependently arisen, such a thing does not exist. Therefore a non-empty thing does not exist."[15]

Co-Dependent Arising

According to Nāgārjuna, the "own nature" (*svābahva; svā* means "own" and *bhava* means "being") of what is said to be such has never been seen in its foundation. There is no separate substance that is the cause of itself to be found anywhere: everything exists in relation to something else, thanks to something else, or dependent on something else. Everything co-arises and is co-dependent. Something arising independently cannot even be imagined, and nothing is grounded in itself but always in something else. However, the moment we name something, we surreptitiously imply its independent existence out there. In phenomenology, it is a matter of suspending faith in a transcendent, pre-given world that common sense and naive realist science has taught us to posit being as out there, independent from us. The following passage by Husserl could have been written by Nāgārjuna to clarify the notion of dependent arising:

> Reality, the reality of the physical thing taken singly and the reality of the whole world, lacks self-sufficiency in virtue of its essence (in our strict sense of the word). Reality is not in itself something absolute which becomes tied secondarily to something else; rather, in the absolute sense, it is nothing at all; it has no "absolute essence" whatever; it has the essentiality of something which, of necessity, is only intentional, only an object of consciousness, something presented in the manner peculiar to consciousness, something apparent.[16]

Husserl speaks of overcoming any positing of transcendent objects. To undermine faith in the existence of self-independent objects, one must go beyond traditional language because language is the very vehicle through which reification happens; it is sympathetic to a world made of objects. The substantializing tendencies hidden within language are neutralized for Nāgārjuna through a linguistic device: the Buddhist *tetralemma,*[17] the *Catuṣkoṭi,* the four-cornered system of argumentation (P; not-P; both P and not-P; neither P nor not-P). Through this logical figure, the dualistic Aristotelian view of the *tertium non datur*—the idea that things either correspond to state P or to state not-P—is called into question. Nāgārjuna's use of the *Catuṣkoṭi* is generally understood to "provide an enumeration of four exclusive and exhaustive logical alternatives, all of which are then shown to be deficient and rejected"[18] and thus to conceive of a state of things that does not correspond to P, not-P, both, or the negation of both. It is in the *Vigrahavyāvartanī, The Dispeller of Disputes,* that Nāgārjuna seeks to chase away and dispel [*vi-graha*] these misconceptions and misunderstandings [*vyāvartanī,* "counter-movement"]. He wants to undermine readers' faith in what they have heard about but have never actually seen. The interesting thing is that Nāgārjuna avoids granting any substantial existence even to his own words, which are empty of inherent substance, just like everything else. For this reason, the objection of an imaginary critic concerning an alleged contradiction in his argument can find no grip on Nāgārjuna's thesis, as attested by the following kārikās:

> "This speech does not exist substantially, therefore there is no destruction of my position." [. . .] "I do not negate anything, and there is nothing to be negated. To this extent you misrepresent me when you say 'you negate.' "[19]

When Nāgārjuna argues that "we do not speak without assenting to the conventional truth,"[20] he is implying that as long as we continue to use language, we are moving within a realm of conventional or relative truth. But by highlighting the limits of language, we can point toward another dimension that is beyond it and its reifying tendencies, because, as the *Mūla-madyamaka-kārikā* relates, "The Buddha's teaching of the *Dharma* is based on two truths: a truth of worldly convention [*saṃvṛti-satya*] and an ultimate truth [*paramārtha-satya*]."[21] Heidegger points in a similar direction when he distinguishes between the point of view of being-there [*Dasein*], the ontic and existential dimension, and the point of view of Being [*Sein*], the ontological and ultimate dimension. The former remains valid within the natural attitude but is partial and provisional, like conventional truth, while the latter is the standpoint of the one who has overcome the objectifying and dualistic view of reality. In fact, the object is precisely what is believed within the natural attitude to exist inherently and independently.

In the *Mūla-madyamaka-kārikā*, the idea of an independent existence is discarded regarding practically everything: things and their attributes, causes and effects, even emptiness itself. However, Nāgārjuna warns that "by a misperception of emptiness a person of little intelligence is destroyed. Like a snake incorrectly seized or like a spell incorrectly cast."[22] Nāgārjuna's rhetorical strategy is to engage in a dialogue with an imaginary detractor who asserts the nonemptiness of things and to show how this starting point leads to untenable conclusions: "If all this were nonempty, as in your view, there would be no arising and ceasing. Then the Four Noble Truths would become non-existent."[23] He cites the very clear example of suffering: "If not dependently arising, how could suffering come to be? Suffering has been taught to be impermanent, and so cannot come from its own essence."[24] Nāgārjuna objects to his virtual opponent that if things are substantial, suffering would also have a substance. But if it had a substance, an intrinsic existence, why would it arise? Because things arise and cease only through dependence on others: "If there is essence [own nature], the whole world will be unarising, unceasing, and static. The entire phenomenal world would be immutable."[25] Realizing the emptiness of inherent existence is like realizing a net of interconnectedness in which everything arises and ceases like the sparks of light coming from shimmering gems woven into Indra's net:

> Far away in the heavenly abode of the great god Indra, there is a wonderful net which has been hung by some cunning artificer in such a manner that it stretches out infinitely in all directions. There hang the jewels, glittering like stars in the first magnitude. . . . If we now arbitrarily select one of these jewels for inspection and look closely at it, we will discover that in its polished surface there are reflected all the other jewels in the net, infinite in number. Not only that, but each of the jewels reflected in this one jewel is also reflecting all the other jewels, so that there is an infinite reflecting process occurring.[26]

Indra's net can be read as an image of Nāgārjuna's emptiness or dependent origination: "Whoever sees dependent arising also sees suffering and its arising and its cessation as well as the path."[27]

Figure 5.1. Indra's net. *Source:* Myriams-Fotos, Pixabay.

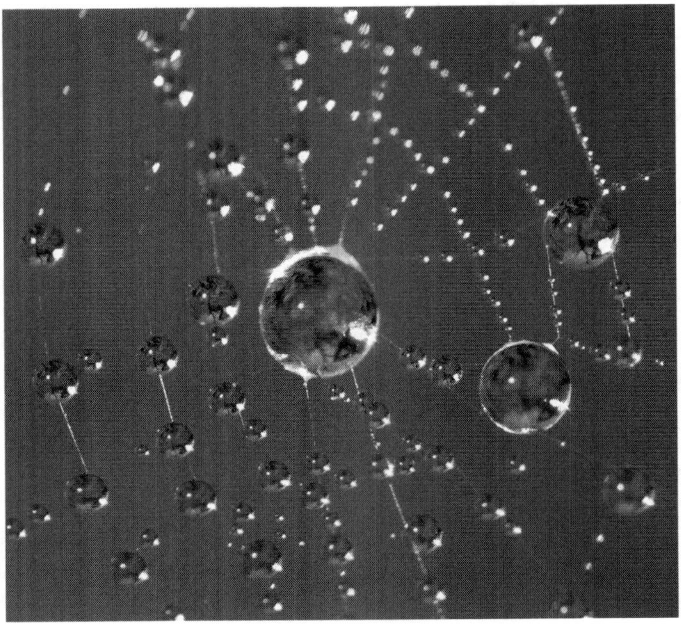

Not only are the Four Noble Truths empty of inherent nature, but even the Buddha is to be understood as empty of substance. The Buddha that Nāgārjuna venerates and in front of whom he bows is Buddha Śūnyatām, "The one who taught emptiness, dependent origination, and the Middle Way as one thing, the incomparable Buddha."[28]

Heidegger's Being and Emptiness

Nāgārjuna's notion of emptiness [*śūnyatā*] has a strong affinity with Heidegger's notion of Being and Nothingness,[29] and the influence of Eastern thought on Heidegger is known.[30] He had a profound exchange of views with Shūzō' Kuki, a Japanese writer and poet who had studied with him and to whom he addresses a grateful memory in "A Dialogue on Language."[31] This text, included in *On the Way to Language*,[32] unfolds as a dialogue between Heidegger and a Japanese interviewer, Tomio Tezuka, who elicits Heidegger's memories about Count Kuki, in which important issues about not only language but also the connections between West and East are addressed. Heidegger mentions the controversial question he had discussed with Kuki of the extent to which "Eastasians" (such as Tezuka, a professor of German literature at the Imperial University of Tokyo) should study and "chase after the European conceptual systems"[33] and refers to the danger "hidden in language itself" of, as the interviewer guesses, "shifting everything into European."[34] After having assessed that "Europeans presumably dwell in an entirely different house than Eastasians," Heidegger leaves a narrow opening for the existence of this "nearly impossible dialogue." The Japanese interviewer rushes to add, "You are right to say 'nearly.' For still it was a dialogue and, I should think, an exciting one, because Count Kuki, in the workshops he held with us at Kyoto University, came back again and again to those dialogues with you."[35] Heidegger at one point states that "emptiness" is the same as "nothingness," which is the same as the essential Being,[36] and the interviewer makes clear that "to us [Easterners] emptiness is the loftiest name for what you mean to say with the word 'Being.'"[37] But in which sense is it possible that nothingness ultimately coincides with Being? Because just like Buddhist emptiness, Heideggerian nothingness [*Nichts*] does not mean absolute nothingness or inexistence but the nothingness of the entity [*Seiende*]; in other words, the nothingness of objects. *Nichts* is the nonentity par excellence.[38] And what is first and foremost the space of the nonentity? It is Being, which is empty of an objectlike and inherent nature.

In his biography of Heidegger, Heinrich Petzt recalls a passage from the dialogue between Heidegger and the Thai Buddhist monk Bikkhu Maha Mani, who was familiar with Heidegger's philosophy, and says the following: "Nothingness, however, is not a 'null,' but the opposite: the fullness [*die Fülle*]. Nobody can name it. But it is, nothing and all, the full realization [*Erfüllung*]." Heidegger replies as follows: "This is what, in all my life, I have said."[39] For this reason, Heidegger's notion of Being can be connected to Nāgārjuna's notion of emptiness [*śūnyatā*] and co-dependent arising [*pratītya-samutpāda*], which are exemplified by the image of Indra's net. Moreover, in the previous chapters of this book a connection between this notion of Being and Husserl's transcendental background horizon consciousness has been established. Further elements in support of this are found in Patañjali's claim, discussed above, that the state of *samadhi* in which consciousness unfolds in the "loftiest way" is a fundamentally empty condition in which the mind is devoid of its own form [*svarūpa-śūnyam*]. It becomes clear what this actually means reading Nāgārjuna's Rātnāvali where it is said that "The Buddha in fact preached to some the law so that they could be freed from sin [. . .] to other the laws based on a duality. To some others he preached the laws beyond duality, deep, terrifying those who are afraid."[40] The fact that emptiness might describe the dimension of transcendental consciousness is further confirmed in Milarepa's teachings, as we see below:[41] the Buddha Mind is described as the space of *Dharmakāya*,[42] a "great illuminating void awareness."[43] This is the space of transcendental consciousness [prajñā] in which nondual and nonlinguistic ultimate truth is foreshadowed:

> But in [the realm of] absolute truth Buddha himself does not exist; there are no practices nor practisers, no path, no realization, and no stages, no Buddha's bodies and no wisdom. There is then no *nirvāṇa*, for these are merely names and thoughts. Matter and beings in the universe are non-existent from the start; they have never come to be. There is no truth, no innate-born wisdom, no karma, and no effect therefrom; *Saṃsāra* even has no name. Such is absolute Truth.[44]

No Difference Between *Samsāra* and *Nirvāṇa*

The Hundred Thousand Songs of Milarepa [*Mila Grubum*], one of the masterpieces of Tibetan literature, has been taken as the "biography of a saint, a guide book for devotions, a manual of Buddhist Yoga, a volume of songs and poems, and even a collection of Tibetan folklore and fairy tales."[45] As the text has no attribution, the identity of its compiler is not clear but might be the fabled and mysterious yogi Tsangnyön Heruka, a Kagyu master in the lineage of Milarepa's disciples.[46] Vajrayāna Tibetan Buddhism (the third turning of the *dharma* wheel)[47] owes the philosophical framework of its inquiry to Nāgārjuna's Madhyamaka, adding to it a profound emphasis on esoteric tantric teachings in both theory and yoga practices.

Drawing on Nāgārjuna,[48] Milarepa makes clear that the notions of emptiness and dependent origination prominently describe the nature of transcendental consciousness that might be accessed "by realizing the awareness of Light-Void" because "the nature of Mind is the Light and the Void."[49]

This dimension of consciousness is called Dharmakāya. Just as Patañjali's *vṛttis* are neutralized in the absorption, Milarepa's "errant thoughts are liberated in the Dharmakāya; the awareness, the illumination, is always blissful."[50] Milarepa is reminiscent of Patañjali but can also be viewed as anticipating the nonreifying vocation of phenomenology when saying, "Should your wavering thoughts vanish in the *Dharmakāya,* never think of them as real entities."[51]

The emphasis in Buddhist Tibetan yoga is on realizing the identity between *saṃsāra* and *nirvāṇa* and on overcoming the duality between an alleged spiritual realm and a material, sensory, and transient one: "The non-differentiation of manifestation and Voidness is the Dharmakāya, in which Samsāra and Nirvāna are felt to be the same. It is a complete merging of Buddha and sentient beings."[52] Milarepa had of course absorbed Nagarjuna's lesson, which is essentially a milestone for all further tantric traditions: "There is not the slightest difference between cyclic existence [*saṃsāra*] and *nirvāṇa*. There is not the slightest difference between *nirvāṇa* and cyclic existence."[53] Milarepa repeatedly returns to this point, as when he says, "Let me help you to the last realization that the *Dharmakāya* and all forms are one!"[54] and when claiming that "the embodiment of all the Buddhas is the *Dharmakāya* in itself."[55] But how can dualism be overcome? Because the faith in an inherent substance has been broken, if there is no inherent substance, there is no intrinsic purity and impurity: thus everything, including the embodied dimension, can become a door into the nondual space. Exchanges[56] between tantric Buddhism and Kashmir Śivaism milieus are likely to have taken place since a similar revaluation of the senses and of the body is attested in both. Tantra (which literally means "weaving" or "intertwining") refers to a heterogenic system of texts, practices, and teachings in which a nondual approach to reality is central. Tāntrikas do not exclude one part of the world in favor of another. The Indologist André Padoux cites Madeleine Biardeau to claim that the doctrinal aspect of Tantra is "an attempt to place *kāma*, desire, in every sense of the word, in the service of liberation . . . not to sacrifice this world for liberation's sake, but to reinstate it, in varying ways, within the perspective of salvation."[57] Several tantric schools broke with the traditional rules through nonconventional secret practices because they sought a way out of the dichotomy of pure and impure, as summarized in the words of Śaiva philosopher Abhinavagupta (10th–11th centuries CE): "Here there is no purity nor impurity, nor discussion on what can be eaten, no duality nor non-duality . . . everything is here prescribed and prohibited. This only is mandatory . . . that mind be steadily directed towards true reality, all the rest doesn't count."[58]

Just as the phenomenon is the only reality—Being itself and not a representative of a true thing placed somewhere beyond it—the cornerstone that qualifies tantric approaches is the idea that facing manifold reality does not consist in being confronted with an illusionary world [*maya*] that has to be negated and overcome in favor of another world that is beyond it: true, eternal, and blissful. On the contrary, "The joy of *Samādhi* is the bliss in the world [*lokānandaḥ samādhisukham*],"[59] as stated in the *Śivasūtra* by Vasgupta (8th–9th centuries CE), and "the yogin shall focus his mind wherever it finds satisfaction,"[60] as is said in the *Vijñānabhairava Tantra,* a text of the Kashmir school of Trika (7th–8th centuries CE), in which the term *Vijñāna* stands for consciousness, like the Tibetan *She-Pa*. An additional passage from the *Vijñānabhairava Tantra,* "for the one who meditates that, all the body and the universe are essentially consciousness, thanks to a thought lacking all differentiated representations, the supreme awakening arises,"[61] mirrors the following verse by the Buddhist Milarepa: "Happy is the yoga in which I identify the *Dharmakāya* with apprehensions! The words and writing, the dogmas and the logic I absorb in the realm of illuminating consciousness."[62] Milarepa confirms the primacy of intuitive embodied experience over discursive analytical knowledge: "All forms then become the *Dharmakāya*. Happy am I without those foolish books."[63]

Clear Light Consciousness

The Dharmakāya is identified with a clear light that shines forth. The photism that is to be found at the dawn of the Western world in the myth of Phanes is also a major emphasis in Eastern traditions, especially in Tibetan Tantra, in which the expression "clear light"[64] [*'od gsal* in Tibetan, *prabashvara citta* in Sanskrit] comes to indicate something close to the transcendental consciousness of phenomenology. Milarepa indicates the moment following death [*Bardo*][65] as the favorable point at which to access this dimension of all-pervading luminous consciousness for practitioners who have devoted themselves to this realization during their lifetimes: "When at death the Transcendental Wisdom of the *Dharmakāya* shines."[66] Though Milarepa repeatedly mentions the *Bardo* path,[67] more detailed instructions on the intermediate state of the *Bardo* are given in the *Bardo Tödöl Chenmo,* a scripture attributed to *Padmasambhava* [*terma*],[68] which translates literally as the "liberation through hearing during the intermediate state"[69] but is more widely known by the term that Evans-Wentz chose in his 1927 translation: *The Tibetan Book of the Dead.* This text contains a prescription to recognize[70] in the final moment the luminous-conscious-empty principle and to allow oneself to be reabsorbed within it. In this intermediate state[71] between death and rebirth, what is most important is not to allow oneself to be scared away by the dazzling light and the terrifying apparitions that follow, which are produced by one's own mind.[72]

If the practitioner manages not to be distracted by these mental projections, the mental energy in the individual state [*Sem* in Tibetan] becomes reabsorbed in the "clear light" consciousness, and the cycle of transmigration is over: "Do not be distracted. This is the dividing-line where buddhas and sentient beings are separated."[73]

In Tibetan Buddhism, the "yoga of clear light" is considered a preparation undertaken in life of this recognition in order to facilitate it in life's final moment. The Dalai Lama lists several moments in life that are particularly favorable for accessing the dimension of this state of transcendental consciousness. Referring to the Kālacakra tantric tradition, a lineage that can be traced to the teachings of Nāropā,[74] master of Marpa and root-master of Milarepa (Marpa's direct disciple), Tenzin Gyatso states the following:

> Even on the ordinary level there are certain occasions in which we naturally have slight experiences of the subtle level of mind called clear light or the non-conceptual state. These occasions are during sleep, sneezing, fainting and sexual climax. This shows that we have within ourselves a certain potential or seed that can be developed further. Among these four naturally occurring states, the one that accords us the best opportunity to generate the experience of clear light is during sexual climax. Although we are using this ordinary term "sexual," the reference should not be taken in an ordinary way.[75]

This indication recalls what appears in the *Vijñānabhairava Tantra*, confirming the mutual exchanges of views between tantric Kashmir Śivaism and tantric Tibetan Buddhism: "standing above a deep hole or well and looking steadily downward, into the abyss, lacking discursive thinking, immediately arises the dissolution of the mind . . . at the beginning and end of sneezing, in terror, in sorrow or in confusion, in front of an abyss, when fleeing from a battlefield, in excitement of desire, at the onset or appeasement of hunger, that state is the eternal existence of Brahman."[76] These words might also be astonishing to hear from a practitioner accustomed to considering the embodied standpoint as a flaw from which one is to be freed as soon as possible. The tendency to think of the path of yoga as a way to gradually emancipate oneself from the bodily dimension has its roots in the basic ambiguity of how to interpret the notions of "body" and "senses."

Phenomenological Experience vs. Mental Object

In the traditional texts, starting from the Vedanta tradition, there are many warnings regarding the body [*śarīrasyā*] and the senses [*indriya*]. However, one must read in these cases, thanks to the phenomenological key, "body-object"[77] instead of "body" and "sense-object" instead of "sense." The passages of the *Chāndogya Upaniṣad* that discuss the body as a true chain for *prāna* are of course well known[78] and use terms similar to the prison of the Platonic soul. The *Upaniṣads* in general overflow with admonishments that appear to concern the fallibility of the senses that, if not properly reined in, risk behaving like runaway horses [*duṣṭāśvā*], according to the metaphor in the *Kaṭha Upanishad*[79] and make us confuse "snakes with ropes,"[80] to cite a classic example from the *Māṇḍūkya Upaniṣad.* Yet these cases do not actually refer to the dimension of the body in unalloyed terms but to a domain of the body already heavily structured by the reifying mental level. This is the meaning of the contactless yoga [*asparśayoga*], which is hard to obtain but advocated by Gauḍapāda in his commentary on the *Māṇḍūkya Upaniṣad.*[81] The contact at stake has nothing to do with touch; what needs to be suspended is contact with reified mental objects. In these cases, unlike with sensory experience, we are dealing with mental representations built over the phenomenological experience and is for this reason betrayed as such. In the *Kaṭha Upanishad* example, the unbridled horses are to be compared to the objectified senses, not to sensory experience itself. As stated in the *Vaiśeṣikasūtra* (4th century BCE), the problem comes from mixing raw sensory experience with mental representation: "Pleasure and suffering [arise] as a result of the drawing together of the sense organs, the mind and objects."[82]

When explaining Tibetan Buddhist epistemology in the 1920s, writer and explorer Alexandra David-Néel, the first woman to reach Tibet, employs terms that are very close to the phenomenological arguments with which Husserl has made us familiar:

> Do not we ourselves add, on our own authority, various accretions for which our senses are in no way responsible? Let us see: You happen to be in a vast, bare plane, and in the distance you see a fleck of green standing out on the yellow sand. . . . To say that you have seen a tree in the distance is incorrect. Your eyes did not show you a tree with leafy branches able to shelter you from the sun's rays. The idea of the tree and of its representation in your mind are the results of mental activity which has been set in motion by the sight of the tiny flecks of green. . . . Other green spots seen in similar conditions have led to the finding of a tree at the end of a plane. This has been remembered. . . . Nevertheless these are ratiocinations.[83]

From this point of view, the fifth limb of Patañjali's *ashtanga yoga*—the withdrawal of the senses, *pratyāhāra*—also does not require withdrawing from sensory phenomena but rather from the mental representations built on purely phenomenological data. By the way, it is worth mentioning that the concept of "phenomenon" developed by phenomenology radically differs from the one we frequently come across in translations of Eastern texts, where the words "phenomenon" and "phenomenal" are often used to translate something that is far from truth or reality. This could cause the reader some confusion. It should be remembered that this latter use, which highlights a fundamentally dualistic approach, is not technical, as in phenomenology, and thus includes in the "phenomenon" its mental and conceptual representation.

As already recalled, in yoga the body and senses are not in themselves considered something from which to be purified but quite the opposite: "From *tapas,* on account of the removal of the impurities, rises the perfection of the senses and the body [*kāyendriyasiddhir*]."[84] However, the mind is always trying to get hold of not only sensations but also of emotions, seeking to organize and often crystalize them. When emotions are made mental rather than being physically and fluidly experienced, the body is no longer able to absorb them and release them like water wrung from a sponge. It is only in these cases that emotions become obstacles. In other words, what needs to be suspended is a level of sensitivity that is already deeply structured by the discriminating mind.

The Dalai Lama highlights the distance that exists between these philosophical teachings and the ordinary prescriptions given, for example, in the Vinaya, the book of discipline of the monks.[85] But why are these secret tantric indications so different from the ordinary ones connected to the conventional truth? The answer is that between the two lies the profound understanding of the notions of emptiness and dependent origination.

Yoga Tantra

Only the practitioner who has internalized the meaning of emptiness can successfully use the body and the connected touch dimension without running the risk of reifying and transforming it into an object. One must first undermine one's own faith in the inherent existence of the ego [*asmitā*] and consequently of everything else; only then can the tantric yogic techniques, of which *Haṭha* yoga is a spinoff, be approached without risk. This is what "initiation" in such contexts is about: making sure that the candidate approaching certain practices and techniques is in the condition to understand what is at stake because misunderstanding is always round the corner and, as Nāgārjuna warns, "by a misperception of emptiness a person of little intelligence is destroyed. Like a snake incorrectly seized or like a spell incorrectly cast."[86] In the Kālacakra tradition,[87] the precondition to be initiated to any higher teaching is the *bodhicitta* resolution on the part of the practitioner to be devoted to reaching awakening [*bodhi*] for the sake of all beings.[88] This being said, a few foundation stones of this tradition, might, in the light of such disclaimers, be tackled to realize how bodily practices, especially those concerning the sexual domain, represent the gateway to the realization of the transcendental clear-light consciousness.

The *Sekoddesa*, the summary of the initiation,[89] the dialogue between the mythical king of Śambala, Sucandra, and the Buddha, the Blessed one, contains a commentary by Nāropā, master of Marpa and Milarepa and abbot of Nalanda University. This text deals with liberation in life through the experience of the highest pleasure or bliss [*ānanda*].[90] From a conventional point of view, the advice offered by the Buddha to the king is striking, as it consists of continuing the desiring experience for as long as possible: "there exists no greater sin than the lack of desire, there exists no greater merit than pleasure, therefore, oh King, you must apply the mind continuously to the unmoved pleasure."[91] The experience of pure pleasure and desire [*sukha* and *icchā*][92] for the one who has understood and is ready has nothing to do with craving objects [*rāga*], the affliction of which Patañjali speaks of; rather, it is an all-encompassing experience that saturates the space of the mind-stuff, *citta*, and silences the fluctuations of the drunken monkey mind that clings to and then jumps from one object to another, as the *Sutta Pitaka* describes the Buddhist triple basket: "Just as a monkey, swinging through a forest wilderness, grabs a branch. Letting go of it, it grabs another branch. Letting go of that, it grabs another one. In the same way, what's called 'mind,' 'intellect,' or 'consciousness' by day and by night arises as one thing and ceases as another."[93] Whereas Saṃsāra is dominated and perpetuated by alternating periods of desire and nondesire, the yogin must avoid this swinging because during the phases in which desire stops, the natural attitude toward reality might be reestablished, and a tendency toward the objectifying attitude might recur. In addition, sentimental feelings, in so far as they are creations of the mind (i.e., reified through mental processes), are in Nāropā's view impediments to be burnt: "passions, etc., are in fact creations of the mind . . . from the fire of knowledge the stain is burnt, not the luminous mind."[94] In the Kālacakra teachings, after a description of the initiations[95] performed in the *mandala*, a six-limbed [*sadāṇga*] yoga is described.[96] At the center of this yoga is a gesture of union, initially performed physically and eventually symbolically, called *Mahamudra*: "The union of emptiness and compassion is the non-emitted bodhicitta."[97] The practice of breathing techniques, such as the retention of the breath, and of visualizations gradually enables both male and female practitioners to avoid emitting the sexual fluid [*bindu*], which symbolizes the *bodhicitta*, the resolution of awakening:[98] "From the stopping of the wind, the *bodhicitta* is stopped, from the stopping of the *bodhicitta*, the emission is stopped . . . [and the practitioner] will reach unmoved pleasure [*sukha akṣara*] and will be freed from transmigration bonds."[99] It is called *binduyoga*,[100] *vajrayoga*,[101] and *Yuganaddha* ("two in one"), for through these physical [*Karmamudrā*] and figured practices, the practitioner realizes the union of emptiness [*śūnyatā*] and compassion [*karuṇā*].

The Six Yogas of Nāropā

Tzong Kapha Chenmo, the founder of the Gelug school and holder of teachings dating to Nāropā,[102] wrote a commentary on *The Six Yogas of Nāropā* that are closely linked to the tantric teachings of the Kālacakra on which Nāropā comments. As a matter of fact, these six yogas are even considered higher teachings to be accessed by the practitioner only when the public teachings concerning emptiness and codependent origination have been internalized, mostly contained in Tzong Kapha's imposing text on the stages of the path, the *Lam Rim*.[103] The yogin is asked to confront the preliminary practices such as the initiations referred to above that are true empowerments[104] and the resolution of the *bodhicitta*.

For the purpose of the path followed thus far, a thorough analysis of all six yogas[105] is not of primary concern, but it is useful to highlight some aspects concerning the dimensions of heat and purification, which are at the heart of both the yogic and phenomenological stances. The practice of *tummo* (*gtûm-mö* in Tibetan, *chandali* in Sanskrit) is the creation of internal heat and entails a combination of specific *haṭha* yoga practices,[106] such as bodily postures, breathing techniques like retaining the breath, and visualizations of energetic channels and centers associated with specific mantra syllables.[107] Through specific practices such as vase breathing,[108] a "blazing inner fire"[109] is kindled that promotes the melting of the drops [*bindu*] of consciousness [*bodhicitta* or *bodhi mind*] and the experience of the "four blisses"[110] [*ananda*]. This is the first yoga described by Nāropā and leads to the emergence of the first signs of the clear light consciousness, which is an experience "beyond conceptuality consciousness."[111] However, a more profound experience of the clear light consciousness in which a fusion with the *Dharmakaya* takes place needs to be preceded by the realization of the emptiness, on which Tzong Kapha places particular emphasis and that, according to Nāropā, should be prepared by the "yoga of the illusionary body."[112] In this yoga, a distancing from the ordinary conceptualization of the everyday objects is trained: the practitioner realizes that other than the ego, there is a crystallized concept of the body, which, in phenomenological terms, is called the concept of the body-as-object [*körper*]. The illusionary nature of the body refers to this concept of the body, to the mentalized body, and not to the body as lived-through experience, which Husserl calls the *Leib*. To understand these kinds of practices, one must understand the unobjectifiable nature of emptiness. Only from the bliss stemming from the *mahamudra*, the meditation on emptiness and codependent existence, can one approach the yoga of clear light, the highest or *anuttara* yoga tantra.[113] Even in this final stage, the practice is still gradual, entailing the retention of clear light, first during wakeful periods and finally during sleep, including dream yoga, in which "one meditates on how all these appearances are empty of a true self nature, yet manifest as illusions."[114] The intensity of this light varies in degree. For example, the experience of "utter emptiness and clear light" is described as a "sense of clear light like that of the sky at dawn, when there is neither sun, moon or darkness"[115] and is an intermediate stage compared to the "inseparable ecstasy and void"[116] that also enables overcoming the limited vision of the karmic law,[117] which still belongs to the level of conventional truth.

Lama Yesce, a contemporary monk in the tradition of Tzong Khapa, has dedicated a text to the bliss of the internal fire, which he considers the heart of Nāropā's teaching, and urges a nondual[118] view according to which one should not "reject pleasure, but rather utilize it"[119] in view of realization, since "difficulties come from the mind, not from the body":[120] "a sense of bliss arising from the secret chakra will indicate that you are making progress. . . . This experience is beyond concepts, beyond words."[121] Following Tzong Khapa's commentary on *The Six Yogas of Nāropā,* Lama Yesche, after having detailed the preliminary procedure[122] for vase breathing turns to lighting the internal fire: as a consequence of the retention of the breath and the visualizations, the "inner fire explodes limitlessly and fills your entire body."[123] The *Sekoddesa* to the Kālacakra also refers to the moment in which "the yogin sees the *chandali* inflamed at the navel, thanks to the retention":[124] "This power of the vital wind, halted at the navel, similar to the lightning, raised in the form of a stick, shall ascend light and plane, driven through the central channel from wheel to wheel, until it comes to reach violently the opening at the crown of the head, as a thorn on skin."[125] This powerful experience of the descent and ascent of the *bindu* is accompanied by the experience of the blisses. David-Néel, in a report on her trip to Tibet a century ago, describes how the tantric disciple initiated into the *tummo* is capable, through the production of physical and psychic heat, of warming up cloths that have been deliberately soaked in ice water and wrapped around the body several times on freezing Tibetan nights: "I saw some hermits seated night after night, motionless on the snow, entirely naked, sunk in meditation, while the terrible winter blizzard whirled and hissed around them!"[126] In describing this practice, she adds that the disciples "on the shore of a lake or a river in the heart of the winter, dried on their bodies, as on a stove, a number of sheets dipped in the icy water!"[127] David-Néel also recounts this practice from the first-person perspective: "Yet my mind continued to be concentrated on the object of the thumo rite. I soon saw the flames rise around me—they grew larger and larger, they engulfed me, their red tongues arching over my head. I soon felt an exquisite wellbeing come over me. . . . I felt the fire come out of my head, arise from each of my fingers."[128]

As noted above, in the Tibetan Kālacakra tradition, the philosophical framework is offered by Nāgārjuna and his Madhyamaka: emptiness is considered to be the mother of everything, wisdom [*prajña*], and compassion is considered to be the father of everything, the skillful means [*upāya*].[129] Emptiness and compassion are two sides of the same coin. Nāgārjuna had taught that emptiness is not a dry and cold intellectual realization but brings peacefulness: "Whatever is dependently arisen, such a thing is essentially peaceful. Therefore that which is arising and arising itself are themselves peaceful."[130] As Jay Garfield argues in reference to Nagarjuna's view, "If one reifies phenomena—including such things as one's own self—and if one thinks that things either fail to exist or exist absolutely, one will be unable to attain any peace. For one will be subject to egoism, the overvaluing of oneself and one's achievement and of material things."[131] By contrast, when one realizes that nothing has an independent existence, one realizes the essential interconnectedness of everything and the impossibility of disentangling oneself from the world. This is why compassion stems from the understanding of emptiness as a natural consequence.

Chapter 6

Mapping the World Without Independent Essences

Interdependency and Quantum Physics

The idea of reality as an intertwining or weave [*tantra*] that the concepts of emptiness and co-dependent origination suggest adopting, appears to have something in common with what physics has been facing for the last century.[1] A similar impossibility on the part of the subject to subtract itself from the field of observation or the impossibility of disentangling[2] from the studied dimension has been encountered by quantum physics, as highlighted by Niels Bohr: "While we previously thought that the properties of any object were determined, thus neglecting the interaction between that object and the others, quantum physics shows us that interaction is an inseparable part of the phenomena themselves. The nonambiguous description of any phenomenon requires including all the objects involved in the interaction in which the phenomenon gives itself out."[3] At this point, it is easy to understand why physicist Carlo Rovelli brings into the discussion no less a figure than Nāgārjuna:

> I am not a philosopher, I am a physicist. . . . To this vile mechanic who deals with quanta, Nāgārjuna teaches that I can think of the manifestation of the physical objects without having to ask myself what the physical object is, independent of its manifestations. . . . Nāgārjuna offers us a tremendous conceptual tool to consider the

> relationality of the quanta: one can think of interdependence without independent essences that would eventually start relating to one another. By contrast, interdependence demands forgetting about independent essences. Physic's long quest for the "ultimate substance" that crossed matter, molecules, atoms, fields, elementary particles . . . has sunk into the relational complexity of the quantum theory of fields and of general relativity. Could it be that an ancient Indian thinker offers us a conceptual tool for unravelling?[4]

But does phenomenology not also work with manifestation, regardless of the existence or inexistence of a transcendent object that is normally posited as out there? Phenomenology is interested in how something is given in the space of consciousness, independent of any theory about the alleged object in itself. Rovelli notes the dialogue across fields (philosophy and physics) that took place in the early decades of the twentieth century: Werner Heisenberg and Wolfgang Pauli "had followed the discussions on the relation between reality and experience that spanned Austrian and German philosophy at the beginning of the century. Ernst Mach, who had a profound influence on Einstein, preached the necessity of basing knowledge on observations alone, breaking free of any implicit 'metaphysical' assumption."[5]

While the phenomenologist rigorously sticks to what is given, to the fundamental data of experience within the limits in which they are given, quantum physics deals only with the fundamental data of experimental work, "only to what is observable": that is, the laws that connect different systems or apparatuses of measurement, without assuming the existence of objects.[6] A reduction of hypostatizing interpretations takes place in both phenomenology and quantum mechanics,[7] because they both avoid doing any metaphysics. In Eastern traditions, it is the concept of emptiness that serves this purpose and fulfills that antidogmatic role. The phenomenologist Maurice Merleau-Ponty, to whom the last part of this book is devoted, engages with quantum physics in a few writings that make clear that "the meaning of physics is to make us make 'negative philosophical discoveries.'"[8] Merleau-Ponty claims that "the physical beings, as mathematical beings, are not 'natures' anymore, but 'structures of whole of operations'"[9] and that through the indeterminism that is characteristic of quantum physics, "we admit that probability enters into the fabric of the real."[10] Citing the founder of quantum physics, Merleau-Ponty adds, "As Niels Bohr said, it's not by chance, if there is harmony between the descriptions of psychology (we would say: of phenomenology) and the conceptions of contemporary physics,"[11] because "the world perceived is a world in which there is discontinuity, probability, and generality in which every being is not subject to a unique and actual placement."[12] So in this sense, we can say that physics gives us tools, conceptual charts, and theoretical models that lead to obtaining efficient predictions,[13] thus allowing us to enact and shape a world that is also shaping us.

When it comes to relation, one approach is to think about preexisting elements or poles that are put into communication through relation. This is the traditional view. Thanks to phenomenology, however, we have become acquainted with a different scenario. It is no longer a matter of positing different elements that would eventually start interacting but of imagining the relation itself as shaping both poles of this interaction, which can only be singled out retrospectively but do not preexist.[14] Phenomenology is not interested in an independent content, in what philosophy calls a transcendent object and in yogic terms is known as an "inherent nature." It is interested in how this content is given within the space of consciousness. This givenness of the world within consciousness is the first relational data with which we are confronted. The independent object is just a derivation, an abstraction, and from this point of view entails a misrecognition of the genealogical process that led to it.

Scientific Idealities and Being-in-the-World

Martin Heidegger provides important insights into how the idealities of science, which are often taken to be the starting points of scientific inquiry, are actually the ultimate output of an abstraction of a fluid embodied process.[15] In order to emphasize the centrality of praxis, Heidegger offers very simple examples: "The forest is a forest of timber, the mountain a quarry of rock, the river is water power, the wind is wind 'in the sails.' "[16] Nature is encountered for the first time in the surrounding world [*Umwelt*] as a means [*Zeug*] in everyday practical dealings with the world; only afterward, by abstracting from this encounter the practical implications (known as the "handiness" of the means), the mere objective presence [*Vorhandenheit*] arises: "The botanist's plants are not the flowers of the hedgerow, the river's 'source' ascertained by the geographer is not the source in the ground."[17]

Mere objectivity, according to both Husserl[18] and Heidegger, is something that at the conclusion of an idealizing and stabilizing procedure, is placed in front of the hand (and thus is no longer at hand), grasped by conceptual analytical thinking which makes a representation of it,[19] and pinned under the gaze of the subject as an "ob-ject," literally "thrown [*jectum*] against, in front [*ob*]." This objective presence is taken as an independent self-sufficient entity from a theoretical viewpoint because its genesis in the lived world in which it is first encountered as a tool at hand [*zu-hand*][20] has been stripped away and thus disregarded.[21] Genealogically, Heidegger reconstructs the development of the mere objective presence as something that might occur when the means at hand turns out to be unfit for the intended purpose: "When we come upon something unhandy, our missing it in this way, again discovers what is at hand in a kind of only being present."[22] The mere objective presence results from the entity or means being unfit, lacking, or unusable; this process opens up a more abstract kind of consideration.

We have seen that through the phenomenological reduction, mere objectivity is suspended in favor of the givenness of experience within the space of consciousness, and this space of consciousness in which the world gives itself out is an embodied dimension. We are not speaking of an abstract concept of consciousness, but of a consciousness that matches the space of our bodily presence and action. The primacy of the embodied experience and of the lifeworld [*Lebenswelt*] over any reminiscence of metaphysics is at the heart of Husserl's late period. Starting with the *Crisis*[23] but especially in his last, unedited writings, Husserl makes clear that the domain of the transcendental consciousness is grounded in nothing more than the flowing present moment of the shared lived experience.

Varela's En-action and Structural Coupling

The centrality of embodiment, action, and the inextricable interconnectedness between subject and world is the starting point of Francisco Varela's analysis. Deeply imbued with the entire phenomenological lineage, Varela's direct reference point is Maurice Merleau-Ponty, the thinker among Husserl's students who most concentrated on the embodied dimension of experience. A biologist and neuroscientist, Francisco Varela founded, together with the Dalai Lama and Adam Engle, the Mind and Life Institute in 1987 to foster dialogue between interdisciplinary scientific research and contemplative practices. Varela is convinced that our "being in the world" changes the world:

> We come to reflect on that world as we grow and live. We reflect on a world that is not made, but found, and yet it is also our structure that enables us to reflect upon this world. Thus in reflection we find ourselves in a circle: we are in a world that seems to be there before reflection begins, but that world is not separate from us. For the French philosopher Maurice Merleau-Ponty, the recognition of this circle opened up a space between self and world, between the inner and the outer. This space was not a gulf or divide; it embraced the distinction between self and world, and yet provided the continuity between them. Its openness revealed a middle way, an *entre*-deux. . . . Science (and philosophy for that matter) has chosen largely to ignore what might lie in such an entre-deux or middle way.[24]

Varela is trying to question the traditional scientific viewpoint, according to which a pregiven independent subject is studying a pregiven independent world, in favor of the idea that subject and world are mutually constituted through their relating to one another; he calls this "structural coupling." Thanks to this codetermination, a mutual production of world and mind takes place moment after moment, which is how understating and knowledge occurs: "Organism and environment enfold into each other and unfold from one another in the fundamental circularity that is life itself."[25] Referring to this fundamental circularity, Varela introduces the term en-action: "We are claiming that organism and environment are mutually enfolded in multiple ways, and so what constitutes the world of a given organism is enacted by that organism's history of structural coupling."[26] Varela treasures the analysis that his French teacher had offered in the direction of moving beyond the split between subject and object toward this "fundamental correlation";[27] in fact, Merleau-Ponty had claimed that "consciousness is in the first place not a matter of 'I think that' but of 'I can'"[28] and that "the world is inseparable from the subject, but from a subject which is nothing but a project of the world, and the subject is inseparable from the world, but from a world which the subject itself projects."[29]

This is why, for Varela, all knowledge is fundamentally action: "Cognition consists not of representations but of embodied action."[30] This enactment happens mutually, both on the side of the subject and on the one of the world: "We propose as a name the term enactive to emphasize the growing conviction that cognition is not the representation of a pregiven world by a pregiven mind but is rather the enactment of a world and a mind on the basis of a history of the variety of actions that a being in the world performs."[31]

Varela questions the still dominant representationalist model in the cognitive sciences, according to which the mind is a box in which contents are represented to an alleged internal and mysterious spectator. This idea is often referred to as the *homunculus* argument. But who is this little man inside the brain watching the movie on the screen? Of course, any number of questions arise on the nature of this viewer and on the infinite regress of this argument.[32] A variation of this theory is called the Cartesian theater, a term coined in derision by the materialist Daniel Dennett: "Cartesian materialism is the view that there is a crucial finish line or boundary somewhere in the brain, marking a place where the order of arrival equals the order of 'presentation' in experience because what happens there is what you are conscious of. . . . Many theorists would insist that they have explicitly rejected such an obviously bad idea. But . . . the persuasive imagery of the Cartesian Theater keeps coming back to haunt us—laypeople and scientists alike—even after its ghostly dualism has been denounced and exorcized."[33]

Varela's review of different standpoints within cognitive science, though dating to the 1990s, singles out a few trends that have persisted in the intervening decades and for this reason must be noted here. Neuroreductionism or eliminativism holds that consciousness is fully explainable and reducible to biological mechanism, as summarized by this provocative statement by DNA pioneer Francis Crick: "You are nothing but a pack of neurons."[34] Functionalism has been the most prevalent view in recent decades and entails the idea that consciousness is an emergent phenomenon and can be explained through the unification of modules of individual cognitive functions.[35] There are other positions that Varela regards as emphasizing the intrinsic limitations of the means through which knowledge of the mental is acquired and thus claim that the hard problem of consciousness is unsolvable; for this reason, they are "resigned to mystery."[36] The fourth group identified by Varela is phenomenologically inspired and is concerned with firsthand experience as a "basic fact."[37] After having listed all these options, Varela concludes that the representationalist model of knowledge remains widely used across the theoretical spectrum:

> Practically since its inception cognitive science has been committed to a very explicit set of key ideas and metaphors which can be called representationalism, for which the inside-outside distinction is the center piece: an outside (a feature-full world) represented inside through the action of complex perceptual devices. In recent years there has been a slow but sure change towards an alternative orientation, one that I have contributed to and defended for many years. This orientation differs from representationalism by treating mind and world as mutually overlapping, hence the qualifying terms embodied, situated or enactive cognitive science.[38]

Furthermore, most cognitive theories share the idea that consciousness in general terms correlates to specific faculties and is present when cognitive content is also present. For this reason, consciousness is generally associated with the sense of some kind of "I"; that is, with *self*-consciousness. What phenomenology and yoga are now contributing to this issue is the idea that if mind and world are not separate and independent entities with their own natures but overlap, then consciousness in broad terms is not necessarily localized in the skull of the subject or even inside the skin but is more likely at the threshold between subject and world. In fact, consciousness in Eastern traditions is never located inside the individual but, as we have seen, envisaged as a dimension that overflows the borders of the individual and flows out at the intersection between the inside and the outside. Through a simultaneously vigilant and relaxed examination of experience, one can realize the existence of this dimension of consciousness beyond any empirical "I."

Difference between Psychological Introspection and Phenomenological Reduction

Varela recommends that anyone examining the mind should master some basic assets of phenomenology: "My proposal implies that every good student of cognitive science who is also interested in issues at the level of mental experience, must inescapably attain a level of mastery in phenomenological examination in order to work seriously with first-person accounts."[39] More specifically, he points out the importance of distinguishing within mental content between a "what" and a "how": "The point is to turn the direction of the movement of thinking from its habitual content-oriented direction backwards towards the arising of thoughts themselves."[40] Here, Varela valorizes Husserl's suggestion that we "establish a consistent universal interest in the 'how' of the manners of givenness."[41] The space of attention in which every object gives itself out turns from a means to direct oneself toward objects into an end in itself.

Intuition is a fundamental ingredient to achieving this aim. According to Varela, Western researchers in particular need to become acquainted and even intimate with this alternative gaze on reality: "This gain in intimacy with the phenomenon is crucial, for it is the basis of the criteria of truth in phenomenological analysis, the nature of its evidence."[42] The kind of intuition to which phenomenology refers to is vastly different from intuition in a psychological sense, which is associated with a name inserted into an associational biographical chain and mixed with linguistic links and suggestions. Husserl makes this point very clearly when he states that "the psychological phenomenon . . . is not a truly absolute datum."[43] For this reason, the phenomenological method is not merely a psychological method like introspection, and its actuation requires a difficult effort [*mühsamer Betätigung*].[44] Just as the transcendental subjectivity, which Husserl also calls the "reduced I" or "transcendental ego," is not a psychological "I," the eidetic intuition is not contingent but essential; that is, it rigorously singles out the invariant features of a course of perceptions [*Verlauf von Perzeptionen*].

Husserl repeatedly stresses that the suspension of the natural attitude caught up in the objects of the world is a difficult task; this strenuous effort recalls the kind of discipline needed when it comes to yogic practices:

> That we set aside all hitherto prevailing habits of thinking, that we recognize and tear down the intellectual barrier with which they confine the horizon of our thinking and now, with full freedom of thought, seize upon the genuine philosophical problems to be set completely anew made accessible to us only by the horizon open on all sides: these are hard demands. But nothing less is required. Indeed, what makes so extraordinarily hard the acquisition of the proper essence of phenomenology, the understanding of the peculiar sense of its problems, and of its relationship to all other sciences (in particular to psychology), is that, for all this, a new style of attitude is needed which is entirely altered in contrast to the natural attitude in experiencing and the natural attitude in thinking.[45]

Referring to the "uncritical introspection" of Wilhelm Wundt and Edward Titchener, Varela states that "this manner of mobilizing reflexive capacities still falls into the natural attitude for a phenomenologist, for it rides on the wave of previous elaborations and assumptions."[46] By contrast, Varela defines phenomenological intuition as follows: "It cuts short our quick and fast elaborations and beliefs, in particular locating and putting in abeyance what we think we should find, or some expected description. Thus phenomenological reduction is not a seeing inside, but a tolerance concerning the suspension of conclusions that allows a new aspect or insight into the phenomenon to unfold. In consequence this move does not sustain the basic subject-object duality but opens into a field of phenomena where it becomes less and less obvious how to distinguish between subject and object (this is what Husserl called the fundamental correlation). . . . In this context, intuitive capacity does not refer to some elusive, will-o-the-wisp inspiration."[47] Furthermore, Varela emphasizes the fact that "intuitive evidence must be inscribed or translated into communicable items"[48] and that a long training must be fostered within the scientific community to develop and refine these abilities: "It implies a disciplined commitment from a community of researchers. . . . In the West we have not had a rich pantheon of individuals gifted for phenomenological expertise (with notable exceptions, such as Husserl or James) rendering their investigations public to an attentive community . . . we shall need subjects whose competence in making phenomenological discriminations and descriptions is accrued."[49]

Neurophenomenology

Varela's proposal is to take advantage of neuroscientific imaging techniques and measures regarding neuro-activation and combine them with accounts of first-person experience: "On the one hand we have a process of emergence with well defined neurobiological attributes. On the other, a phenomenological description which links directly to our lived experience. To make further progress we need cutting edge techniques and analyses from the scientific side, and very consistent development of phenomenological investigation for the purposes of the research itself."[50] Varela's highly demanding objective is that the two domains be linked with reciprocal constraints:[51] "a large-scale integration mechanism in the brain such as neural synchrony in the gamma band should be validated *also* on the basis of its ability to provide insight into first-person accounts of mental contents such as duration. . . . The novelty of my proposal is that disciplined first-person accounts should be an integral element of the validation of a neurobiological proposal."[52]

An interesting example that Varela proposes is the one on time and more specifically on the consciousness of the present time. When it comes to contemplative practices, one of the basic instructions is to tune in to the present moment and avoid lingering over anticipations of the future and memories of the past. Phenomenological analysis helps determine what this present moment, which William James calls the "specious present," actually amounts to.[53] Husserl shows that the present is continually infiltrated by both present and past[54] and that the ordinary image that we have of time—as a single point on a vector—is an abstraction from classical physics representations of the world. Varela correlates Husserl's view about the present (overflowing the conceptual instant to which it is traditionally confined) with a measurement made from a third-person point of view, the one of the minimum time required for the emergence of a neural event, confirming Husserl's intuition:

> A basic three-part structure of the present with its constitutive threads into past and future horizons, the so-called 'pretentions' and 'retentions.' In fact, these structural invariants are not compatible with the point-continuum representation of linear time we have inherited from physics. But they do link naturally to a body of conclusions in cognitive neuroscience that there is a minimal time required for the emergence of neural events that correlate to a cognitive event. This non-compressible time framework can be analyzed as a manifestation of the long-range neuronal integration in the brain linked to a widespread synchrony.[55]

Another notable example concerns the distinction between transcendent object and phenomenon. From a neural point of view, there appears to be a difference between directing attention to the object taken as a transcendent entity, as in the natural attitude, or on the phenomenon intended as how the object is given in the space of consciousness, as with the phenomenological method: "In fact the neuronal data on filling-in seem to correlate well with what phenomenological reduction had concluded some time ago: there is an important difference between 'seeing as,' visual appearance, and 'seeing what,' a visual judgment."[56]

Varela explicitly acknowledges the influence that Eastern traditions have had in orienting his inquiry: "We explicitly draw from Asian traditions, Buddhism in particular, as living manifestations of an active, disciplined phenomenology."[57] The traditional *Weltanschauung* equipped with self-sufficient and independent entities that grounds knowledge in certainty leads to losing the connection with the lived world (as Husserl points out in his last book, the *Crisis of European Sciences and Transcendental Phenomenology*) and to the creation of an impressive structure that ultimately means very little from an experiential point of view. However, such a foundational enterprise in traditional science is reassuring for the individual who feels solidly grounded within it, even if this ostensible grounding always comes to mean less than is hoped. By contrast, settling on a phenomenological and yogic view according to which there is no inherent nature whatsoever means that everything is grounded in something else; this makes it impossible to treat consciousness as an object and to assign it a definite location and creates what Varela defines as a "Cartesian anxiety."[58] The need to face uncertainty is the outcome of both a phenomenological standpoint and of contemplative practices, in so far as the practitioner is asked to become grounded in this very emptiness of inherent and substantial existence. Reconnecting his own research to venerable wisdom, as Varela does, helps with confronting the Cartesian anxiety, because Eastern traditions have trained the enquirer to desire something other than objects for centuries. What is at stake is letting go of the search for an ultimate ground, and of any foundationalist project, which of course is also the core of Husserl's enterprise. His initial goal was actually to refound science. However, this initial intention would eventually fade away in the face of more significant discoveries from a phenomenological point of view, such as the surfacing of the dimension of the transcendental. Varela brings the Madhyamaka doctrine into the heart of his approach and states that "groundlessness [*śūnyatā*] is the very fabric of dependent coorigination."[59] Indeed, according to Tzong Kapha, the incessant search for grounding, which translates into reification, is what ties human beings to suffering: "Essentialist schools reify many different things. When you negate the referent of ignorance's cognitive process, you completely stop all of these tenet-driven reifications, as though you cut a tree at its root. . . . You see that living beings are bound in cyclic existence by a wrong conceptual consciousness."[60] In his text on the stages of the path, the *Lam Rim*, where basic and public teachings are stored, Tzong Kapha points to the importance of "overcoming the reifying view of the perishing aggregates" (which depends "upon developing the wisdom that knows that the self, as thus conceived, does not exist"),[61] quoting Candrakīrti (one of the greatest masters in Madhyamaka and a spiritual disciple of Nāgārjuna) and his emphasis of this point: "Reality is the total extinction of the conceptions of both the self and that which belongs to the self. . . . In their minds yogis perceive that all afflictions and all faults arise from the reifying view of the perishing aggregates. And, knowing that the self is the object of that view, they refute the self."[62]

Chapter 7

The Transformation of Perception in Yoga

On the Misunderstandings around the Notion of Body

The importance of avoiding hypostatization is particularly important when turning toward the dimension of *haṭha* yoga, the yogic path that specifically works with bodily postures, sealing gestures, purifying acts, visualizations, and breathing techniques. It is the path that considers the practitioner's body as the gateway to the realization of consciousness. The wandering yogin Saraha of the *mahāmudrā* tradition, one of the founders of Vajrayāna Buddhism, claimed that he had not seen a place of pilgrimage and an abode of bliss like his body.[1] The body of the practitioner is impure only if it is substantialized and experienced as a crystallization of the past and a receptacle of the old. The habits of everyday life are transmitted and reflected in the body in terms of postural customs and physical stiffnesses, which recursively nourish the mental stiffness of the natural attitude. There is a tendency to bind oneself not only to habitual bodily patterns that in time become ossified but also to specific groups of densities within the muscles and even to anatomical and emotional imbalances. A surreptitious attachment also takes place regarding discomforts and pains, which became reassuring in their apparent certainty and thus get stabilized and almost solidified within. Only in this sense is the body impure, in as much as it is territorialized by the mind and must be purified by the burning flames of *haṭha* yoga.

The flames of *tapas* are directed toward the senses, the emotions, and the body as altered by the intellect. The *Yogabija*, a *haṭha* yoga text of the fourteenth century, is clear on the topic: "When egoism has dissolved, how can there be hardness in the body? Omniscient, omnipotent, free, with cosmic form, the yogi becomes liberated while alive [and] wanders the world at will. . . . When [the yogi] becomes undifferentiated then he is said to be liberated [*mukta*]. Bodies and senses are made of consciousness; when they become undifferentiated then [the yogi] is said to be liberated."[2] What must be suspended through what one could call, with all due caution, a "phenomenological reduction" is a level of sensory perception that is already deeply structured by the objectifying mind. This is the only way we can make sense of the general encouragement to discard the body and the connected sensory realm that are to be found, as previously noted, in the Upanishadic philosophy and in many canonical Buddhist texts.

This problem has grown, especially when these texts have been transferred to a Western context, imbued with dualistic tenets. What is particularly problematic is the widespread tendency in English translations to render the second meaning of *dharma*[3] [*dhamma* in Pali] as "phenomena" instead of "objects." In these translations, the term "phenomena" is meant in a nontechnical way[4] and refers to the ensemble of the mundane events, taken in the ordinary "un-wise manner" as objects; thus, it usually has a negative nuance, especially when the advice along the path amounts to overcoming "phenomenality" in favor of an allegedly deeper essence to be accessed. For this reason, when in such instances one finds the term "phenomenon," one must think of the opposite of what it means within phenomenology, where nothing is deeper than what surfaces moment after moment.[5] An example of the use of *dharma* in reference to the context of the objects appears in Gauḍapāda's commentary on the *Māṇḍūkya Upaniṣad*. Referring to the knowledge of the awakened [*buddhasya jñānam*], Gauḍapāda cautions that it does not relate to any object [*dharmeṣu*].[6] In a case like this, translating *dharmeṣu* with "phenomena" instead of with "objects" would be misleading.

Schopenhauer's intercession in the nineteenth-century Western reception of Hinduism and of Eastern philosophies more generally has been particularly misleading. The celebrated Upanishadic sentence *Tattvamasi*,[7] "you are that," which is typical of the master pointing out at the world before him (the dimension of the nondual consciousness) and suggesting to his student where the true self can be found, is misunderstood by Schopenhauer, who mistranslates the sentence as meaning "you are this"[8] instead of "you are that." On one occasion, this sentence is even rendered as "this living one, you are,"[9] meaning: "You are your neighbor," accompanied by a Christian concept of compassion in the prescription to "love your neighbor as yourself."[10] Of course, for Schopenhauer the identification with a personal "I" is also an illusion. Yet, the quote above shows that he does not seem to entirely overcome the notion of "I." More generally, Schopenhauer presents a reading of soteriological traditions as offering salvation from the alleged "will" of bodily natural existence. What Schopenhauer appears not to have understood is that the vitalism that for him needs to be hindered through spiritualizing practices is simply the other side of the coin of the dualism between matter and spirit. The blind vital dimension is a creation of the conceptual mind and has nothing to do with the bodily, perceptual dimension, toward which phenomenology leans as such. It is the dominant controlling action of representation that puts the world at a distance and turns it into a counterpart of this intellectual volition. For this reason, a number of Eastern traditions, contrary to Schopenhauer's interpretation, do not aspire to suppress the naked phenomenality and depth of the living world but rather the dominant intellectual tendency of the categorizing mind that turns the fluid and everchanging sensory dimension into a hypostatization and a fetish. In *Haṭha* yoga the purifying heat of the practice does not entail "burning" the body, which is the fundamental tool to realize our continuity with the world, but rather entails "burning" the "I" that wants to compete with the world in order to come back to the pure evidence of a thickness that is shared with the world.

Discarding Habit and Discovering Awe

It is a matter of discarding the preexisting conception of the body through the fire of yoga[11] and opening new spaces of awe in the joints and the automatism of compulsive thinking. If in the Vedic myth the enemies were the demons who hindered the unfolding of manifestation and, thanks to the burning flames of *tapas*, were turned to ashes, who are these enemies for us, metaphor aside? If not from the material, the senses, the bodily dimension, from what kind of evil is one to be purified? The evil is that which has robbed us of the awe and the capacity of letting ourselves be astonished and amazed at the miracle of existence and of remaining within the beginner's look, the truly virgin look of the one who remains open-mouthed. Though initially present in everyone, this ability is as fragile as fine crystal and sooner or later ends up being chipped and in many cases shattered because of the constant threat of habit: the crushing grip of routine that sorts and categorizes every aspect of existence before we are even able to experience it. Boredom and repetition, day after day, wear away our ability to marvel at what is given in the present moment. Though everything is, in its essence, unique and unrepeatable, in the context of ordinary alienation (and in more severe terms in cases of psychological suffering) it seems to be crushed under the weight of the already-seen and already-known, to the point at which darkness falls, and nothing more is able to emerge.

The operative dimension that claims to make the most of every second given is the enemy of surprise. At the origin of this lies a view of knowledge that sees the exhaustive systemization of reality as the ultimate value. Intellectual understanding has developed under the logic of taxonomy: a tendency to classify things, according to which reality is placed at a distance, under the lens of a microscope or a telescope, dissected into the smallest of parts, and lost in terms of genuinely lived experience. The paradox of this logic, which came to a head in the last century in the crisis of Western sciences, can be detected in the ideal to which students aspire: far from cultivating the value of awe, they strive endlessly not to be floored by any circumstance, repeatedly reassuring themselves with a silent: "Yes, I knew that." This concept of knowledge is blended with the dimension of power: the less surprised and taken aback one is by a new event, the less vulnerable one is to the other subjects involved. It is a conception diametrically opposed not only to Husserl's "philosophical amazement,"[12] but also to Plato's view of wonder: "For this is an experience which is characteristic of a philosopher, this wondering: this is where philosophy begins and nowhere else. And the man who made Iris[13] the child of Thaumas was perhaps no bad genealogist."[14] Wisdom means existing in a state of perpetual awe for Indian philosophers as well: in the tantric *Śivasūtra* by Vasgupta, it is said that the stages of yoga are "stages of wonder,"[15] while the commentator Kṣemarāja refers to the amazement produced in the great yogin "in touch with the various manifestations of knowable reality."[16] In yogic traditions, it is not a matter of hoarding knowledge or accumulating it as if culture could be weighed in pounds. Instead, it is a matter of burning it at every moment so as not to undermine the experience that is yet to come and that needs virgin soil in which to root as something new. Experiencing the amazement of the "beginner's mind" is at the base of all yogic practices. A similar enhancement of the "virgin look on reality" and of doubt can be found in Buddhist yogic techniques as recalled by Alexandra David-Néel: "Examine [the facts] attentively and at length, putting aside all preconceived ideas, empty your mind of all the opinions which it has harbored concerning these facts; doubt that which you have mechanically admitted up to the present; look as you would look at quite new things, those which form your physical environment; you will then investigate the mental reactions to which they give rise."[17] The *ṛṣi*, the Vedic sages, were fully aware of the fact that "to know one must burn. Otherwise, all knowledge is ineffective. One must therefore practice *tapas*. *Tapas* means ardor—it means the heat within the mind."[18] Conceiving knowledge in these terms means being ready to set off on an adventure that will change the inquirer irremediably. Phenomenologist Michel Bitbol, speaking of the quest to know consciousness that is the very enterprise of the yogin, warns that "the questioner [*questionnant*] will not be the same after having walked with a question like the one of conscious experience. The question will have reinvented its own questioner. She surely will not have anything essential to lose in the adventure, but she still does not know."[19] We are at the antipodes of a vision that thinks of culture as an ornament to be shown off, a status symbol that may offer a competitive advantage in society but that must be kept at a distance, for example, by making it an object of specialized study in order to avoid the risk of being overwhelmed and irremediably transformed by it. Instead, those who burn to understand know that they will never gain greater certainty and security. An endeavor motivated by the purifying fire leaves scorched earth around itself and permanently changes the seeker, who is forced to make a kind of leap into the void and never again be the same because it is the seeker's own "I," which Patañjali called the *asmitā* and in the Yogācāra tradition is referred to as the afflictive consciousness [*kliṣṭamanovijñāna*],[20] that has been sacrificed in the process.

If in the ordinary attitude one is exposed outside oneself, following dreams, fears, and ghosts, both the phenomenological and the yogic purification direct one inward toward an internal recollection. The difference between being-out and being-in is symbolized—at the extremes—by the shaman on the one hand and the awakened on the other. Mastery over fire and the creation of mystic heat connect yogic and shamanic techniques. More specifically, some rituals typical of fakirism, such as the rope trick[21] in which a shaman initiate is cut with knives so that he can be resurrected in a new body, closely recall the primordial sacrifice and dismemberment of the Vedic deity Prajāpati. However, there is a fundamental difference between these two dimensions, of which *tapas* is an essential component. In shamanism, *tapas* is used to favor possession by a spirit, while in yoga one is dispossessed by means of purification even of one's own self. In ecstasy (from the Greek *ek-stasis*, "standing outside oneself"), one is thrown outside. In the higher stages of *samādhi*, on the other hand, an *enstasis* takes place, a being-within, which, given the homology between the microcosm and the macrocosm, also encompasses everything outside, including the entire universe:[22] "The joy of his *samādhi* is bliss for the whole universe."[23] While the shaman may be possessed by different spirits, the yogin is possessed not even by his own spirit; he is in everyone's and no one's land.

It is the fire that, after having scorched the earth around our conceptions, ghosts, and fetishes, allows us in a second phase to gather ourselves in an experience that is given only when we are capable of becoming aware of and guarding it. Postures in *haṭha* yoga, as I show below, are therefore a constant attempt to become displaced from what one believed to know about oneself, in as much as the conceptual mind had delimited a perimeter within the continuum of everchanging experience.

Haṭha Yoga

As is the case for phenomenology, for Vedic literature, Patañjali's *kriya* yoga, and both Tibetan and Nath *haṭha* yoga, it all comes down to purification. And this is not by chance: *haṭha* traditions, of which we have quite late written texts, have incorporated different layers of teachings. On top of the early layers, which likely date to the Indus Valley Civilization of Mohenjo-Daro and Harappa[24] (thirtieth to twenty-fifth centuries BCE), more recent layers have local influences from the Vedanta and elements of Patañjali's *rāja* yoga blended together. What is of particular interest is the recent discovery of a Buddhist Vajrayāna substratum (c. eighth century CE onward) in specific *haṭha* yoga contexts of the Nath tradition, a tradition that can be traced to famed masters like Matsyendranāth and his disciple Gorakṣanātha.[25] Sanskritist James Mallinson claims that the first written occurrence of the *haṭha* yoga is to be found in Buddhist texts like the *Amṛtasiddhi* (eleventh century CE),[26] upending the traditional attribution of *haṭha* yoga to exclusively Śaiva milieus. According to Mallinson, the Kadri monastery in Mangalore is where "the appropriation from Vajrayāna Buddhists by the Saiva Nāths of not only practice and terminology, but also the Kadri monastery itself" occurred[27] and where the demise of Buddhism in India took place: "The evidence presented suggests that the Kadri Vajrayāna Buddhist tradition was not destroyed or expelled, but absorbed into that of the Nāths, and provides a possible model for how Buddhist teachings survived elsewhere in India, after Buddhism's demise there as a formal religion."[28] This helps explain why the terms used in the subtle physiology in the Vajrayāna Kālacakra context are also present among Nāth tantric texts like the *Haṭhayogapradīpikā*, *Śivasaṃhitā*, and *Gheraṇḍa Saṃhitā*, to note the best-known cases. Among these, the one with the strongest influence on subsequent literature is the *Haṭhayogapradīpikā*,[29] literally "the lamp on *Haṭhayoga*," which was compiled by Svātmārāma. According to it, yogic physiology is made up of subtle channels [*nāḍī*-s] through which vital energy [*prāṇa*] is taken to flow and knots or plexa of such channels in the form of wheels [*cakrā*]: "There are 72,000 *nāḍī*-s throughout the cage of this body. Suṣumnā is the Śāmbhavī, the remaining *nāḍī*-s are unimportant."[30] (figure

Figure 7.1. Subtle physiology. *Source:* https://archive.org/details/dli.ernet.536500/page/n4/mode/1up.

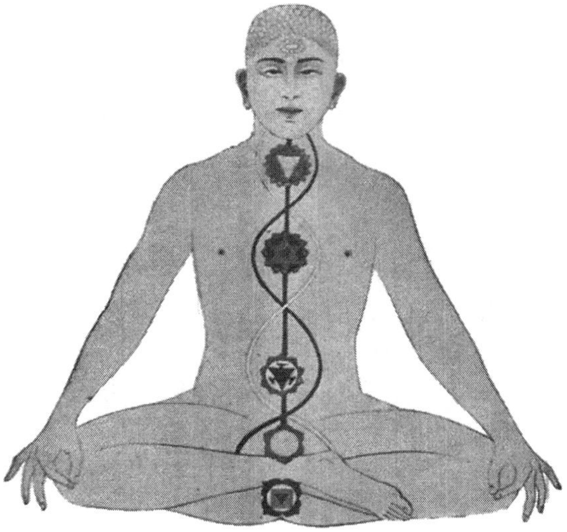

7.1). This vital energy takes different names according to direction and quality of its movement or the winds [*vāyus*], which are the airs, winds, or vital breaths that move both in the outside world and in the body of the practitioner. Even in the *Atharva Veda*[31] an initial reference to the different directions of the moving breaths appears; in the *Praśna Upaniṣad*, these winds moving in the body were connected to the internalization of sacrificial fires "of prāna [vital energy] which remain awake in this city [of the body]."[32]

The ultimate goal of the practice, deeply engaged and uninterrupted,[33] is to enable the vital energy to enter the central channel [*suṣumnā*];[34] this leads to a blissful experience of liberation similar way to what we have seen occurring in tantric Tibetan teachings with the arousing of the Chandali in the central channel [Avadhuti]. According to the *Haṭhayogapradīpikā*, what blocks this process are impurities disseminated in the seventy-two thousand more peripheral channels (the same number appears in the *Bṛhadāraṇyaka Upaniṣad*),[35] which therefore must be cleansed through all the purifying acts and procedures that make up the practice [*sādhanā*]: "When all the *nādī*-s and *cakrā* which are full of impurities are purified [*śuddhim*], then the yogi is able to retain *prāṇa*.[36]" While five airs are listed,[37] the most important are *prānavāyu*, which regulates the intake and assimilation of energy and is linked to the process of inhaling or welcoming the new, and *apānavāyu*, which governs the capacity of exhalation and the expulsion of all moods and waste substances produced by the body, and thus helps free one of the old: "Raising the *apāna* upward and bringing the *prāna* down from the throat, the yogi becomes free from old age."[38]

In breathing, the relation between *prānavāyu* and *apānavāyu* is described by twentieth-century *haṭhayoga* teacher T. K. V. Desikachar[39] in these terms: "On inhalation the breath moves toward the belly, causing a draft that directs the flame downward, just like in a fireplace; during exhalation the draft moves the flame in the opposite direction, bringing with it the just-burned waste matter. . . . Certain physical positions are beneficial for the meeting of fire and rubbish. In all inverted postures, the agni is directed toward the *apāna*"[40] (figure 7.2). When these two complementary airs meet—one expressing its action upward [*prānavāyu*] and the other downward [*apānavāyu*]—the gastric air is kindled

Figure 7.2. (left) Shoulder Stand, *Sālambasarvāngāsana*. *Source:* Photo by the author. If you have high blood pressure, heart conditions, brain diseases, glaucoma and cervical spondylitis this posture is better to avoid. The information provided in this book here and elsewhere is not a substitute for medical advice or guidance of a qualified yoga teacher. Yoga (including *āsana*-s and *prāṇāyāma*) must always be practiced under the supervision of a qualified teacher who can also help determine which variations of a pose are suitable for your particular case.
Figure 7.3. (right) *Viparīta-karaṇī*. *Source:* Photo by the author.

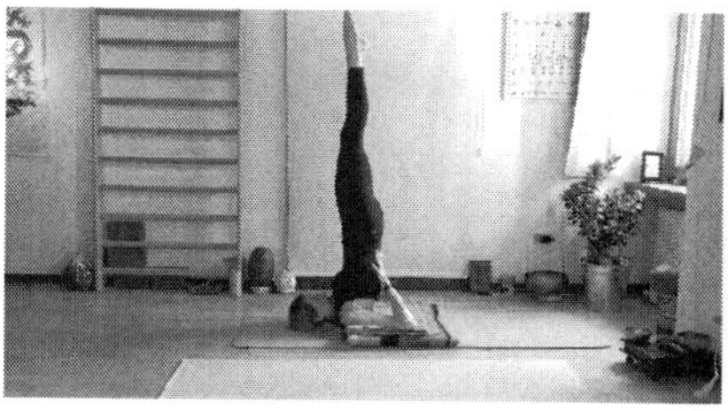

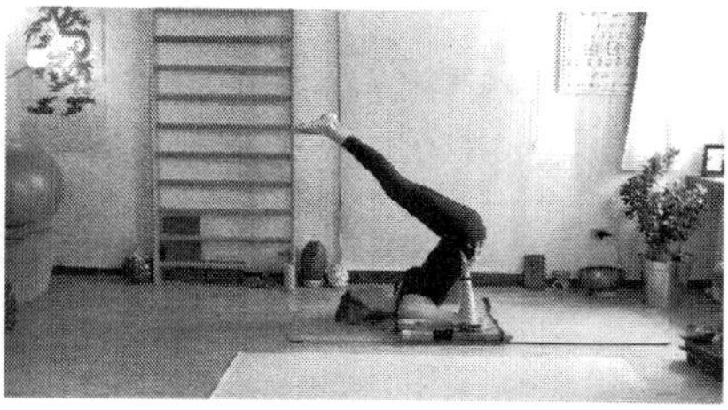

in the form of a fire at the center of the body [*samānavāyu*] that regulates the metabolism and governs the processing of food into energy: "When one is able to hold the *vāyu* according to one's will, the digestive power [*analasya*] increases. With the *nādī*-s purified, thus the inner sound or *nāda* awakens and one is free from disease."[41] The gastric air lights the spark of the interior flame, which some texts depict as the *manipūra cakra*,[42] at the center of the body, roughly where what Western anatomy calls the solar plexus is located:

> *Apāna* moves up into the region of fire (*manipūra cakra*, the navel centre) [*vahnimaṇḍalam*], then the flames of the fire grow, being fanned by *apāna vāyu*. Then, when *apāna* and the fire meet with *prāna*, which is itself hot, the heat in the body is intensified. Through this, the sleeping *kuṇḍalinī* is aroused by the extreme heat [*santaptā*][43] and it straightens itself just as a serpent [*bhujaṅgī*] beaten with a stick straightens and hisses. Just as a snake enters its hole, so *kuṇḍalinī* goes into Brahmā *nādī* [Suṣumnā *nādī*]. Therefore the yogi must always perform *mūla* bandha.[44]

There are three major internal locks or seals [*bandha*] that are to be created in order to contain and direct the subtle energy to the central channel and awaken the *kuṇḍalinī*: the root lock [*mūla*] at the perineum, the abdominal lock [*uḍḍīyāna*], and the throat lock [*jālandhara*].[45] Other than internal locks, there are a number of other purifying acts[46] connected to the idea of overcoming the habitual body and mental attitude, such as the six purifying actions [*ṣaṭ-karma*][47] and the *mudrās*, which are specific positions of parts of the body[48] or of the whole body. Today, the most famous components of this purification methodology of *haṭhayoga* are the renowned postures or *āsana*-s which in the *Haṭhayogapradīpikā* are said to number 84: "Of all the eighty-four postures [*pīṭha*-s literally, stools],[49] the perfect posture [*siddhāsana*] should always be practiced [*abhyaset*]. It cleans [*śodhanam*] the impurities [*mala*] of the 72,000 *nādī*-s."[50] The distinction between *āsana*-s and *mudra*-s is vague; for example, the *mahāmudrā*[51] referred to in the *Haṭhayogapradīpikā*, which entails a retention of the breath combined with the creation of internal locks, has the outer shape of the head-to-knee posture [*jānu śīrṣāsana*]. In addition, specific actions such as the inverted action [*viparīta-karaṇī mudra*] fall in the domain of bodily postures. The goal of this inversion, which resembles the better-known shoulder stand [*sālamba sarvāṅgāsana*], reconnects to what was said in the Tibetan tantric traditions regarding the drops of *bindu*[52] melting from above as drops of *bodhicitta*, drops of consciousness. It is not by accident that the Buddhist text containing the term *haṭhayoga* is titled *Amṛtasiddhi, amṛta* being another term for the nectar [*rasa*] or drops [*bindu*] leaking from the crown of the head, where the moon is symbolically located. A large part of the terminology and notions used in Vajrayana Buddhism are also in the *Haṭhayogapradīpikā*, including *rasa, bindu,*[53] and *amṛta*. In the *Haṭhayogapradīpikā*, this nectar or juice is visualized as stemming from a "moon" [*candra*] located at the crown of the head, whereas the "sun" [*sūrya*] is the well-known flame of the gastric fire located at the navel. The importance of the two poles of sun and moon is one possible origin of the term *Haṭha* itself; this para-etymology with "*ha*" meaning sun and "*ṭha*" moon, is to be found explicitly in the fourteenth-century *Haṭhayoga* text *Yogabīja:* "The sun is denoted by the syllable *ha* and the moon by *ṭha.* Because of the union of the sun and moon it is called haṭhayoga."[54] According to Jason Birch, however, it is in the meaning of *haṭha* as "violent" and "forceful" that the connection with *haṭhayoga* must be found; more specifically, it would refer to the forceful [*haṭha*] upward moving of the *kundalini* through the central channel.[55] After the lit *kundalini* has melted the nectar, this same juice must be preserved from the blazing flames of the gastric fire, as instructed by the *Haṭhayogapradīpikā*. For this reason, the inverted postures are of particular interest: "That nectar [*amṛtam*] which flows from the moon has the quality of endowing enlightenment, but it is completely consumed by the sun, incurring old age. There is a wonderful means [*karaṇam*] by which the nectar is averted from falling into the opening of the Sun [*sūryasya mukha-vañcanam*]."[56] This means or action is the inverted posture that hinders, for reasons of simple gravity, the descent of the nectar into the fire and its consequent extinction: "With the navel region above and the palate below, the sun is above and the moon below. It is called *viparīta-karaṇī*, the reversing process. When given by the guru's instructions it is fruitful."[57] The role of initiations and resolutions of Tibetan tantra is covered here by the role of the teacher, who selects the candidate and the right moment to offer a specific learning.[58] Unlike with Patañjali's first limbs of the practice, in Nāth yoga no preliminary teachings or prescriptions [*nyama*] are established.[59] The antidogmatic tendency of this approach is attested by the inclusion of these prescriptions in a list of elements that destroy the method [*sādhana*]: "Overeating, exertion, talkativeness, adhering to rules [*nyamāḥ*], being in the company of common people and unsteadiness (wavering mind) are the six (causes) which destroy yoga."[60]

The techniques described on the way to the final absorption [*samādhi*] lead to empowerments [*siddhi*]: the powers—the capacity to penetrate the past, the future, and the minds of others—often confer the ability to see clearly. Clairvoyance [*vidyā*], which should be understood literally as "seeing clearly," is closely linked to the destruction of impurities understood as sediments and encrustations that prevent a limpid vision. If one has not turned to the flame of *tapas* to purge the tendency to interfere massively in the unfolding experience, one ends up projecting distortive filters onto it, without even realizing it: this makes one blind not only to the future but also and more importantly to the present, to what is actually happening. If one burns instead, one becomes a Seer, just like the phenomenologist who puts intuition into practice and becomes "a seer of all things."[61]

These powers, however, must not be misunderstood and objectified by the unready and unwise practitioner. For this reason, the teacher's task is to impart the right teaching to the right student, while the practitioner's task is to keep the secret undisclosed: "Hatha yoga is the greatest secret [*gopyā*] of the yogis who wish to attain perfection [*siddhi*]. Indeed, to be fruitful, it must be kept secret; revealed it becomes powerless."[62] Only the one who is capable of realizing the meaning of emptiness *śūnyatā* and of nonduality [*a-dvaita*][63] is ready to train in these techniques using them as means without inherent nature and avoiding the risk of reifying them while remaining subject to the dual conceptual mind: "The entire world is only the fabrication of thought. Play of mind is only created by thought. By transcending the mind which is composed of constructed thought, definitely peace will be attained."[64] In fact the door of liberation [*moksha*] opened by *haṭhayoga* is a door that in the text is described as the mind beyond mind [*manomanī*], the mind devoid of mind [*unmanī*], the *samādhi*, the nondual [*advaita*], the *rajayoga*, the fourth state [*turīya*], and the emptiness [*śūnyatā*], which in the *Haṭhayogapradīpikā* are considered interchangeable.[65] In phenomenology, they correspond to the dimension of appearing as such and more specifically to the dimension of the transcendental consciousness in Husserl, of Being in Heidegger and the structural coupling between mind and world in Varela. In the *Haṭhayogapradīpikā,* the very detailed descriptions of the subtle physiology and consequent perfections or empowerment [*siddhi*] is to be considered with the emphases on the deconstructing notion of emptiness, symbolized by the purifying power of the fire; even the central feature of the *prāna* must be deconstructed in terms of emptiness: "When the Mahāśakti is aroused [*prabuddhāyām*] by the various *āsana*-s, *prāṇāyāma*-s and *mudra*-s, the *prāna* dissolves into *śūnyā*."[66]

Although it is seldom acknowledged by modern commentators, Patañjali also devotes a number of aphorisms to the subtle physiology, as when he suggests directing the attention to the solar channel,[67] the moon,[68] or the navel-plexus [*nābi-cakra*][69] to obtain great powers. However, he warns strictly against the risk of empowerments being taught to the wrong person, the one who might take them for the goals of the practice itself: in such cases, instead of contributing to smoothing the boundaries of the "I," they could produce the opposite effect. Powers turn into daunting obstacles when instead viewing them as side effects of the ardent path, the practitioner confuses them with ends in themselves: "From this, intuition as well as higher hearing, touch, vision, taste and smell are born. These powers are accomplishments for the mind that is outgoing but obstacles to *samādhi*."[70] This is true of many mages and the like who turn their powers, including therapeutic ones, into ends in themselves and risk becoming lost in a process in which the "I," instead of emptying, becomes increasingly full of itself and cumbersome. Those practicing *haṭha* yoga risk something similar by confusing the reinvigorating and strengthening effects of yoga on the body and mind with the purpose of the practice itself. Yoga is not a means to a slender, athletic body, to a peaceful or meek disposition, or a self-image toward which to strive; rather, it is a "detector of the *here,* how it could be no longer encountered because of too much knowing."[71]

The Methodological and Deconstructive Role of Subtle Physiology

From this perspective, the subtle physiology also must not be subject to an overly naïve reading and thus objectified. There is a risk of taking the indications of the subtle physiology too literally and thinking that one should come to terms with the many descriptions of the energetic body to determine once and for all which is the most credible or authoritative indication between the different variations of the subtle body that are found in the yogic lineages of the different traditions. This is how diatribes, controversies, and conflicts between different schools, even in the same tradition, are fostered, with never-ending arguments over the precise location or function of a certain energetic channel or a specific chakra. It is also how the yogic dimension risks becoming riddled with superstition, dogmatic faith, or New Age ideology. For this reason, after having described in some detail the miniature body in the different tantric sects of the Buddhist and Saiva matrix, I turn now to the importance of reflecting on how misleading and flatly wrong it would be to accept the descriptions of the miniature body provided by the texts uncritically and dogmatically: one should not take these suggestions as if they were describing realities within the human body that are somehow truer than the ones provided by Western anatomy and physiology, for example. It is not a question of replacing alleged realities with others that are held to be truer. One must bravely go beyond positivist or mechanistic conceptions that unconditionally consent to the reified model of reality provided by science as if it were a description of how things actually are in themselves. For the same reason, an uncritical ascent to an alternative but equally reified approach should not be granted: a mystery-revelatory view that allows for an unreserved acceptance of a narrative passed down by a text-based tradition or an esoteric teaching. What is suggested is, on the contrary, to settle down toward a phenomenological view, which is essentially a pragmatic approach, according to which the point is not to determine what exists objectively and somehow independent of a given context but rather to realize that what exists comes into being only and always in a context-dependent way. What matters from a phenomenological point of view is to understand what kind of effects a phenomenon produces, within the first-person experience, as it gives itself out. The Eastern world is teeming with dimensions and entities that cannot be objectified but are nonetheless evident to the one who is engaged in practice. Therefore, what is given to rigorous perception within the limits in which it presents itself does, to a certain extent, exist. This is the phenomenological view upon which we have been leaning in addressing the yoga world. Edwin Bryant, in his commentary on the *Yogasūtra,* acknowledges the validity of a phenomenological approach to yoga, noting that "phenomenology does not require the acceptance of the truth claims as necessarily true, but attempts to suspend and avoid judgements on issues of validity or historicity or scientific accuracy," adding that "some approaches in phenomenology stress empathy, and even participation, bracketing one's own personal preconceptions as to what is real or true."[72] This is the empirical and experimental core that yoga shares with phenomenology.

Plunging into the subtle physiology plays a basically deconstructing role and thus carries a methodological meaning. This move is capable of deconditioning[73] from the objectifications that have crystalized over the years as a result of what Husserl calls the natural attitude and includes not only a mental stance but also a bodily one that has developed along with a specific lifestyle and with peculiar postural habits. Past environmental conditions, specific events, and even traumas all powerfully affect the kind of experience one can have within the body. The very practical fact of sitting for a long time on a certain type of chair, for example, or sleeping on a hard or a soft surface creates an internal delusional representation of the body which in time becomes crystalized; one becomes sensitive to some parts of the body while others are forgotten. The habit of noticing certain groups of muscles to the detriment of others and specific forms of stiffnesses and peculiar weaknesses becomes established. Even discomfort and pain are automatically attributed to certain areas of the body; over time, they turn into true blockages that the mind cuts out of the fluid continuum of the bodily experience. Above all, one has to add the map offered by modern anatomy, which to a certain extent creates another layer of objectivity, overlapping the one of the individual bodily pattern. The chances of inhabiting the body are therefore restricted within very specific limits and coordinates and bound to this kind of tight conditioning.

The yogic physiology of the body evolved very differently from the Western one. While the latter developed from the surgical dissection of corpses, the former emerged in terms of "inner empiricism";[74] that is, it developed from a firsthand and first-person experience harbored by the yogin in the "lived body." This is why, thanks to the constellation provided by the yoga practices, the certainties of the usual bodily pattern are displaced, and a new experience of the body can be accessed. This is the methodological value of entering into representations that differ from the habitual; it is like undermining the faith in the previous existing ones and thus counteracting the theft by the conceptual mind to the detriment of the lived body; ultimately, this means opening spaces of freedom. However, one must be careful not to turn these temporary means, which lack inherent existence and will eventually also be burned in the very purifying process they have triggered into fetishes and new idols, as if they represented true metaphysical realities. Once the geography of the subtle body has emerged through these supports [*ādhāra*], the ladder that brought the practitioner to this point must be burned. In order to allow for the empty space to come into view, an indication of getting rid of the ultimate traces (the deeply fascinating narratives on subtle or pranic dimensions) is clear. As in the case of Wittengenstein's propositions, when the reader "has used them—as steps—to climb up beyond them. (He must, so to speak, throw away the ladder after he has climbed up it.) He must transcend these propositions, and then he will see the world aright."[75] In Eastern texts, the recourse to the notion of emptiness [*śūnyatā*] and the insistence on not reifying the appearing world, not only in Buddhist texts but also in the *a-dvaita* Vedanta tradition, Patañjali's *Yogasūtra*, and the Śiva Nath texts, fulfill this purifying function.

The Body-As-Object and the Lived-Body

In discussing the difference between the body intended as a fabrication of the conceptual mind and the raw, prereflective experience of the body, a brief account of Husserl's distinction of the body-as-object [*Körper*] and the lived-body [*Leib*] is in order. In some instances, Husserl's analysis of the transcendental consciousness relies on the image of the "purely theoretical spectator,"[76] which might lead to a disembodied interpretation of this dimension, and Merleau-Ponty's criticism of his teacher centers on precisely this point.[77] However, it must be stressed that as early as the *Ideas* Husserl felt the need to develop an inquiry into the embodied character of the transcendental consciousness that belongs to a "vital horizon."[78] The transcendental consciousness or psyche does not stem from an immaterial dimension but from the bodily kinesthetic orientations in space. It inheres to a living and flowing horizon [*Horizonthaftigkeit*][79] "belonging to one's own living body with its two-sided character (internal kinesthesis, external physical-real movements)."[80] "The psyché has a Body"[81] because it is "related back to correlative multiplicities of kinesthetic processes having the peculiar character of the 'I do,' 'I move' (to which even the 'I hold still' must be added)."[82] Therefore, the classical representation of space as seen from an eye above is an abstraction. This third-person point of view is in fact a no-person point of view, a virtual point of view, the one that God might have of the world, and that is not Husserl's standpoint. Husserl points out that anything that appears in the space of consciousness appears from a situated perspective: "The things appear and do so from this or that side, and in this mode of appearing is included irrevocably a relation to a here and its basic directions. All spatial being necessarily appears in such a way that it appears either nearer or farther, above or below, right or left."[83] The reference point from which the world is opened is the body: "The 'far' is far from me, from my Body; the 'to the right' refers back to the right side of my Body, e.g., to my right hand."[84] The lived-body takes over the transcendental function[85] due to its "unique distinction of bearing in itself the zero point of all these orientations;"[86] "I have all things over and against me; they are all 'there'—with the exception of one and only one, namely the Body, which is always 'here.' "[87]

Husserl's embodied view of consciousness, attested by claims like the one that "all sensings pertain to my soul [psyché],"[88] is not contradicted by cases of apparent phenomenon of disembodiment or out-of-body experiences. The case of phantom limbs[89] shows that proprioception, even when transferred to an altered system of visual coordinates, maintains a situated and embodied character.

Advanced meditators may report an experience of a fading of the border that separates them from the environment or a sense of loss of belonging, in terms of ownership, to their own body; however, everything still takes place within a global sense of embodiment, despite being altered.[90]

Husserl's analysis of the body rests on the distinction between the lived experience of the body and the body as conceived by the conceptual mind, which takes it as an object among others. Whereas the latter body-as-object [*Körper*] entails an external, third-person perspective on the body, the lived-body [*Leib*] entails a first-person point of view and is the "matter," as it were, that makes up consciousness: "Hence the Body is originally constituted in a double way: first, it is a physical thing, matter; it has its extension. . . . Secondly, I find on it, and I sense "on" it and "in" it: warmth on the back of the hand, coldness in the feet, sensations of touch in the fingertips. I sense, extended over larger Bodily areas, the pressure and pull of my clothes."[91]

When the body is not considered as a material entity but is lived from within, it turns into the abode of sensations. Sense perception (being the original manner of givenness) has absolute primacy in Husserl's view, with touch in particular having a constitutive or transcendental role. But why is touch different from every other sense? The sphere of touch, which is of enormous importance in yoga, has something unique that does not belong to the other senses. Sight, hearing, taste, and smell are like openings to what is outside that enable us to collect information about the world, but they do not tell us much about ourselves. The eye, in particular, can survey a scene but can never see itself: there is a fundamental blindness of the eye vis-à-vis itself. By contrast, when one touches something one discovers, together with the perceived object, something about the sensing hand. For example, if one lightly touches something very smooth and delicate, one may notice the roughness and cuticles of some parts of one's own fingers. Touch is the only sense that gives back information about oneself while scanning the outside world. Small children, in particular, use objects and external space to feel their own shape, to get to know their own bodies. The sensation produced through touch is thus twofold because it is oriented toward both the world and oneself: "My hand is lying on the table. I experience the table as something solid, cold, and smooth. Moving my hand over the table, I get an experience of it and its thingly determinations. At the same time, I can at any moment pay attention to my hand and find on it touch-sensations, sensations of smoothness and coldness, etc. In the interior of the hand, running parallel to the experienced movement, I find motion-sensations, etc."[92] What Husserl is suggesting here is that while touching, one is also touched, as if from the outside: "I do not see myself, my Body, the way I touch myself. What I call the seen Body is not something seeing which is seen, the way my Body as touched Body is something touching which is touched."[93] Husserl uses the example of the paperweight and the possibility of tuning the tactile attention to the external glass-object or the touch sensations in the fingers that linger even after the contact with the external object has ended: "in order to bring to perception here the tactual thing, paperweight, I touch it, with my fingers, for example. I then experience tactually the smooth surface of the glass and the delicate crystal edges. But if I attend to the hand and finger, then they have touch sensations which still linger when the hand is withdrawn. Likewise, my finger and hand have kinesthetic sensations."[94]

Touch places itself in the middle of the distinction between world and subject, which happens only retrospectively once the sensation has begun, by deciding to direct attention to one direction or the other: "In the case of the hand lying on the table, the same sensation of pressure is apprehended at one time as perception of the table's surface (of a small part of it, properly speaking) and at another time produces, with a 'different direction of attention,' in the actualization of another stratum of apprehension, sensations of digital pressure."[95] When a person's two hands touch, the phenomenon unfolds in a more complex way: "In the case of one hand touching the other, it is again the same, only more complicated, for we have then two sensations, and each is apprehendable or experienceable in a double way."[96]

Āsana

In yoga through posture, *āsana* (literally, the "seat"), the body is repeatedly brought in touch with itself by folding and twisting the limbs. The lingering touch sensations mentioned by Husserl and discussed above, are of enormous importance to yoga practice; they work as traces to which attention is tuned as the outer action comes to an end but continues virtually through these bodily imprints. They are slowly uncovered and become noticeable, as if stemming from some undetermined background or horizon. In these moments, something that was concealed is disclosed. In Heideggerian terms, one could call this a moment of truth in the sense of the *aletheya*, the coming into view of what was invisible.

Patañjali's *Yogasūtra* has just a few aphorisms about the *āsana* but nonetheless offers some enlightening elements on this theme.[97] Descriptions of the different *āsana*-s are missing because they are practical cues intended to be given privately by the teacher,[98] thus avoiding the risk of misunderstanding any indications on the practitioner's part. Vyāsa and Vāchaspati Miśra, both commentators on the *Yogasūtra*, add lists of different *āsana*-s ("thirteen and more" in the case of Vyāsa); in Vāchaspati Miśra's gloss, a bare sketch of the *āsana*-s is offered that does not provide many clues about how to actually practice them. One can, however, deduce that some of the *āsana*-s mentioned stand for whole classes of postures (whose overall number thus increases sharply) and that within the "sitting postures" are included a number of postures linked to the animals, which recall a group of postures that exceed the classical ones that involve sitting cross-legged: "The *Krauñchniṣādana* and others of the same class are to be imitated from the sitting postures of the *Krauñchā* [crane], the elephant, the camel, etc."[99] In reference to the "and more" added by Vyāsa to the list of *āsana*-s, the commentator Vijñānabhikṣu states that "the word '*et cetera*' refers to the Peacock Posture, *et cetera*. This is a summary of the fact that there are exactly as many postures as there are kinds of living beings."[100] Furthermore in Śankara's early commentary, *Yogasūtrabhasyavivaraṇa*, a more detailed description and an explanation of their execution are offered. Some very interesting practical cues are given, with supported postures and props even mentioned: "The One with support [*sopāśraya*] is with a yoga strap [*yogapaṭṭa*] or with a prop such a crutch."[101]

But it is in the *Haṭhayogapradīpikā* that a detailed description of the place where the practice should be carried out is offered,[102] together with a more precise explanation of 15 of the 84 (the canonical number) *āsana*-s mentioned. These thorough descriptions, however, do not provide the practitioner with enough indications to practice without the guidance of the teacher; this is quite deliberate, since "by proper practice of *prāṇāyāma* etc., all diseases [*roga*] are eradicated. Through improper practice all diseases can arise."[103] Though the sitting posture *siddhāsana* is particularly valued, the fifteen postures explained[104] include a number of non-seated postures, such as backward folds (*dhanurāsana*),[105] forward folds (*paścimottānāsana*),[106] arm balances (*kukkuṭāsana, mayūrāsana*),[107] the corpse pose (*śavāsana*),[108] and the inversion (*viparīta-karaṇī*),[109] which are strongly emphasized.

There is a contemporary scholarly trend that considers any posture other sitting as a recent discovery. Singleton's claim, defended in his *Yoga Body*, that the performance of a wide range of *āsana*-s is characteristic of "modern yoga"[110] and that traditionally only a small number of bodily postures were covered in yogic practices, is called into question not only by the quotes cited above and by the proliferation of *āsana*-s in late medieval texts[111] but also by the very existence of architectural testimony like the medieval Mahuḍī Gate.[112] This monument in Dabhoī, Gujarāt, is a gigantic arch deeply engraved and rich with sculptures and reliefs that both Vijay Sarde and James Mallinson date to around the late thirteenth century CE. Indeed, some of these sculptures portray yogis practicing highly complex and physically demanding postures such as the headstand [*Śīrṣāsana*] and other inversions like the scorpion posture [*Vṛścikāsana*] (Figs. 7.4–7.6), twists, and effortful postures like the head-to-knee balancing posture [*Ūrdhva Mukhapaścimottanāsana*] (Figs. 7.4–7.6):[113] "There are thirteen images of Nātha-yogīs in the third row. There are six images of Nātha yogīs starting from the south to north corner of the western wall of the gate and seven images are on the Eastern wall. Out of thirteen images, Ādinātha, Matsyendranātha, Gorakṣanātha, and Chauraṅginātha are clearly identified by U. P. Shāh."[114] If these *āsanas* were celebrated on an important monument like the Mahuḍī Gate (but there are many other sites singled out by Vijay Sarde, especially in the Indian region of Maharastra, depicting yogis and yoginis [female practitioners][115] performing *āsana*-s), one must assume that they were already an important part of living *haṭha* yogic traditions. Before attaining public celebrity and the kind of institutionalization represented by being literally carved in stone, these *āsana*-s must have been practiced for a long time.[116] For this reason, not only can one agree with Jason Birch when he says that "it is clear that more than eighty-four *āsana*-s were practised in some traditions of *haṭha* yoga" and that "the majority of these *āsana*-s were not seated poses, but complex and physically-demanding postures, some of which involved repetitive movement, breath control and the use of ropes,"[117] one can also subscribe to Birch's view that these *āsana*-s belong to a period placed "before the British arrived in India" and go even further in ascribing their belonging to local traditions dating centuries before that, as demonstrated by the Mahuḍī Gate and the reliefs on the pillars of Vijayanagara temples at Hampi analyzed by Seth Powell:

> The depictions of non-seated *āsana*-s carved onto the pillared reliefs at Hampi are striking for their complexity and variation. The reliefs include standing postures, inversions, and unique "pretzel-shaped" balancing postures. Based on inscriptional evidence dating to the early 1500s CE, these sculptures represent important and overlooked early visual evidence for the practice of advanced non-seated postures in late-medieval South India. Moreover, a number of images bear a marked similarity to certain non-seated *āsana*-s featured in more modern postural yoga systems, and might represent some of the earliest evidence of their existence—visual, textual, or otherwise.[118]

Figure 7.4. Headstand—*Śīrṣāsana — relief of the Mahudi Gate. Source:* Photo by Dr. Vijay Sarde, from his paper: 'Yoga on Stone': Sculptural Representation of Yoga on Mahuḍī Gate at Dabhoī in Gujarāt, *Heritage: Journal of Multidisciplinary Studies in Archaeology* 5 (2017): 656–75. Used with permission.

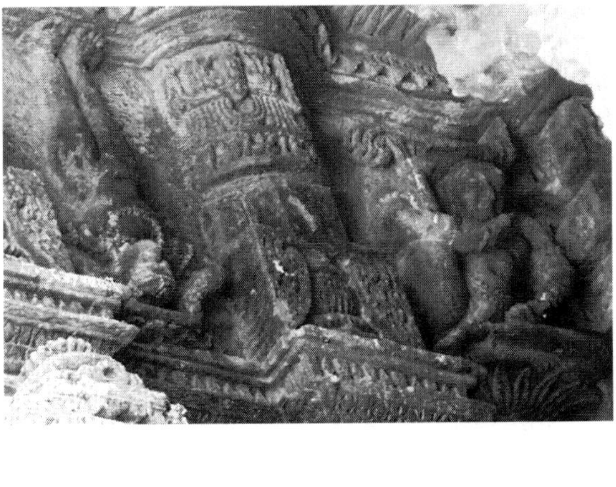

Figure 7.5. Scorpion pose—*Vṛścikāsana — relief of the Mahudi Gate. Source:* Photo by Dr. Vijay Sarde, from his paper: 'Yoga on Stone': Sculptural Representation of Yoga on Mahuḍī Gate at Dabhoī in Gujarāt, *Heritage: Journal of Multidisciplinary Studies in Archaeology* 5 (2017): 656–675. Used with permission.

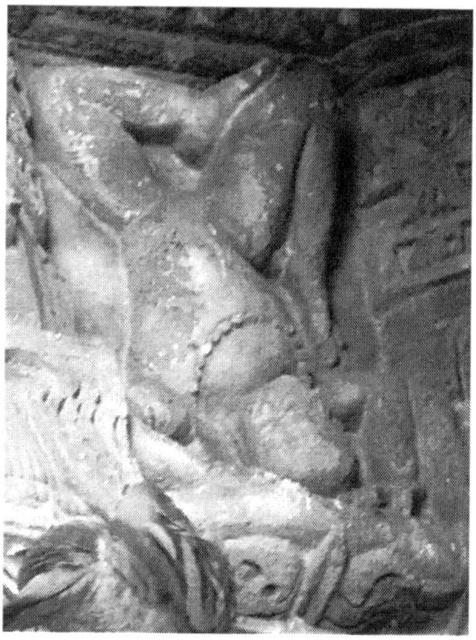

Figure 7.6. *Ūrdhva Mukhapaścimottanāsana* (head-to-knee balancing posture). *Source:* Photo by Dr. Vijay Sarde, from his paper: 'Yoga on Stone': Sculptural Representation of Yoga on Mahuḍī Gate at Dabhoī in Gujarāt, *Heritage: Journal of Multidisciplinary Studies in Archaeology* 5 (2017): 656–75. Used with permission.

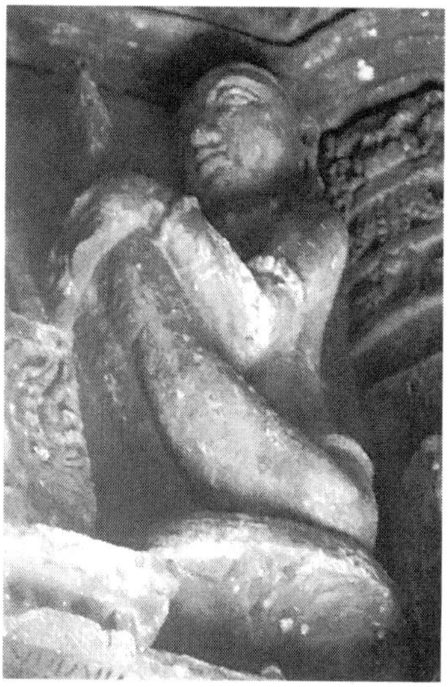

Chapter 8

A Phenomenological Approach to Practice

Doing and Letting Happen

But what is the yogic value of performing physical postures? According to Patañjali, the central point is combining two dimensions that seem to be an unsolvable duality, steadiness [*sthira*] and ease or comfort [*sukha*]: "the *āsana* should be steady and comfortable."[1] In everyday life, one is used to considering these two terms as opposites that exclude one another: the steady engagement of the body appears to bring with it a certain inevitable dose of stiffness, tension, and discomfort, while what is normally meant by comfort is assumed to be accompanied by a kind of laid-back and even lazy sloppiness typical of collapsing onto a couch. The *āsana,* however, trains us to bring these two opposite attributes and dimensions into a kind of accord. The dynamic that enables achieving this combination consists in the expression of an initial effort that later ceases "by relaxation [*śaithilya*] of effort [*prayatna*] and by absorption in the infinite [*ananta*]."[2] In this sutra, Patañjali is speaking of two phases, with "effort" preparing the ground for the "relaxation" that follows to be more fully experienced;[3] when entering the pose a certain degree of directed effort[4] is required, but once the body has become acquainted to the new setting, it can start releasing the initial tension and soften, with the posture becoming more and more comfortable while retaining its shape. Vyāsa makes clear that the "posture becomes perfect when effort to that end ceases, so that there may be no more movement of the body,"[5] and the commentator Vijñānabhikṣu refers to "the slackening of effort as the way to this [steadiness]."[6] What differentiates an *āsana*, a yogic seat, from an ordinary physical action taken from the domain of physical activity or gym is precisely the fact that it is not just a matter of a "vigorous doing," as in sports, but also a question of a comfortable "letting happen": a moment of bodily engagement and effort, be it a contraction or an extension of the muscle areas, opens the space for the subsequent and consequent moment of de-contraction and release. In the first phase, the stagnating body juices are squeezed out of the fibers and cells; in the second phase, when the body relaxes within or releases the posture, freshly oxygenated blood and lymph are invited to flow back into the involved areas. The passage between these two phases is what is beneficial and invigorating from the gross-body perspective; that is, according to the narrative of Western physiology.

One can connect these two moments regarding the *āsana* outlined by Patañjali with what he says at the beginning of the *Yogasūtra* about yoga itself, stemming from the suspension of the fluctuations of the mind on the one side and from the revealing of consciousness in terms of the seer on the other.[7] The "nirodha" is an active phase that breaks with the ongoing mental associations and habits through an intentional effortful restriction. Physical effort has a similar function; it breaks with the habitual bodily patterns and stances that are above all mental patterns and stances. When one is asked to face physical intensity, one notices the mental schemes falling apart and crumbling: this is the value of a bodily engagement.

The abode of the seer is a receptive stance in which one becomes porous to the world in its shining forth and comes into contact with the domain of the transcendental consciousness. This second phase matches the moment of relaxation in the *āsana*, when, Vyāsa notes, "the mind is transformed into the infinite, that is, makes the idea of infinity its own," which "brings about the perfection of posture."[8] Patañjali repeatedly[9] comes back to this fundamental twofold dynamic in other passages of his *Yogasūtra*, as when introducing the already mentioned distinction between "reiteration" [*abhyāsa*] and "non-attachment" [*vairāgya*].[10] Reiteration refers to the practice as a whole but can also denote the determination and steadiness required when entering the *āsana*, whereas nonattachment equals the absorption in the infinite that follows the relaxation of the effort. This twofold dynamic is the essence of purification from the origins onward: *tapas* also has an active-burning phase and a subsequent welcoming-brooding one that was previously inaccessible. Purification is also the essence of phenomenology, as we have come to know it through Husserl and Heidegger. It is precisely the methodological key singled out in phenomenology of the two-phase dynamic of the *epoché* (the suspension of the natural attitude) and the consequent unfolding of the space of transcendental consciousness or Being, that has favored un-concealing what happens in yoga. Thus, as with the fire, it is a question of learning to do something (to suspend or burn more specifically), but also of letting be, of letting happen.

The two-fold dynamic typical of the phenomenological stance[11] that in turns and through a virtuous circle has gained in form and detail thanks to contributions from yoga is the gate to the preordained dimension of consciousness. The contrast between the moments of doing and of letting happen offers access to the domain of the background consciousness because this reveals itself precisely in Gestalt terms, as seen in the second chapter. It was precisely the dynamics of figure-background, determined-undetermined, and clear-unclear that allowed Husserl to realize that there was something other than the figure to be considered when inquiring into the nature of consciousness. For phenomenology, it is the unseen that becomes visible only through a contrast, like the distant horizon or horizon consciousness, that harbors the greatest significance.

Realizing the Horizon

Within a yoga practice, entering and molding the *āsana* creates a laboratory in which forms and shapes are taken and left, to realize in this passage that there was an underlying background. This transparent canvas on which the yogin depicts and erases forms, releasing the *āsana*, has the function of a *mandala,* a space in which shapes are created and destroyed so that the empty space can be revealed. This condition of the possibility of all things can be compared to the silence that comes before music, without which the sound would not exist. Through this dimension, one becomes receptive to the simple fact that the lights are on, as it were: there is a kind of stage on which the singular forms of existence are traced and erased.[12] There is a space of wide-open awareness prior to all thought and to the very awareness that we can have of ourselves and our individual situations. This space is an empty space—an intertwining, a relational space—that absolutely must not be substantialized but understood as a weft, a *tantra*.

In this immersion in what comes into view and dissolves back into the horizon, the personal experience of being an individual "I"[13] ceases, and one tunes into what underlies and comes before any other thing. For it is precisely the "I" that opposes with all its might the contemplation of this weave, and that is secretly in competition with the unlimited manifestation. The "I" is the one who feels as if it is vanishing in front of the vastness of the relational empty space and who, as the scene is stolen from it, suffers deeply. The "I" identifies with thought.[14] In the West, at least since the seventeenth century, we have all become Descartes's heirs without even knowing it. Descartes's identification of being with thought is widely taken for granted: *cogito ergo sum*, I think therefore I am. This means that within the ordinary attitude, one believes that one exists only to the extent to which one is a "thinking thing" [*res cogitans*]. This axiom has burrowed so deep in many people's bones that they hardly conceive of existence, or at least conscious existence, outside of thought, inner chatter, and rumination. And this is why so much contemporary debate tends to identify consciousness with self-consciousness or with conscious executive dimensions entailing cognitive faculties while overlooking the question of a prereflective and pretheoretical consciousness, overflowing the boundaries of what Husserl called the empirical "I."

Contemporary research on mind develops from everyday experience of scholars and researchers, most of whom are imbued with a surreptitious Cartesian faith, according to which only object-directed or content-directed consciousness matters: once the flow of thoughts stops, everything disappears, everything ceases. But is it really the case that when thinking stops, everything comes to and end? Or might it be quite the opposite? According to yoga, everything truly begins when discursive thought stops. For a moment, there is the simple evidence of being-in-the-world: this certainty is experienced within a space of presence, of consciousness, and not of an individual consciousness, of being a particular person. Rather, the space is a horizontal continuum of consciousness.

One of the last of Husserl's pupils, the Czech philosopher Jan Patočka, stresses the importance of developing phenomenology toward a-subjectivity. The "a-subjective phenomenology" of perceptive experience [*wahrnehmende Erfahrung*][15] proposed by Patočka in the 1970s focuses on the question of the appearing of what appears [*l'apparaître de l'apparaissant*]; according to him, this is "the fundamental problem of phenomenology."[16] The space of appearing is irreducible to human enterprise or initiative and like Heidegger's dimension of Being, another thinker by whom Patočka was heavily influenced, comes as a "pure givenness" or "donation": "appearing" is there thanks to Being.[17] "This world belongs to the specific dimension of Being that could be called manifestation. The rules and the structure of manifestation are not the ones of the manifested entities. The being of manifestation is not the work of men; the time it presupposes is not created by existence. Manifestation envelops man, needs him, but also other things. In the end, it is about manifestation, the being of the phenomenon to which, in my opinion, phenomenology aims."[18]

There is a horizon, a "giving itself out" of the world, even before it takes on the meanings we attribute to navigate within it, and thus even before we can call it "world." While Husserl, as we have seen, in his later texts had begun to speak of a horizon consciousness, it is Patočka who repeatedly returns to this theme: "The consciousness of horizon [. . .] is not an intention that can be filled. The horizon remains always the same as a totality [. . .] The horizon is the background for a particular foreground; everything that is actual can and must emerge from the inactuality only to return to lose itself in it."[19] At times, he expresses this in terms of the "indefinite": "The indefinite not as the inaccessible absolute, but as that which continuously responds to us and renders possible the appearing as such."[20] To break free from the subject-centric logic in which we are deeply entrenched, leading us to objectify even consciousness, considering it as just another object, there is a need to speak of a fundamentally impersonal "giving itself out" of consciousness, without owners; the appearing is there thanks to being and cannot be explained through the existent: "The world is not primarily given as a collection of things, that is, it is not given according to the mode of consciousness in which individual things and their sets are intuited and given; there exists instead a more original consciousness of totality and of a more broadly inclusive, indeed all-comprehensive totality: the consciousness of the world"[21]

Overcoming Husserl's notion of the "transcendental ego," still overly compromised by Cartesian subjectivism, Patočka considers the subject a moment of manifestation itself, giving "back to phenomenology, along with Husserl's original intention, the meaning of an investigation of appearing as such."[22] The transcendental in Patočka's view is the world itself, which is not the totality of things; rather "the transcendental, *id est* the subjectivity previous to existent, is the world."[23] He refers to an absence of specific content, an "empty intention" [*intention vide*] and to a "spatial as such [*le spatial en tant que telle*]" as the "condition of possibility of the visible."[24] In order to be realized, this "backdrop" [*toile de fonde*] or "ultimate horizon" requires a modification of the gaze and an overturning of normal experience, a change of attitude within the human being. What interests Patočka is the structure of appearing that is tightly bound to the lived body but treasures an autonomy and independence from human intention and agency: "What is the difference between subjective phenomenology and asubjective phenomenology? The level of explanation of subjective phenomenology is situated in the subject. . . . In asubjective phenomenology, the subject in its appearing is a result to the same extent as everything else. There must be rules *a priori* of my entrance into appearance as well as of the appearing that I am not."[25] Patočka's a-subjective phenomenology is an "exterior phenomenology" in which an autodonation takes place; this autodonation, or givenness of appearing has an anonymous character.[26] Patočka moves in the direction of envisaging consciousness in terms of relation rather than of substance when intending "appearing" as the relative inaccessibility of all that appears; this proves to be very close to Merleau-Ponty as well, for whom "the invisible is 1) what is not actually visible, but could be (hidden or inactual aspects of the thing—hidden things, situated 'elsewhere'—'Here' and 'elsewhere') 2) what, relative to the visible, could nevertheless not be seen as a thing."[27]

If scholars and researchers are not exposed to the possibility of experiencing the world at this level of consciousness, how are they supposed to bring it into the discussion and mapping of the mind? The moments of spontaneous tuning in with the horizon-consciousness that can occur in front of a natural scene or on specific occasions might give a clue of this unseen dimension but are generally not by themselves sufficient to create an ongoing feel for the existence of this possibility. These instances of casual revelation—as when "standing above a deep hole or well and looking steadily downward into the abyss, lacking discursive thinking,"[28] the dissolution of the mind arises—are not enough to undermine the identification with the "I" that has gained strength and stabilized over time. This is for the simple reason that one has dedicated a large part of one's own life to providing a sense of constancy to this unified pole of cognitive material that philosopher of neuroscience Thomas Metzinger calls the "ego tunnel," in which one is virtually trapped.[29]

Only what one practices can one discover: if the unseen dimension of consciousness must be acknowledged theoretically, it must first be experienced. For this reason, it is essential that people engaged in studying the mind confront and become involved theoretically and especially practically in yoga and contemplative practices.

Changing Shape

What the practice of *āsana*-s offers is the chance to experiment with what one could call a middle stage in the process of undermining the identification with the "I": postures are opportunities to take up a provisional identity that differs from the usual one. Sooner or later, every practitioner has come up with the question about why the world of *āsana*-s is so densely populated, beyond the geometric figures, by sages, heroes, animals of all sorts, plants, planets, and even insects. Why is it that through practice one dives into this caravansary?

The answer has to do with trying on a different character. More precisely, in order to burn one's delusory identity, one can first train in meeting experience with a different filter or through a different lens and feel the space as, for instance, an animal might when stretching its back and extending its paws. It is not simply a question of doing the "dog" pose or the "cow" pose but rather of provisionally shifting into these beings and embodying not only their moves but also their attitude and temper. For example, by plunging into the cow pose to the extent of starting to exude placidity and docility out of every pore, one can forget for a while about one's miseries or successes; before one can begin identifying with this new character, the practice offers a new transfer, perhaps into the electric, crackling body of a locust poised to jump. After that, one might embody the strength of a warrior or the vulnerable resistance of a tree. By taking seriously the world of beings invoked through the practice, one can dissolve into them. This is the purifying methodological strategy through which the *āsana* prepares the ground to undermine and shake the faith in the "I." In other words, in order to accomplish the utmost sacrifice and recognize what Varela called the circular continuity between the subject and the world, one might first train in becoming something other than one thought of being.

It is easy to agree with Mark Singleton about the idea that the mechanical and repetitive execution of sequences of *āsana*-s typical of many forms of modern yoga are very likely the result of the influence of Western fitness trends. The automatic approach to sequences of power yoga, imparted like military training, which is now very common leaves no space for the practitioner to either realize the shift of identity discussed above or to carry out the second step, which is realizing the undetermined horizon underneath all those figures in a figure-background dynamic. Today, the practitioner often ends up on an assembly line, waiting for the next order from the instructor to leave this posture and move to the next one, without any engagement in becoming aware of the states of consciousness that are being crossed (because there is literally no time for that). In such cases, the practitioner is paradoxically driven into autopilot mode, in which one might start thinking about many different things (such as what to add to the shopping list or a recent conversation) while one is supposedly dedicated to the practice. When "habit" takes over, a submergence in what phenomenology calls the "natural attitude" takes place, and thus one is very far from being able to do the *epoché* or the *nirodha* or to establish the conversion of the gaze and the stance.

For these reasons, the practice of the *āsana* needs to burn all previous executions and thus encounter the *āsana* each time with the beginner's mind. The practice of the *āsana*-s gives birth to a laboratory in which the practitioner trains with postures that have been, in some instances, repeated unchanged for centuries but that need to be experienced differently and in an unexpected way every time they are done, burning every memory of what has been experienced before. This same tenet will then be applied to everyday life, for lives repeat, seemingly unchanged, for years: wake up, put on one's socks, make tea, have a shower, travel, work, shop, cook, do the dishes, brush the teeth, and sleep. Life can become dramatically alienating if taken as a routine. But it is precisely the neutralization of habit, trained through practice, that can lead to living this rhythm as the expression of endless musical variations on a single theme. There is a recurring theme that will always come back because life is rhythm. At the same time, however, these variations on the theme differ from one another; they never repeat because they are always essentially new and unsettling. It is within this logic that one can interpret the gradual [*krama*] progression that occurs in practice. Doing more advanced and difficult *āsana* cannot be considered a goal to reach in any absolute sense. While it is true that simple postures evolve in more challenging ones over time, this happens as an inevitable consequence of an ardent practice and is not an end in itself; it happens as a secondary effect of a practice in which, instead of labeling discomfort and crystallizing it, one surrenders to something new, capable of displacing previous certainties. For this reason, interruption and contrast are at the heart of the phenomenological approach to yoga.

Delving into the essence of yoga means experiencing the two phases of purification: both the burning flame and the brooding warmth; both the suspension of the fluctuations and habitual patterns of the mind and the revealing of the Seer; both the *epoché* and the letting be. It takes ardor and surrender, and it also takes the awareness to notice switching between the two levels.

Why is it necessary to emphasize this aspect? Because today, on the one hand, there is an alleged form of yoga that has been turned into fitness that leaves no space for work on the mental level to be done; on the other hand, there are many meditative approaches that entail a detailed inquiry into the state of mind but overlook bodily involvement. And yet the indication in the *Haṭhayogapradīpikā* is clear: "There can be no perfection if *haṭha* yoga is without *rāja* yoga or *rāja* yoga without *haṭha* yoga. Therefore, through practice of both, perfection is attained."[30] Patañjali describes the three limbs of *āsana, prāṇāyāma,* and *pratyāhāra* as preliminary stages to be encountered on the way to the final stages known as *samyama.*[31] This exploration of the physical, sensory dimension is even more crucial for Western practitioners, who, due to their sedentary lifestyles, are increasingly hostage to bodies that have become fully alien and are only felt when in pain. Nonetheless, people often tend to polarize their habits and idiosyncrasies, accentuating them over time; they also seem to get on well with separate competencies when it comes to yoga. All involved choose what suits them best and are at no risk of being questioned on their choice. Those who are philosophically engaged but perhaps not inclined toward physical effort will choose a form of yoga that is not demanding on the practical side. Others might try to use physical activity to fill in the empty spaces of listening rather than facing the way their own minds work; they might end up lost in effort and unable to express any contemplative intensity at all. However, as has become increasingly clear, yoga is not a tool for reassurance of past trends but a means to unsettle them, to neutralize habit and the past more generally and to open the door to transformation [*pariṇāma*]:[32] this is the essence of the fire, which philosopher Gaston Bachelard describes as "less monotonous and less abstract than flowing water, even more quick to grow and to change than the young bird we watch every day in its nest in the bushes, fire suggests the desire to change, to speed up the passage of time, to bring all of life to its conclusion, to its hereafter."[33] This means that once steadiness and vigor have been expressed, one must be able to stop the drive toward compulsive agitation and learn to dwell in the pose within a vigilant rest. This change of pace from action to attentive stillness is an enormous effort for our one-sided temper and an authentic expression of the purification at stake. If when entering the *āsana,* a strong intention to open a passageway in the old body pattern and the physical resistances (which are not different from mental ones) is required through a moment of muscular engagement, at a certain point this phase must come to an end and leave room for a moment of receptive quietness and careful observation in which to let go of everything that was brought in through the initial intention. At this point, it is about stopping and holding still, noticing everything that is given to perception once all that is supposedly one's own has been removed. It is about becoming aware of what is happening in this intertwining between the lived body as a sensing element (feeling the floor, the air, the other parts of the body) and as a sensed one (by the surrounding space), about which Husserl was speaking. Ultimately, one can decide to deepen the posture further, with a new active phase through which to intermingle more deeply between the folds of the world or to definitively release in the corpse pose [*śavāsana*].

The shapes and forms that have been entered one after the other and then left are still virtually present as traces and confer a feeling of full availability, not only regarding the shapes one has actually gone through during practice, but also and quite bewilderingly to all possible ones, as if through an endless potentiality, as if one had become both every man's land and simultaneously no man's land. This availability comes together with the coming forward of a tactile sensitivity, located in particular at the periphery of the body, unknown to the domain of ordinary perception.

What Happens During an Inversion

Let us take the inverted posture shoulderstand as an example; it has already come up from the perspective of the subtle physiology. This posture, beneficial to all the limbs [*sālambasarvāngāsana*],[34] entails an active phase in which the lower part of the body reaches up against gravity as high as possible, like a flame, and a subsequent quiet phase of calm brooding. In other words, after the last intentional cues have been brought about—perhaps in order to activate the point between the shoulder blades for better support and to place the feet right above the shoulders, without engaging the neck—one deliberately dismisses action and delves into what is going on within: blood and lymphatic juices are moving downward, and the weight increases in the perception, especially in the shoulders. Instead of fighting this process, one can surrender to it, allowing oneself to be overwhelmed by this unprecedented flow. A sensation of filling up in the lower part is counteracted by a sensation in the upper part of something gradually emptying. By directing the attention precisely toward the feet, ankles, and legs, in the process of becoming lighter and lighter, one might discover a new tactile field opening at the edge of the skin: the surface of the skin appears to be slightly brushed as by a virtual feather, and the border between the supposed inside of the body and these light, caressing touches can no longer be determined.

Coming out of the inversion or another posture the body is released in the supine corpse-pose [*śavāsana*]; by this passage, the opportunity of realizing the inextricable intertwining of body states and mind states is offered. This time the exercise consists in scanning the body, district after district, in order to switch off the activity of the muscles that had been engaged in performing the previous *āsana* and enable a full release in the different areas to take place. As soon as the hidden contractions (which usually remain within the body even after a given bodily motion has ended)[35] are appeased by directing the field of attention toward that area and trying to remove any intention, a new experience of the body surfaces: from the relaxed limbs, a bubbling ferment arises; from the depth of the flesh a vibration starts unleashing itself, like a swarm buzzing delicately deep within. This pleasant and satisfying tingling sensation is the experience of the body not as one is used to considering it from the intellectual level—that is, from the outside—but from the inside.

Turning off the arms and hands muscles and abdicating their manipulative capacities, a micro-tactility within the upper limbs arises. As the hands let go of their grip, they become receptive as antennas and can detect the slightest pulsing sensation: a hidden perceptive universe slowly manifests. Yet, the movements undergone through the previous practice are still dwelling within according to a form of existence that one could call "intermediate." For example, one might notice at the base of the neck a thickness, a density, a kind of warmth similar to the one experienced performing the shoulder stand. We are not used to paying attention to this kind of sensation because once something is considered to be done, we turn to something else in the wrong conviction that everything was finished. . . . Nonetheless, these simple traces that remain when all seems to be over are the ones that carry the experience of the body de-territorialized by the mind.

In yogic terms, this is the experience of the subtle or energetic (*pranic*) body. In phenomenological terms, one could call this, on a first approximation, the experience of the lived-body, but it is something more in respect to what Husserl refers to when speaking about the *Leib*. It is the experience taking place once the discursive mind has been deactivated and moved out of the way, thanks to the pulverizing effect brought about by the previous active phase. It really shouldn't be called an experience of the body because what is normally called the "body" is a creation of the categorizing mind. Once that level of the mind has been dismantled, there is also no more body left. The mind-body dualism that is an artifact of conceptual thought has been overcome, and what is left is no more body than mind. It is an experience that takes place within the limitless field of acceptance of the present moment. As Maurice Merleau-Ponty puts it, "In the present and in perception, my being and my consciousness are at one."[36] However, it is directing the attention to what we are used to calling the body that has led the experience to this point. Before the dualism has been overcome (through a nonconceptual experience), there is of course a "body" and a "mind." Being immersed in a world of conventional truth as we are, the starting point for us is this separation; so one needs to start working on the body. We are born within a body, and our consciousness from the start is an embodied consciousness that runs through every pore of our skin. Only after a process of progressive abstraction and disembodiment does one start believing in a dimension of consciousness conceptually separable from the body. Once this process has come to the point of creating the pervading mind-body dualism we all experience, to overcome it one needs to take this separation as the starting point and direct the attention to the pole of the alleged body.

Turning our attention back to the supine posture, once the spotlight of attention directed to different places has reached the head, one notices an interesting thing happening on the brow. Allowing one's usual facial expression to collapse by relaxing the face muscles one cultivates the occurrence of a certain internal movement in the skin of the forehead. The procedure needs to start from the eyeballs under the closed lids that are invited to widen slightly toward the temples; the eyebrows also go through an analogous process of divergence from one another, with the connected feeling of something opening up from the center toward the temples. These extremely subtle motions might well not be perceivable from the outside but are definitely felt from within, and that is what matters. Turning to the forehead, a similar motion should be cultivated by the practitioner from the center of the forehead toward the sides, as if an invisible hand were smoothing the skin of the forehead that is usually furrowed in the middle, especially when one is concerned about personal issues concerning the "I" or is trying to intellectually grasp a problem. One should mentally visualize one's own forehead in great detail, with all the wrinkles that cross it, and then imagine evening out those lines, from the center to the periphery. This creates at the top of the forehead a soothing sensation, as if the space of the mind-stuff had been cleared of clutter; mental constipation is gradually relieved as this subtle action happens on the edge of the skin. At once, the knots of mental events appear to loosen, and an empty, luminous space slowly opens up. What is striking about this little experiment that the reader might want to try out, after lying down, is that these experiences occurring in the space of awareness are triggered by a very simple bodily gesture: cultivating the feeling of the skin of the forehead smoothly stretching toward the temples.

None of this will come as a surprise to the practitioner who knows to set aside the physical eyes (which are closed) when resorting to the legendary third eye, located according to the subtle physiology in the center of the forehead, just above the eyebrows. This is the *ājñācakra*, the archetype of the capacity of penetrating reality not with ordinary sight but through a vision that does not pin reality to categories but treasures its wide and spontaneous revelation.

What happens on the epidermis is capable of determining what occurs to the mind. In fact, as long as one monitors the released condition of the skin, one realizes the concrete impossibility of conceptually grasping any determined object and conversely being in the condition of tuning in with an open field of presence that spans all 360 degrees and is usually out of reach. The condition of the skin correlates, in Varelian terms, to the experience of what through phenomenology we have learned to call the horizon-consciousness, the background, distant consciousness or, using a different terminology, the dimension of Being. This can be confirmed by a counter-experiment. At the cost of exiting the conscious dimension previously attained, one can try to grasp a determined element (i.e., coming back to the natural attitude) and realize by doing so that a subtle furrowing reappears on the brow. The conclusion is that the experience of smooth skin and a wide internal space at the forehead is incompatible with object-directed thinking. On the contrary, this bodily stance favors entering another field of experience that is beyond concepts or words, as affirmed by Patañjali who refers to the one who has attained the *āsana* as the one who "is not afflicted by the dualities [*dvandva*] of the opposites."[37]

The fish pose, *matsyāśana* (figure 8.1), is an interesting posture for experiencing upward causation starting from the cellular level: lying supine, bring your arms underneath your back, placing your hands beneath the pelvis with the palms facing down; pressing through the elbows and leveraging them, arch the chest as much as possible, as if drawing it into a bow. The neck extends backward until the crown of the head touches the ground beneath, while the thighs relax.

The unfolding and extension of the throat induces a kind of purification: it is as though we are cleansing ourselves of everything we have been taught about the world, or that we believe we know. We let go of all theories and knowledge, as our open eyes observe the surroundings from an unfamiliar upside-down vantage point—recognizing minor details in the space behind that we would otherwise never have noticed. From here, we may begin to cultivate the beginner's gaze—as if seeing the world for the very first time. We remain suspended in this dimension of pure presence, floating in the waters of wonder, for as long as it is comfortable. Then, we gently release and return: drawing the chin in and allowing the arms to slide to the sides, back to *śavasāna*. Lying supine on the ground, we are offered the opportunity to notice the profound calming effects of this posture. The surprise that awaits us is the sensation—not only of quiet stillness—but of a particular, unexpected sense of appropriateness and adequacy: a feeling of being in the right place without striving. The heels seem to rest exactly where they belong, the calves melt perfectly into the floor, the arms are released precisely where they should be—and we feel no desire to change a single detail. Unlike in daily life, where we so often experience dissatisfaction with how things are and strive relentlessly to improve them, here we are met with the opposite experience: everything appears fitting, adequate, enough and fulfilling, exactly as it is. A deep sense of peace and serenity—initially perceived on a purely cellular plane—arises on all levels.

Only when the distinction between body and mind has been undermined through the *āsana* can one start devoting oneself to the breath work [*prāṇāyāma*]: "when that [*āsana*] is accomplished, *prāṇāyāma* [follows]. This consists of the regulation of the incoming and outgoing breaths."[38]

Prāṇāyāma and Constraints between Breath and Mind

In *prāṇāyāma* it is a question of rescinding the habitual irregular motion of the breath [*vṛitti*] and distributing it evenly between breathing in, breathing out, and suspending the breath and to modulate it in terms of duration, number, and quality.[39] Just as there is a correlation between the bodily posture, even in the state of the skin, and the mind state, there are reciprocal constraints between the state of affairs in breathing and in the mind. The ordinary fluctuations of the breath [*vṛitti*] are to be yoked and confined through a restricting action [*gativiccheda*], just as the fluctuations of the mind [*vṛitti*] are to be controlled [*nirodha*]. This double binding dynamic between mental events and breath is also confirmed in the *Haṭhayogapradīpikā* where it is said that a disturbed breath brings with a disturbed mind-space [*citta*], whereas a steady breath leads to a steady mind-space.[40] For this reason, it is reminded, the yogi should train in controlling [*nirodhayet*] the air [*vāyu*].[41] In the *Haṭhayogapradīpikā*, the same term that Patañjali uses in reference to the stilling of the fluctuations of the mind refers to the uneven swirling breaths that should be stilled [*nirodha*] through the yoking action of the *prāṇāyāma*. Mind and breath are bound together by reciprocal constraints: when the mind is unquiet, the breath becomes unquiet, but the opposite is also true, for when the breath is quieted, the mind becomes quiet. By intervening in the breath, the mind state can be changed. In other words, there is both a top-down dynamic and a bottom-up one. The existence of the latter is particularly interesting because it means that by modifying the breath-body patterns one can modify the states of consciousness.[42] This very special form of upward causation that recent experiments in neuroscience are exploring[43] was already known at the time of one of the most ancient *Upaniṣads*, the *Chāndogya* (eighth to sixth centuries BCE): "the mind is bound (*pranabandhanam*) to the *prāṇa*,"[44] and the *prāṇa* is moved around the body thanks to the breath: "the one who has mastered the vital energies . . . should exhale the breath through the nose [*nāsikā*]."[45]

Breathing also entails a Gestalt dynamic figure-background to be realized. At the beginning, just as in the case of the posture, one needs to perform the *epoché*: withdrawing the attention from the habitual mental objects (figures in the foreground) that in the natural attitude usually catalyze it and reorienting it toward the unseen silent background that enfolds them. By tuning more deeply in the direction of this invisible horizon, one notices its progressive un-concealment. After a while, what had previously been detected as an empty silent space upon closer inspection appears to be filled with sound, like distant music that at first is scarcely recognizable and progressively becomes more audible. Among the various sounds that make up this sort of horizon soundtrack (the chirping of birds and perhaps a distant barking mixed with the sound of a car engine turning over), one can start to distinguish the sound of one's own breath. It is a soothing sound, like the sound of the ocean, that becomes more audible by tucking the chin slightly in and delicately reducing the passage of air at the height of the glottis, thanks to what is called the "throat lock" [*jalandhara bandha*]. This sound was present before, but it was concealed by the ordinary apprehension, which is directed exclusively to the world of objects (be they physical things or concepts); only now, as the *epoché* has been established, does the background start revealing itself. But this is not all. After the surrounding soundtrack has come into view, one realizes the different moments of this breathing pattern. At first glance what appears are just the inhalations [*pūraka*] and exhalations [*recaka*],[46] which appear to switch continuously from one into the other. But at a more careful glance sustained over time, one starts noticing that there is something else that had been invisible: a kind of background of the breathing pattern itself. This second-order background is the natural pause that establishes itself spontaneously between one inhalation and the subsequent exhalation and again between the exhalation and the next inhalation. As before, the reader is invited to try what it feels like to notice these spontaneous halts. Without any need to lengthen these entirely natural interruptions, one simply hangs on to them for a moment and discovers that by slightly leaning into them, the next breath unwinds more easily and evenly. These pauses in which the breath is naturally retained are similar to the instant in which a swing becomes still, at the top of the excursion. One can thus invert the normal way of thinking about breathing and consider these moments of stillness as the actual salient features of the whole pattern, with inhaling and exhaling being simply natural oscillatory consequences or corollaries of these pauses. This happens both in normal breathing and in alternate nostril breathing.[47] In yogic texts, these retentions are divided into external [*bāhya*], the pauses following exhalation, and internal [*antara*],[48] the pauses following inhalation; with time and increased skill, they are gradually prolonged and become the very heart of the breathwork.[49] Retention becomes the primary means through which the digestive fire is lit [*śarīra-agni*].[50] But why are these retentions [*kumbhaka*][51] so important from a global perspective? Because if one is careful enough during those pauses, one might realize that the mind stops working in its usual way: no objects can be grasped during these pauses. One could say that the practitioner is faced with a conscious state in which there is perfect wakefulness but no specific content; even the content "I" is surprisingly absent. Thoughts and concepts are missing, the identification with the alleged self is missing, and even the separation of a so-called inside from an alleged outside is lacking. However, as surprising as it may sound to the person unfamiliar with yogic practices, darkness has not fallen onto the scene; precisely the opposite is the case. The lights are on, and shine more brightly than ever.

In the natural attitude, one often has the feeling of being immersed in a kind of personal bubble (made of one's wishes, fears, anticipations, and memories) that somehow dulls the evidence of being there, of being in the world. One is trapped in one's own personal movie, in a kind of constant daydreaming. It is this kind of dreaming that in the state of consciousness at stake comes to an end. The feeling is of awakening to the world for the first time. The Buddha is the awakened, and the *buddhi* is the ability of awakening to the thickness and intensity of the world, a world that is not opposed to the experiencing subject but rather overflows the boundaries between inside and outside. Referring to the state in which the advanced yogin dismisses breathing *tout court* for long periods,[52] the so-called fourth state [*caturtha* or Turīya] (other than inhale, exhale, and retention),[53] Patañjali expresses it this way: "Then the covering [*āvaraṇam*] of the illumination [*prakāśa*] is weakened."[54] Similarly, Heidegger's revival of the ancient Greek notion of *aletheya* is centered on the idea that the moment of truth is given as a dimension in which the layers of concealment that prevent the open space from shining forth are unhidden, allowing the Clearing to come into view.

Through these "impossible translations" between different yogic dimensions, which of course have their specific meanings and times but nonetheless seem to point in the same direction, this book is trying to confront another recent widespread scholarly tendency: the fashionable trend of arguing for the fundamental inexistence of yoga as such. According to this view, because of the changing forms it has undergone, the term has become devoid of any meaning, as if it were an empty shell ready to be filled in any possible way. The author, however, is convinced that the efforts should be directed in showing that yoga, even as used in different worldviews and practices and across the centuries, does point toward a common essence. It is precisely phenomenology that teaches how to distill, within the multiple variables through which a phenomenon[55] can give itself out, the so-called invariant: that is, the common core that recurs through the endless variations. The ultimate core to which the different Eastern yogic traditions point, each in its unique and irreducible way, is a purification process leading to the recognition of the space of the appearing as such. Within the framework of this volume, there is of course no intention of exhausting the field of yogic approaches, which would be impossible given the vastness of the field. On the contrary, a specific choice of field has been made: taking into account a number of yogic paths that train overcoming duality[56] by plunging into the unalloyed field of perception in order to realize "the compound of the world and of ourselves that precedes reflection,"[57] as Husserl's student Merleau-Ponty describes it. It is precisely Merleau-Ponty's contribution that is going to help in carrying out the final lap in this inquiry because, according to him, phenomenology is a "philosophy for which the world is always 'already there' before reflection begins—as an inalienable presence; and all its efforts are concentrated upon re-achieving a direct and primitive contact with the world, and endowing that contact with a philosophical status."[58]

Figure 8.1. Simple version of the Fish posture, *Matsyāśana*. Source: Photo by the author.

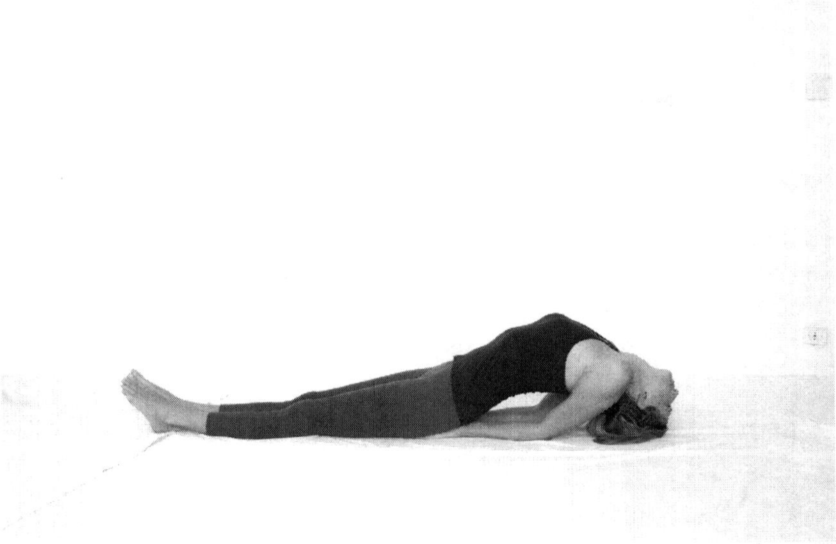

Chapter 9

Merleau-Ponty and Undoing the Mind-Body Split

The Role of Attention

Maurice Merleau-Ponty, who with the exception of Martin Heidegger, is the most prominent heir of Husserl's phenomenology, deeply influenced Chilean neuro-phenomenologist Francisco Varela in his development of the concept of an embodied mind. Just as Heidegger had imprinted a profoundly individual twist on phenomenology, Merleau-Ponty modifies Husserl's phenomenology in important ways, placing even more emphasis on the domain of the transcendental: "That is why phenomenology, alone of all philosophies, talks about a transcendental field. . . . It is also why phenomenology is phenomenology, that is, a study of the advent of being to consciousness."[1]

In his major work, *Phenomenology of Perception* (1945), Merleau-Ponty claims that exploring consciousness in its prereflective life is the role of philosophical thinking. This exploration of consciousness takes the form of a theory of attention:[2] "The first operation of attention is, then, to create for itself a field, either perceptual or mental, which can be 'surveyed.'"[3] Using attention to open up a perceptual field is also the first move in yoga. The insistence in the *Haṭhayogapradīpikā* on the necessity of uninterrupted practice, "by thus practicing [*abhyasa*], night and day," is equaled by the emphasis placed on avoiding automatism [*manovṛtti*] during practice and of fostering a constantly concentered mind [*manoyuktaṁ*]:

"All the pranayama methods are to be done with a concentrated mind. The wise man should not let his mind be involved in the modifications [*vṛittis*]."[4] Only in such a way do mind [*manas*] and breath [*vāyu*] come to adhere to one another.[5]

Merleau-Ponty offers enlightening hints on the theme of attention by making clear that attention overflows the subjective pole and gives itself out as a structure or field that encompasses both subject and object, which can only emerge retrospectively: "Attention first of all presupposes a transformation of the mental field, a new way for consciousness to be present to its objects."[6] The structure of attention is "presence," whereas subject and object can be taken "as two abstract 'moments' of this unique structure which is presence."[7] According to Merleau-Ponty, this contrasts with the widespread view characteristic of both empiricism and rationalism, which holds that "attention creates nothing, since a world of impressions in itself or a universe of determining thought are equally independent of the action of mind."[8] This approach, from which Merleau-Ponty distances himself, imagines a state of affairs as follows: things exist out there, independently from any observers. These observers might or might not consider them through attention, but this occurrence does not change anything on the side of the things (or on the side of the subject), which are believed to remain exactly the same, regardless of whether they are enclosed in the field of attention. However, after having followed the phenomenological path to this point—and especially after having internalized Nāgārjuna's analysis on the codependent arising and emptiness of intrinsic nature—this widespread view no longer appears convincing. Relational interpretations of quantum physics undermine common sense, as Rovelli notes: "Schrödinger's ψ (*Psi*), the wave function, is a tool of calculation that tells us the probability that something is going to happen. . . . The wave ψ evolves in time following the equation written by Schrödinger, as long as we don't look at it. When we do look at it, poof! It concentrates into one single point, and there we see the particle, as if the mere fact of observing were sufficient to modify reality."[9] The dimensions of the yogic subtle physiology appear to behave in the same way. They produce noticeable effects only in as much as they are embraced in the space of consciousness; the moment the concentration fades, they stop existing at least as they existed before. From this perspective, there is no difference between the vital energy [*prāṇa*] and consciousness: "*Prāṇa* is that which is known as the breath [*vāyu*]. . . . It is seen to be indivisibly united with consciousness."[10] For this reason, the myths tell us that "the *ṛṣis* [ancient sages] hence 'see' or meditate upon certain aspects of reality and by doing so actually bring these realities into concrete existence."[11]

Merleau-Ponty's initial concern is showing that "the miracle of consciousness consists in its bringing to light, through attention, phenomena which re-establish the unity of the object in a new dimension at the very moment when they destroy it."[12] Here, Merleau-Ponty is deeply indebted to Husserl's intuitions on the figure-background dynamic and to Gestalt experiments: "the perceived 'thing' is always among other things and is always a part of a field";[13] "to pay attention is not merely further to elucidate pre-existing data, it is to bring about a new articulation of them by taking them as figures."[14] After analyzing famous cases of optical illusions and ambiguous figures, Merleau-Ponty comes to the conclusion that "to perceive in the full sense of the word (as the antithesis of imagining) is not to judge, it is to apprehend an immanent sense in the sensible before judgement begins."[15] The difference between asserting and perceiving was, as the reader will recall, Husserl's starting point. Perception does not take place as a sum of data, as with empiricism, but as a whole, and the "Gestalt is recognized as primary."[16] "Thus attention is neither an association of images, nor the return to itself of thought already in control of its objects, but the active constitution of a new object which makes explicit and articulate what was until then presented as no more than an indeterminate horizon."[17]

The Ante-Predicative Life of Consciousness

What Merleau-Ponty emphasizes even more is the idea of an absence of belonging within perception, which happens in his view as "a comprehensive organization of the field"[18] in an "undivided way."[19] The experiencing individual is sucked back within the field of perception that provisionally covers the role of a new subject that subsumes within itself both subject and object and overcomes that ultimately false duality: "I am not myself a succession of 'psychic' acts, nor for that matter a nuclear I who brings them together into a synthetic unity, but one single experience inseparable from itself, one single 'living cohesion' [. . .] I am a field, an experience."[20]

A kind of "global self-organization of the field of experience"[21] takes place before the separation between me and the world. Merleau-Ponty thus establishes a "third way" between empiricism (according to which what comes first is the world) and rationalism (for which the subject comes first). This third is the *entre-deux*, the space between subject and object, the domain of the transcendental: "The figure-ground distinction introduces a third term between the 'subject' and the 'object.' It is that separation [*écart*] first of all that is the perceptual meaning."[22] Varela, having learned Merleau-Ponty's lesson calls this same space the "subject-world circularity" and defines his approach as a "middle way," just like the Buddhist one.[23] In *The Embodied Mind,* Varela quotes Merleau-Ponty on how the domain of the transcendental is envisaged by referring to the world: "The world is not an object such that I have in my possession the law of its making; it is the natural setting of, and field for, all my thoughts and all my explicit perceptions."[24]

Taking the Husserlian baton of returning to the life-world, Merleau-Ponty refers to the domain of the transcendental and says that "we have to rediscover the primordial substrate from which ideas and things are born."[25] He is interested in "our experience of brute being . . . the umbilical cord of our knowledge and the source of meaning for us."[26] Merleau-Ponty intends to bring back to light the "ante-predicative" or "un-reflective life of consciousness,"[27] the only one that can give sense to scientific operations that constantly refer to it: "Experience of phenomena . . . is the making explicit or bringing to light of the prescientific life of consciousness which alone endows scientific operations with meaning and to which these latter always refer back."[28] It is precisely this prereflective layer of consciousness that contemporary debates on the philosophy of mind seem unable to imagine; in other words, before tackling the empirical capacities of a subject positing a world, a world must first be opened.[29]

Varela understands very well Merleau-Ponty's point that "consciousness is in the first place not a matter of 'I think that' but of 'I can' "[30] and that, when it comes to thinking en-action, the traditional distinction between subject and objects fades away in favor of experiences that have, in the words of his teacher, not yet been "worked over" and that "offer us all at once, pell-mell, both subject and object."[31] This is what phenomenology, for Merleau-Ponty, is interested in: "The world is not what I think, but what I live through. I am open to the world, I have no doubt that I am in communication with it, but I do not possess it; it is inexhaustible."[32]

All this can happen because one has a body; not only is the body "our general medium for having a world"[33] but also "existence is a perpetual incarnation."[34] Merleau-Ponty marks the advance from interpretations of phenomenology that still move within empirical and reductionist implications in which "a set of facts (like 'psychic facts')" are "being reduced to others" and from dualist interpretations of phenomenology, in which a sense of "I"-ness is maintained and opposed to the bodily dimension, in favor of the idea of the world as a "woven fabric"[35] made up of inter-communicating facts endowed with boundaries that "run into each other."[36] Woven fabric is also the literal meaning of tantra,[37] as noted above. This shared terminology is particularly striking since Merleau-Ponty did not inquire deeply into Eastern traditions, just as Husserl who, referring to the groundbreaking experience opened up by the *epoché* and the subsequent phenomenological perception, speaks of a method that "creates by itself a new kind of experience [*neuartige Erfahrung*]"[38] and adds that such an "experience before phenomenology was unknown to human life,"[39] thus basically ignoring yogic practices. Merleau-Ponty, however, did edit an anthology on the famous philosophers of the past, *Les philosophes célèbres*, that begins with "two Indian philosophers" (the Buddha and Nammalvar) and "two Chinese philosophers" (Xunzi and Zhuangzi). In his introduction, Merleau-Ponty not only distances himself from Hegel's paternalistic judgments of Eastern philosophies, which he charged with "childishness" and of "being a failure in the same understanding," but also advocates overcoming the boundaries between Eastern and Western philosophies because "pure and absolute philosophy, in the name of which Hegel excluded the Orient, also excludes a good part of the Western past."[40] Although Merleau-Ponty's intention was to challenge "the border that compartmentalizes philosophy and groups it into different camps of philosophy and nonphilosophy,"[41] he did not actually develop a dialogue with Indian traditions. The convergences between Merleau-Ponty's view and tantra-oriented Eastern traditions testify to the idea that, even when beginning from profoundly different starting points, inquiries can come to similar discoveries and conclusions for internal reasons. Reasons that pertain to the matter itself, regarding the embodied nature of the intertwining or woven fabric of the world that ultimately is consciousness. "My body is the fabric into which all objects are woven, and it is, at least in relation to the perceived world, the general instrument of my 'comprehension,' "[42] insists Merleau-Ponty, implicitly echoing insights typical of Eastern tantric traditions, as in Abhinavagupta's words: "Tact dwells at the superior level of energy, intended as subtle ineffable sensation to which the yogin aspires relentlessly; this contact in fact leads to a consciousness equal to the pure firmament that shines with its own light (*prakasha*)."[43] In tantric literature, using the term *Cinmatraśparsa* ("touch of pure consciousness")[44] means referring to the embedding in touch and in perception more generally of the dimension of consciousness.

Body as the Gateway to Consciousness

The body turns out to be the privileged access point to the domain of the transcendental; not the body as ordinarily referred to, not the body "thought" by the conceptual mind. For this reason, "We must therefore avoid saying that our body is in space, or in time" but opt instead for the idea that "it inhabits space and time."[45] According to Merleau-Ponty, "in every focusing movement my body unites present, past and future, it secretes time . . . it creates time instead of submitting to it."[46] Starting from Husserl's premises, Merleau-Ponty points to an even more radical experience of the lived-body when he says that "our bodily experience . . . provides us with a way of access to the world and the object, with a 'praktognosia,' which has to be recognized as original and perhaps as primary."[47] This embodied experience is already no more "body" than "mind" in Husserl, for whom there is an inextricable tangle between the lived body and the psychic life.[48] Merleau-Ponty reaches the point of saying that "sensation as it is brought to use by experience is no longer some inert substance or abstract moment, but one of our surfaces of contact with being, a structure of consciousness."[49] Distancing himself from empiricists' views on perception, Merleau-Ponty states that "perception is not a science of the world, it is not even an act, a deliberate taking up of a position; it is the *background* from which all acts stand out, and is presupposed by them."[50] Perception, when thought radically enough, is an antidote to the innate tendency of substantializing and reifying things, because a "thing is in a place, but perception is nowhere."[51] Instead of increasing the usual identification with the sense of "I," phenomenological perception, which is not a perception of objects as traditionally understood, has a prepersonal and anonymous character in the sense that, when tuned in to this receptive stance, one does not feel one is the intentional agent of it. Rather, one feels like one is being included within perception itself, at the fringes of one's personal life:

> But this activity takes place on the periphery of my being. I am no more aware of being the true subject of my sensation than of my birth or my death. Neither my birth nor my death can appear to me as experiences of my own, since, if I thought of them thus, I should be assuming myself to be pre-existent to, or outliving, myself, in order to be able to experience them, and I should therefore not be genuinely thinking of my birth or my death. I can, then, apprehend myself only as "already born" and "still alive"—I can apprehend my birth and my death only as prepersonal horizons: I know that people are born and die, but I cannot know my own birth and death. *Each sensation, being strictly speaking, the first, last and only one of its kind, is a birth and a death.* The subject who experiences it begins and ends with it, and as he can neither precede nor survive himself, sensation necessarily appears to itself in a setting of generality, its origin is anterior to myself, it arises from sensibility which has preceded it and which will outlive it, just as my birth and death belong to a natality and a mortality which are anonymous. By means of sensation

> I am able to grasp, on the fringe of my own personal life and acts, a life of given consciousness from which these latter emerge, the life of my eyes, hands and ears, which are so many natural selves.[52]

In order to gain access to this realm of experience, one needs to convert one's interest from the objects, including concepts, to the wider scene in which perception takes place, "that primordial layer at which both things and ideas come into being;"[53] to do that, one must resume contact "with the sensory life which I live from within,"[54] letting go of the way in which perception has taken place till that point. As Merleau-Ponty puts it, "We believed we knew what feeling, seeing and hearing were, and now these words raise problems. We are invited to go back to the experiences to which they refer in order to redefine them."[55]

Merleau-Ponty's perception entails no substantial subject, just as in the case of the Indian figurine of the "Goddess as the Void" (figure 9.1).[56] This nineteenth-century bronze statue is not only a modern and timeless image but is also an eloquent representation of the idea of the nonsubstantiality of the subject. In this case, it appears literally as what it is: a void. The goddess is made up of the emptiness of a doorway and has her hands extended ready to touch, her ears clearly visible. It is a void that nonetheless perceives. The idea is that by passing through this "sensing" void, one can become the very threshold between inner and outer, between subject and world. By inhabiting the threshold, one can go beyond the ordinary dual placement and dwell within the prereflective dimension of consciousness. In Merleau-Ponty's words, this "all-embracing adherence to the world"[57] happens through a refinement of the sensory abilities, which is exactly what yoga and contemplative practices are about. Merleau-Ponty does not envisage a systematic training like the one that unfolds in yoga, because, as noted above, he lacked specific knowledge of Eastern methodologies, but the following description qualifies as a full-fledged yoga exercise: "At the very moment when I live in the world, when I am given over to my plans, my occupations, my friends, my memories, I can close my eyes, lie down, listen to the blood pulsating in my ears, lose myself in some pleasure or pain, and shut myself up in this anonymous life which subtends

Figure 9.1. The supreme Goddess as a void. *Source:* Collection of the Asian Civilisations Museum, Singapore. Used with permission.

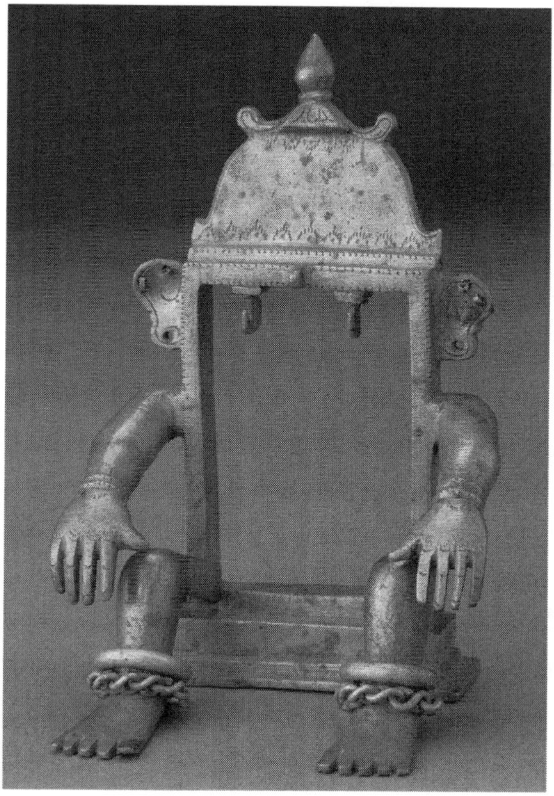

my personal one."[58] The instruction to look for the way within oneself is a recurring theme in yogic practices. This is why the path of yoga is said to be experimental: it does not require any belief or authority except one's own experience. It simply takes full attention and exercise.[59] However, as with the empty space in a bowl, which is really no different from the space outside it, when one descends to the depths inwardly, one finds the world. This is how one comes to understand that the alleged true self within oneself will never be found because it is found elsewhere, on the outside: "I am everywhere,"[60] it is said in the *Vijñānabhairava* tantra. The expression by Ken Wilber, "the more I go into 'I,' the more I fall out of 'I,' "[61] that was widespread in the New Age ideology of the 1970s and 1980s was anticipated by Merleau-Ponty, who died in 1961 and—without the use of psychotropic or psychedelic substances—describes his realization, in his posthumous work *The Visible and the Invisible* (1964), in these terms: "Our flesh lines and even envelops all the visible and tangible things with which nevertheless it is surrounded, the world and I are within one another."[62] The debt that the Beat Generation, who engaged in enquiring nonordinary states of consciousness, owes to Eastern thought is repeatedly acknowledged, whereas their connections with phenomenological insights have rarely been noted.

The Unintended Phenomenological Connotations of Mindfulness

In the 1980s, it was Jon Kabat-Zinn, a molecular biologist with a background in medicine, who brought several basic tenets of Buddhist philosophy to the West and created a defined protocol out of them: mindfulness. He developed a mindfulness-based stress reduction program with the aim of turning this protocol into a therapy to spread in clinical contexts. It draws on both Śamatha[63] and Vipaśyanā meditation,[64] the four foundations of which are to be found in the *Satipaṭṭhāna Sutta* of the Pali canon,[65] and describes the practice as a new way of relating with the experience that is already there and turning off "autopilot mode."[66] But this different way of relating to experience is above all the aim of phenomenology. Is the neutralization of the natural attitude in phenomenology not a way of turning off the autopilot that encounters the world through repetition and habit?

Mindfulness is saturated with phenomenological tenets. The very definition of mindfulness as "the awareness that emerges through paying attention on purpose, in the present moment, and non-judgmentally to the unfolding of experience moment by moment"[67] fits very well with the phenomenological gaze, even if the terminology in mindfulness is less technical and thus more accessible to the wider public. Surprisingly, however, in the elaboration of mindfulness as an expanded awareness of the present experience, hardly any reference is made to the Western phenomenological tradition as a dignified antecedent to it, along with Eastern influences.[68] One of the fringe benefits of the present volume is uncovering how phenomenology had anticipated much of what became the main features of mindfulness[69]; indeed, in the face of the enormous popularity that mindfulness has enjoyed in recent decades, unconcealing the largely unacknowledged phenomenological connotations of mindfulness can no longer be postponed.

Alongside mindfulness, other protocols have been inspired by the dialogue between Eastern contemplative traditions and contemporary psychology, such as the idea of cultivating emotional balance, developed by Paul Ekman, Alan Wallace,[70] and Eve Ekman, which includes several meditations drawn from Buddhism. Within these cross-cultural findings, many exercises entailing bodily and sensory awareness are explored, but there remains a space for practices that emphasize the embodied nature of the conscious experience at stake, such as what one could provisionally call phenomenologically informed yoga practices. It is only by delving deeply into yogic practices on the one hand and the extreme outputs of the phenomenological inquiry on the other that a thorough exploration of the "perceptual consciousness"[71] and how it represents the door to the domain of the transcendental can be carried out, because as Merleau-Ponty notes, "nature and consciousness cannot really communicate other than in us and through our carnal being."[72]

Overlapping Borders: Two Simple Exercises

The domain of the transcendental is the endless circulation between subject and world. According to Varela, "Merleau-Ponty recognized that we cannot understand this circulation without a detailed investigation of its fundamental axis, namely, the embodiment of knowledge, cognition, and experience."[73] When Varela states that "our cognition emerges from the background of a world that extends beyond us but that cannot be found apart from our embodiment,"[74] he acutely understands Heidegger's lesson that Being comes earlier than thinking, and that, as Merleau-Ponty further elaborates, "the world is there before any possible analysis of mine."[75]

But the "sensory fields" that are one's "primitive alliance with the world,"[76] according to Merleau-Ponty, are not to be objectified in terms of *qualia*: "The quality, the separate sensory impact occurs when I break this total structuralization of my vision, when I cease to adhere to my own gaze."[77] Instead, Merleau-Ponty is interested in revealing "a 'primary layer' of sense experience which precedes its division among the separate senses."[78] Sense experience is global and intersensory.[79] It is not an object but a threshold happening in the space between body and world: "It is my gaze which subtends colour, and the movement of my hand which subtends the object's form, or rather my gaze pairs off with colour, and my hand with hardness and softness, and in this transaction between the subject of sensation and the sensible it cannot be held that one acts while the other suffers the action."[80]

It is from this "co-existence of sentient and sensible"[81] that space emerges and spreads, and this can happen because the body is not an object between the others, because it is never really fully displayable in front but maintains an edge of invisibility: "To say that it is always near me, always there for me, is to say that it is never really in front of me, that I cannot array it before my eyes, that it remains marginal to all my perceptions, that it is with me."[82] Here, Merleau-Ponty is recalling the Husserlian analysis of the figure-background dynamic, the dialectic between what is clear and the unclear horizon from which it stems.

Taking up Husserl's example of the hand capable of being both a means through which to inquire about an outer object like a surface and a lived-through element that returns an experience from within, Merleau-Ponty notes that in the case of two hands touching each other, one cannot shift from the third- to the first-person perspective in both hands simultaneously. The attention must take turns in dwelling on them, first on one and then the other:

> My body, it was said, is recognized by its power to give me "double sensations": when I touch my right hand with my left, my right hand, as an object, has the strange property of being able to feel too. We have just seen that the two hands are never simultaneously in the relationship of touched and touching to each other. When I press my two hands together, it is not a matter of two sensations felt together as one perceives two objects placed side by side, but of an ambiguous set-up in which both hands can alternate the roles of "touching" and being "touched."[83]

Merleau-Ponty suggests trying this exercise to explore the reversibility of touch, its lack of full availability, which carries within itself a dynamic of accessibility and inaccessibility or, as Merleau-Ponty calls it in his posthumous work: visibility and invisibility. Once again, the kind of exercise that Merleau-Ponty suggests is nothing more and nothing less than a yoga exercise. The following is an example of how one can develop this insight in yoga practice.

After having gone through an active phase of the practice—thanks to that same effort, tuning in to a deep stillness comes easily—one comfortably lies prone, with the head gently twisted to one side and the cheek resting on the floor [*Advāsana*] (figure 9.2). Without moving, begin noticing the ground underneath, perceiving its density, the hardness or softness of the mat, and perhaps feeling the roughness or evenness of the pattern or the texture of its surface where the cheek touches it. In this moment, things are settled in the traditional way: a perceiving subject and a perceived object (the surface underneath).

After a minute of this way of directing the attention, reverse the scene by switching sides, as with Gestalt images. In order to do this, one must allow oneself first to change attitude and let go of the executive task of scanning the underlying surface of the mat through the bare areas of the skin. Start imagining being held and carried by the floor as if it were the palm of a giant hand. A reassuring sensation of being supported is welcome; the feeling of entrusting the floor to the point of transferring to it full accountability for the situation, with a form of disengagement from personal agency, should be cultivated. At this point, reversing the direction

Figure 9.2. *Advāsana* posture. *Source:* Photo by the author.

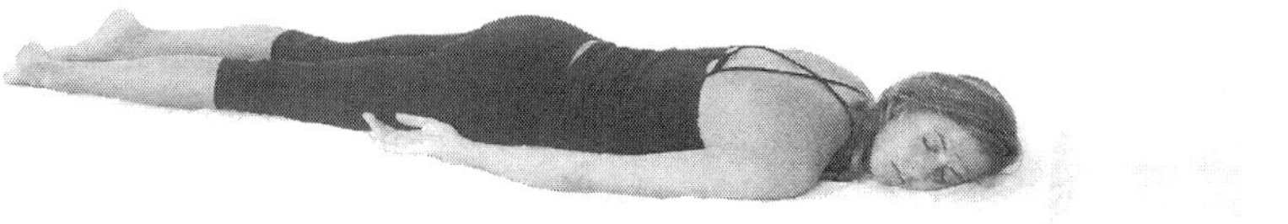

of the attention can take place. Instead of feeling the floor, one can notice how it feels to be felt from it, as if from the outside, as if one had provisionally taken the place of the felt object, whereas the floor had virtually taken up the role of the sensing subject. Through the metaphor of a sensing floor, one can cultivate the experience of perceiving oneself through an external medium, as when the shape of one's own body is felt in someone else's arms. Merleau-Ponty, referring to the experience of touch and its capacity to neutralize and burn any precomprehension of the world, evokes the image of a fire: "Between hand and hand, a blending of some sort takes place—when the spark is lit between the sensing and sensible, lighting the fire that will not stop burning."[84]

Through the exercise described above, the typically forgotten chiastic and reversible nature of touch is realized directly through one's own flesh. From a thorough surrendering to the "body of the world," one can undergo the experience of no longer existing from a subjective dominant standpoint but of being constituted as "touched" from the outside and consequently access that dimension of receptivity and letting be that Heidegger calls *Gelassenheit*. One can then go on to try to shift between these perspectives a few times, from the condition of toucher to the condition of touched, experiencing a sort of mental dizziness every time the realization of the continuity between one's thickness and the world's is made: "The body sensed and the body sentient are as the obverse and the reverse, or again, as two segments of one sole circular course. . . . Where are we to put the limit between the body and the world, since the world is flesh? . . . There is reciprocal insertion and intertwining of one in the other."[85]

Subject-Object Indeterminacy

The experience of indistinguishability is at the base of the homology that the yogin recognizes between the microcosm and the macrocosm, between the body and the universe. According to tantric traditions, the body is not just a map or a cartography of the world. For the practitioner, the body becomes a mandala or the world itself to the point that, as claimed in the *Vishvasāra Tantra*, "whatever is here [in our body] is found elsewhere. But what is not here is nowhere else."[86] There is no difference between one's own body and the body of the world;[87] the yoga body is also provided with a mountain (the back), seas, rivers (energetic channels), islands, sacred sites, wind, fire, water, earth, and planets (along with the sun and the moon), as one can infer from the description of the subtle body found in the Buddhist *Amṛtasiddhi*:

> [Mount Meru] exists in the body, with seven islands, three worlds and fourteen levels. In it are oceans, rivers, regions [and] guardians of the regions; gathering places (chandohas), sacred sites, seats [of deities and] the deities of the seats; lunar mansions, all the planets, sages and holy men; the moon and the sun, moving about causing creation and destruction; the sky, the wind and fire; water and earth; Viṣṇu divided and undivided, [Śiva] the lord of beings (bhūtanātha) [and] Prajāpati. The elements which [exist] in the three worlds are all [found] in the body [and] the elements which are in the body [also] exist elsewhere.[88]

In both *haṭha* yoga and Merleau-Ponty's phenomenology, the "cosmicization" process is triggered by the exploration of the body, which alone "can bring us to the things themselves, which are themselves not flat beings but beings in depth."[89] It is only by entering the depths of the body, which serves as a mandala, that one is able to realize the world. In these Eastern traditions, just as in phenomenology, the separate and dominant subject acting as the protagonist crumbles; as this happens, one realizes the impossibility of disentanglement from the all-pervading continuum of consciousness and consents to being reabsorbed into it, as when at a certain point when looking at the sky, one becomes that very overwhelming blue:

> As I contemplate the blue of the sky I am not set over against it as an acosmic subject; I do not possess it in thought, or spread out towards it some idea of blue such as might reveal the secret of it, I abandon myself to it and plunge into this mystery, it 'thinks itself within me.' I am the sky itself as it is drawn together and unified, and as it begins to exist for itself; my consciousness is saturated with this limitless blue.[90]

This connection between embodied experience and the all-encompassing sky in which, while sensing, consciousness becomes saturated,[91] quite astonishingly is to be found in the *Yogabīja*: "The body is like the sky, [but] even more pure than the sky. It becomes more subtle than the subtle, more gross than the gross, more solid than the solid."[92] It is worth noting that when referring to this nonordinary state of consciousness in which the dimension of transcendental consciousness is accessed, Merleau-Ponty does not say that he thinks about the mysterious blue of the sky but rather that the sky thinks itself within him. Personal agency is dropped, and an attitude of receptiveness toward what is already taking place is cultivated. This is the peculiarity of the phenomenological development of the concept of perception: "So, if I wanted to render precisely the perceptual experience, I ought to say that one perceives in me, and not that I perceive. Every sensation carries within it the germ of a dream or depersonalization such as we experience in that quasi-stupor to which we are reduced when we really try to live at the level of sensation."[93]

The two phases that have been singled out thanks to the contribution of Husserl and Heidegger and that are the essence of yoga—the active-burning phase that clears the space from reifying tendencies and the warm-receptive phase that welcomes the un-concealing of appearing—can be recognized in Merleau-Ponty's development of consciousness through perception. In order for the perceptual communion to happen, the room must have been cleared of the prejudices arising from objective thinking: "Every perception is a communication or a communion, the taking up or completion by us of some extraneous intention or, on the other hand, the complete expression outside ourselves of our perceptual powers and a coition, so to speak, of our body with things. The fact that this may not have been realized earlier, is explained by the fact that any coming to awareness of the perceptual world was hampered by the prejudices arising from objective thinking."[94] This communion or essential indiscernibility of borders and agency can be experienced by simply noticing the breath:[95] every exhalation is an outpouring into the external space, and with every inhalation the external space invades the inside. As the breaths and waves come and go, one realizes that the outer and inner worlds intermingle. The boundaries between inner and outer disappear as if one were to become thinner and thinner, until one might sense turning into a kind of doorway between the alleged self and the world (which keep on redefining each other and changing borders). By offering inhalation to exhalation and exhalation to inhalation,[96] the outside works its way inside, and the inside spreads into the surrounding space. Through the body, one realizes that "inside and outside are inseparable. The world is wholly inside and I am wholly outside myself. . . . I am situated in it and it understands me."[97] By relaxing the reflex to signifying and to decoding the given experience in terms of transcendent objects, one dismisses the natural attitude and the approach to reality based on the premature assignment of meaning. A form of relief is felt from no longer having to worry about how to make things happen and simply bearing the unfolding of experience, moment after moment.

In both phenomenology and yoga, personal boundaries are not fixed once and for all. Through yoga's *prāṇāyāma* breathing, the chest can grow and expand as if touching the ceiling or shrink to the size of a seed.[98] In order to allow such experiences to unfold, one must first make sure to have bracketed what Merleau-Ponty calls "the prejudices of objective thinking;" that is, the tendency to hastily interpret all physical sensations and react to them on the basis of ongoing habit. Another element of postures is the matter of avoiding framing a specific stimulus, perhaps felt at a given spot in the hamstrings as the typical annoying pull from which one should be freed as soon as possible. This kind of stimulus is heavily laden with the weight of past mentalized experiences and should be deconstructed through an archeological process and broken down into "brute perceptions"[99] not yet structured by objectifying mental formations.

Patiently, one begins to observe that which is given within the limits in which it presents itself but no further: is it a clear sensation that we can bring into focus, or is it vague? How broad is its extension? Is the sensation somewhat stable over time, or does it change? In this last case, is it growing or diminishing? Is the sensation still, or does it move? Is it pulsing, tingling, or swarming? Is it light and sharp or dense and heavy? By dint of observing while trying to suspend judgment and interpretation of what is given, it is possible that after a certain amount of time, the previously solid and alarming impulse that urged concluding the posture will dissolve into a surprising new experience. And when the never fully uprooted objectifying tendency does eventually turn this phenomenon into an object, one can restart the process and carry out a further phenomenological reduction, for, as Merleau-Ponty reminds us, "The most important lesson which the reduction teaches us is the impossibility of a complete reduction."[100]

The first move in tackling this phenomenological approach is to tune in to what Merleau-Ponty calls the "thickness" that characterizes perception: "The solution of all problems of transcendence is to be sought in the thickness of the pre-objective present in which we find our bodily being, our social being, and the preexistence of the world, that is, the starting point of 'explanations,' in so far as they are legitimate—and at the same time the basis of our freedom."[101] The experience of this thickness is the gateway to the domain of the transcendental, because it is the common texture through which a world is pregiven to us.

Translating this into practice, it means that after having dwelled in a certain number of postures, one can once more lie supine on the floor, begin to scan from the bottom up the different parts of the body, and gradually start releasing tension. Attention can be directed to the precise point where the body touches the mat, noticing the density of the body and the discharging of the weight; this weight seems to lower and gather at the bottom of the body, like sediment at the bottom of a container held still and filled with liquid. What is happening at the exact point where the vessel of the body touches the floor? What is happening in those spots at the bottom of the heels, in the sacrum, in the elbows, where the body is in direct contact with the floor? The experience can be a discharge of the density and weight of the body into the ground and the converse penetration of the underlying soundness within the perimeters of the body. One's own substance is handed over to the ground, and the ground substance seems to be infusing and diffusing within. There is a mutual exchange after which—if attention is sustained long enough—an experience of indeterminacy arises, along with the impossibility of disentangling oneself from the body of the world. Where one's own body ends and where the underlying body of the world starts can no longer be determined.

This experience of indeterminacy is the gate to the underlying preconceptual dimension of consciousness. Referring to this vanishing of the borders and the impossibility of determining once and for all the threshold between subject and object, Merleau-Ponty speaks of the self as "a fold, which has been made and which can be unmade."[102] The principle of indeterminacy, according to Merleau-Ponty, is not due to some imperfection of human knowledge but is inherent in existence: "Thus there is in human existence a principle of indeterminacy, and this indeterminacy is not only for us, it does not stem from some imperfection of our knowledge. . . . Existence is indeterminate in itself, by reason of its fundamental structure."[103]

This is so because of the fundamentally relational character of existence.[104] As is true for Nāgārjuna, so it is for Merleau-Ponty, when what appears substantial turns out, upon closer examination, to be nothing but a knot of relations: "For we are ourselves this network [*noeud*] of relationships."[105] This integral being is placed at "the intersection of my views and at the intersection of my views with those of the others, at the intersection of my acts and at the intersection of my acts with those of the others."[106] The evidence of the other is possible only thanks to the body,[107] for every relation with Being is a carnal relation, a relation with the "flesh of the visible";[108] "we mean that carnal being, as a being of depths, of several leaves or several faces, a being in latency, and a presentation of a certain absence, is a prototype of Being, of which our body, the sensible sentient, is a very remarkable variant, but whose constitutive paradox already lies in every visible."[109]

From this it becomes clear that the body in virtue of "its double belongingness to the order of the 'object' and to the order of the 'subject' "[110] and its "equivocal status as touching and touched"[111] is the only route through which to realize the dimension of the flesh of the world: "The thickness of the body, far from rivaling that of the world, is on the contrary the sole means I have to go unto the heart of the things, by making myself world and by making them flesh [*la Chair*]."[112] The notion of flesh that Merleau-Ponty introduces into the philosophical discourse for its disruptive and displacing character in relation to metaphysical terminology should not be taken too literally in the physiological sense. Certainly, the starting point for the development of the notion of flesh is the first-person, unobjectifiable experience of the lived-body, but it eventually comes to mean much more than that. Flesh must also not be read for its anthropological or religious connotations.[113] Merleau-Ponty was initially sympathetic to Marxist theory and later became a critic of this ideology but did not embrace any Christian or indeed theological view. The flesh, for him, is the circular course, the cohesion of "the body sensed and the body Sentient,"[114] the "strange adhesion of the seer and the visible,"[115] their "reciprocal insertion and intertwining,"[116] and their reversibility:

> The flesh is not matter, in the sense of corpuscles of being which would add up or continue on one another to form beings. Nor is the visible (the things as well as my own body) some "psychic" material that would be—God knows how—brought into being by the things factually existing and acting on my factual body. In general, it is not a fact or a sum of facts "material" or "spiritual." Nor is it a representation for a mind: a mind could not be captured by its own representations; it would rebel against this insertion into the visible which is essential to the seer. The flesh is not matter, is not mind, is not substance. To designate it, we should need the old term "element," in the sense it was used to speak of water, air, earth, and fire, that is, in the sense of a general thing, midway between the spatio-temporal individual and the idea, a sort of incarnate principle that brings a style of being wherever there is a fragment of being. The flesh is in this sense an "element" of Being. Not a fact or a sum of facts, and yet adherent to location and to the now.[117]

Here we find a version of the "neither this nor that" [*neti neti*] argument that in the *Māṇḍūkya Upaniṣad* applies to the fourth state of consciousness, *Turīya,* which is considered beyond language and beyond duality. Merleau-Ponty makes explicit reference to negative philosophy when he states that "one cannot make a direct ontology. My 'indirect' method (being in the beings) is alone conformed with being—'negative philosophy' like 'negative theology.' "[118] His notion of flesh appeals to the very dimension of consciousness to which this volume points from the start and that has been given many names by different authors. A link can be drawn between Merleau-Ponty's "flesh" and Buddhist "emptiness" [*śūnyatā*] in as much as the relational character of the flesh finds its counterpart in the notion of codependent-arising [*pratītya-samutpāda*][119] (figure 9.3). The "indissoluble link between things and myself"[120] announced by the flesh also has powerful social implications[121] and is the ground for a new, nondogmatic ethics and for a philosophical refounding of ecology.[122]

Merleau-Ponty's intra-ontology opens a new scene not only on the ethical ground but also regarding the understanding of consciousness, as this volume has shown. Since "we are involved in the world and with others in an inextricable tangle,"[123] the knowledge of the world takes the form of an immersion, which Merleau-Ponty calls an "endo-ontology"[124] that is "expressed from the inmost recesses of the process of being."[125] It is situated ontology that entails a "participationist conception,"[126] as Merleau-Ponty explains.

This leads to the fact that the dimension of transcendental consciousness is not something that can be displayed as if it were an object. Is language, with its dual nature, thus banned from this dimension? According to Merleau-Ponty, one should, perhaps through "difficult effort," continue to use "the significations of words to express, beyond themselves, our mute contact with the things, when they are not yet things said."[127]

Figure 9.3. La Chair as weft. *Source:* kjpargeter, Freepik.

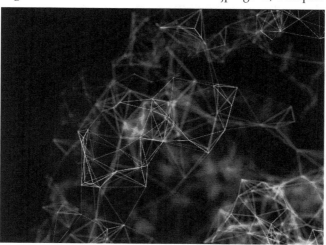

Using language beyond language and its dead ends, and deploying language against its normative structure, can open up through its evocative power unedited space of experience. This is at the base of interviews carried out using micro-phenomenology, when trying to preserve dimensions of experience from the habitual interpretative framework or when preventing them from being territorialized by a pregiven, constricting lexicon and the received view of the world that comes with it.[128] Using words to undo the substantializing tendencies hidden in language and open spaces of freedom is also fundamental to yoga teaching. In order to regain touch with "sensory fields which are," according to Merleau-Ponty, our "primitive alliance with the world"[129] and eventually dismiss tout court the dimension of language, the teacher in yoga and contemplative practices should master a resonant speech to counteract the objectifying tendencies of denotative language and facilitate tuning into other layers of experience. This does not lead to a realm of fluffy stuff and artifacts because there is a constraint imposed by reality that prevents arbitrariness. While some of Husserl's statements might suggest interpreting his view as a form of idealism, despite his insistence on the fact that "just as the reduced Ego is not a piece of the world, so, conversely, neither the world nor any worldly Object is a piece of my Ego,"[130] and despite his eventual dropping of the term "phenomenological residuum," which could convey the idea that only the subjective acts are of interest for phenomenology—to the detriment of the other correlate of the relation, the world[131]—Merleau-Ponty is very clear in excluding any form of idealism, just as he rules out any form of materialism. Merleau-Ponty refers to something in "nature that imposes itself" as an independent condition that he defines as "our problem": "primordial being which is not yet the being-subject or the being-object, and that confuses reflection in every respect."[132] It is that very element that when a theory is being tested in a laboratory, might resist experimental proof and thus call on the researcher to revise the initial hypothesis. Consciousness from a phenomenological perspective, which can provisionally be defined as an experiential fundamentalism, is not reducible to the physical world (in contrast with reductionist theories), but it also does not belong to some proto-psychic, object-like "essence" of the kind found in dualist pan-psychist views. It is more like a threshold, an irreducible gap, a dynamic between visible and invisible, or an ineliminable dialectic between clear and unclear, because it stems from the chiastic reversibility of in and out, from their being enfolded and entangled one into the other.

Future Steps

Above all, the purpose of this volume is to call attention to the fact that next to cognitive, content-directed, conscious dimensions entailing vexing problems like free will, there is another dimension of consciousness—underlying and unseen—that is content-independent and not linked to agency: having carefully explored the world of yoga illuminates this dimension, making it more familiar.

Meanwhile, the phenomenological approach offers a more comprehensive understanding of what is actually going on in yogic states so that this discovery can be included in philosophical discourse. In other words, the path that has unwound to this point has enabled the reader to intuit the existence of this nondual dimension of the appearing, to acknowledge it philosophically, and to understand the twofold dynamic of "doing" and "letting happen" that triggers its revelation. As noted in chapter 1, neuroscientific literature in the best of cases includes this dimension among the "non-ordinary" or "altered" states of consciousness cauldron, despite the fact that in those states nothing is actually altered. By contrast, as has become clear through the path in yoga, those states are considered in Eastern traditions the benchmark of how consciousness can unfold. What is altered and needs to be controlled, according to a yogic perspective, are the swirling fluctuations of the cognitive mind that paradoxically now sets the standard for experimental work. The yogic path enables us to see things from the other way around when it comes to establishing a criterion for what deserves to be considered a conscious state. Yogic states ask us to rethink what an "ordinary" state of consciousness ought to be. When envisioning a space for neurophenomenology, which has thus far dealt mainly with correlations between cognitive tasks and first-person accounts, Varela emphasizes the necessity of reciprocal constraints that entail a double link between the experiential domain and third-person measures developed through scanning techniques. The scenario that could now unfold is beginning to establish a structural correlation between first-person lived experiences and third-person measurements in reference not only to cognitive tasks[133] but also to the underlying continuum of consciousness.

It is worth noting here Zoran Josipovic's neuroscientific research on what he calls the dimension of "consciousness-as-such." Josipovic acknowledges that "for a conceptual mind, attempting to analyze it, nondual, awareness, consciousness as such, can be frustratingly paradoxical," adding that "it is no wonder that researchers, even when curious, have tended to stay away from it" and concluding that "we need to adjust our research focus to include non-dual awareness, consciousness-as-such."[134] Josipovic has conducted research on nondual awareness meditation, reporting a "significant decrease in the anti-correlation between the two networks [extrinsic and intrinsic systems]"[135] and came to "hypothesize that the central precuneus network might be significantly involved in non-dual awareness."[136] He also notes something that could be read in the direction of what has been put forward in chapter 4, regarding the yogic stance being an unnatural attitude: "Discovering and sustaining it [nondual awareness] can take a large investment of energy. [. . .] This is also because initially it requires a de-construction of the self-world model in survival. Hence the evolutionary benefits of sustaining such state are not immediately evident and maybe of a different kind."[137]

What particularly struck me was to find in Josipovic's articles references to neural activity in terms of figure-background: "Nondual awareness can be then hypothesized to function as a background context-frame."[138] As the reader may recall, the first chapters of this book carefully explore the gestalt dynamic in relation to the horizon consciousness. Josipovic also refers to this dimension, if in slightly different terms: "This background awareness appears in meditation to be unitary and unchanging—a cognizance that is in itself empty of content, yet clearly aware and blissful—whereas various sensory, affective, and cognitive contents, and the various states of arousal appear to it as dynamic processes or, as a well-known metaphor states, like images in a mirror."[139] Josipovic's perspective and the one proposed here, however, seem to diverge on the role of embodied experience in mediating access to consciousness as such. While Josipovic maintains that this nondual awareness manifests itself "without a sense of body,"[140] the hypothesis put forward here is that a nondual experience of embodiment is at the base of the recognition of consciousness as such. It was precisely the close examination of phenomenological thought that enabled the distinction of this nonreifiable bodily dimension from the ordinary experience of the body.

Through imaging and scanning techniques, like electroencephalography and functional magnetic resonance, research into the wavelengths detected in neural patterns and brain activity in advanced meditators engaged in different kinds of meditation is underway.[141] The number and scale of such studies should expand in the years to come. Next to different forms of traditional sitting meditations, postural yogic practices (entailing an active phase and a following receptive one) should be carefully examined, precisely because they are so deeply embedded in the perceptual field.

A number of articles discuss recent efforts to test the specific effects of yoga practice.[142] However there is an intrinsic vagueness[143] about yoga itself upstream that runs the risk of undermining the entire attempt. In order to work experimentally on yoga and design an effective model to test the conscious dimensions opened through it, along with its effects on health, it is not sufficient to define it as a science of holistic living or a discipline that is used "for promoting overall growth and harmony."[144] Those definitions only trigger more questions: "What is holistic living?" "What kind of growth is promoted?" By contrast, as has been shown to this point, it is fundamental to be clear about the specific dimensions that yoga deals with and the phases it entails. From that viewpoint, a phenomenological understanding of the core dynamic at play in yoga can also be useful for future experimental work. Unpacking what in yogic milieus is usually presented as a block could eventually also persuade the academic world to begin combining theoretical teachings on the yogic texts with practical classes of yoga as a curricular subject, not only for students of Eastern traditions, but also for students of psychology, neuroscience, and artificial intelligence. Theory is of course important, but it is never enough. It is particularly important that students and researchers working on consciousness and its dimensions become directly acquainted with yogic states in first person and possibly practice.[145]

Heidegger insists that phenomenology can be understood "just by seizing upon it as a possibility,"[146] and Husserl's student and trusted assistant Eugen Fink reinforces that message by claiming that "it is impossible to understand what phenomenology is without being oneself a phenomenologist."[147] Similarly, yoga, according to Vyāsa, can only be known by practicing it and by engaging with it, as he reminds us in his commentary on the *Yoga Sūtra*: "Yoga is to be known by yoga; Yoga goes forward from yoga alone."[148]

Notes

Introduction

1. See Francisco J. Varela, Evan Thompson, and Eleanor Rosch, *The Embodied Mind: Cognitive Science and Human Experience*, 14 (Cambridge, Mass.: MIT Press, 1993).

2. Jean-François Lyotard, *The Postmodern Condition: A Report on Knowledge*, Theory and History of Literature, v. 10 (Minneapolis: University of Minnesota Press, 1984).

3. See, for example, P. Deussen, who nonetheless played an important role in highlighting the value of Eastern thought. *The Philosophy of the Upanishads* (Edinburgh: T. & T. Clark, 1908), 8, 39: "The doctrine, namely, of the sole reality of the Atman, of its evolution as the universe, its identity with the soul, and so forth"; "This identity of the Brahman and the atman, of God and the soul, is the fundamental thought of the entire doctrine of the Upanishads."

4. S. N. Dasgupta, *Philosophical Essays* (Calcutta: University of Calcutta, 1941), 119. "The result is that with most of the old type of Sanskrit scholars, there is a strong tendency not to rejuvenate what appears to be dead but to mummify what is living and pulsating with thought. For the Sanskritist generally starts with the postulate that he is before a dead culture: he has around him nothing but the dead bones: and if anything appear to be living, it must be made to die by the axe of his interpretation, before he can feel himself at ease to work on it."

5. See for example the Dattātreyayogaśāstra: "Whether a Brahmin, an ascetic, a Buddhist, a Jain, a Skull-Bearer or a materialist, the wise man who is endowed with faith and constantly devoted to the practice of [haṭha] yoga will attain complete success." Dattātreyayogaśāstra, 41–42 in James Mallinson, "Haṭhayoga's Philosophy: A Fortuitous Union of Non-Dualities," *Journal of Indian Philosophy* 42, no. 1 (2014): 233.

Chapter 1

1. Cognitive functions are, for example, selective attention, working memory, language, sequential thought, decision making, action guidance, motivation.

2. William James, *The Varieties of Religious Experience: A Study in Human Nature,* Routledge Classics (London and New York: Routledge, 2008), 300. However, in his *Principles of Psychology* James "uses the word thinking [. . .] for every form of consciousness;" William James, *The Principles of Psychology, Vol. I,* The Principles of Psychology, Vol. I (New York: Henry Holt and Co., 1890), 224, https://doi.org/10.1037/10538-000. James identifies consciousness with the "function of knowing" also in his pioneering article of 1904 on consciousness: William James, "Does' Consciousness' Exist?," *The Journal of Philosophy, Psychology and Scientific Methods* 1, no. 18 (1904): 477.

3. According to Zoran Josipovic, consciousness as such is nonrepresentational: "This paper advances a view that the main property of consciousness-as-such, or non-dual awareness is its non-representational non-conceptual reflexivity, knowing itself to be conscious or aware, directly, without relying on conceptual and symbolic representations" (Z. Josipovic, "Nondual Awareness: Consciousness-as-such as Non-Representational Reflexivity," ed. Narayanan Srinivasa, *Progress in Brain Research* 244, ch. 12, Elsevier, 2019, 291.

4. David J. Chalmers, "Facing up to the Problem of Consciousness," *Journal of Consciousness Studies* 2, no. 3 (1995): 212.

5. See Bernard J. Baars, *A Cognitive Theory of Consciousness,* reprint ed. (Cambridge: Cambridge University Press, 1995). According to Chalmers, Baars's theory "is a theory of cognitive accessibility, explaining how it is that certain information contents are widely accessible within a system, as well as a theory of informational integration and reportability" Chalmers, "Facing up to the Problem of Consciousness," 205.

6. Ned Block summarizes the central aspect of the Global Workspace Theory as follows: "Perceptual systems supply representations that are consumed by mechanisms of reporting, reasoning, evaluating, deciding, and remembering, which themselves produce representations that are further consumed by the same set of mechanisms"; Ned Block, "Comparing the Major Theories of Consciousness," in *The Cognitive Neurosciences IV,* ed. Michael Gazzaniga, 2009, 1111, https://philpapers.org/rec/GAZTCN-3. According to Block, the question of why a globally broadcast representation would be conscious remains open within such a theory: "The most neuroscience can do for us according to the global workspace account is explain how a representation can be broadcast in the global workspace, but the task will still remain of explaining why global broadcasting,

however realized, is conscious. In principle, global broadcasting could be realized in an electronic system rather than a biological system, and of course the same issue will arise." See Block, 1114.

7. Bernard J. Baars, "A Scientific Approach to Silent Consciousness," *Frontiers in Psychology* 4 (2013): 3, https://doi.org/10.3389/fpsyg.2013.00678.

8. See Stanislas Dehaene, Jean-Pierre Changeux, and Lionel Naccache, "The Global Neuronal Workspace Model of Conscious Access: From Neuronal Architectures to Clinical Applications," ed. Stanislas Dehaene and Yves Christen, *Characterizing Consciousness: From Cognition to the Clinic?* (Berlin and Heidelberg: Springer Berlin Heidelberg, 2011), 55–85. Stanislas Dehaene, Hakwan Lau, and Sid Kouider, "What Is Consciousness, and Could Machines Have It?," *Science* (New York, NY) 358, no. 6362 (October 27, 2017): 486–92, https://doi.org/10.1126/science.aan8871.

9. See, for example, David M. Rosenthal, "Metacognition and Higher-Order Thoughts," *Consciousness and Cognition* 9, no. 2 (2000): 231–42, https://doi.org/10.1006/ccog.2000.0441.

10. Block, "Comparing the Major Theories of Consciousness," 114.

11. See Daniel C. Dennett, *Consciousness Explained* (Little, Brown, 2017). On the topic Chalmers states: "Dennett's use of 'heterophenomenology' (verbal reports) as the primary data to ground his theory of consciousness appears to rest on the assumption that these reports are what need explaining, or that the only 'seemings' that need explaining are dispositions to react and report" D. J. Chalmers, "Consciousness and its Place in Nature," in *Blackwell Guide to Philosophy of Mind*, ed. S. Stich and T. Warfield (Malden, MA: Blackwell, 2003) 12.

12. Michael A. Cohen and Daniel C. Dennett, "Consciousness Cannot Be Separated from Function," *Trends in Cognitive Sciences* 15, no. 8 (August 2011): 361, https://doi.org/10.1016/j.tics.2011.06.008.

13. Thomas Metzinger, "Minimal Phenomenal Experience: Meditation, Tonic Alertness, and the Phenomenology of 'Pure' Consciousness," *Philosophy and the Mind Sciences* 1, no. 1 (2020): 7.

14. Metzinger, "Minimal," 25.

15. Metzinger, "Minimal," 33.

16. These constraints are: "Wakefulness, Low Complexity, Self-Luminosity, Introspective Availability, Epistemicity, Transparency/Opacity" Metzinger, "Minimal," 7.

17. Metzinger, "Minimal," 9.

18. Metzinger, "Minimal," 36.

19. Thomas Nagel, "What Is It Like to Be a Bat?," *The Philosophical Review* 83, no. 4 (1974): 435–50, https://doi.org/10.2307/2183914.

20. Joseph Levine, "Materialism and Qualia: The Explanatory Gap," *Pacific Philosophical Quarterly* 64, no. 4 (1983): 354–61, https://doi.org/10.1111/j.1468-0114.1983.tb00207.x.

21. Chalmers, "Facing up to the Problem of Consciousness," 202.

22. Chalmers, "Facing," 203.

23. Chalmers, "Facing," 212. It is worth noting that Chalmers departs from other scholars by distinguishing the term "awareness" as the functional phenomenon associated with consciousness and "consciousness" as the experience at stake.

24. Ned Block, "On a Confusion about a Function of Consciousness," *Behavioral and Brain Sciences* 18, no. 2 (June 1995): 230, https://doi.org/10.1017/S0140525X00038188.

25. Block, "On a Confusion," 230.

26. Block, "On a Confusion," 230.

27. Block, "On a Confusion," 230.

28. John R. Searle, "Who Is Computing with the Brain?," *Behavioral and Brain Sciences* 13, no. 4 (December 1990): 632–34, https://doi.org/10.1017/S0140525X00080663.

29. Giulio Tononi, "Consciousness as Integrated Information: A Provisional Manifesto," *The Biological Bulletin* 215, no. 3 (December 2008): 216–42, https://doi.org/10.2307/25470707.

30. *Māṇḍūkya Upaniṣad* I.5, in *Upaniṣad*, ed. Raphael (Milan: Bompiani, 2010), Sanskrit-Italian parallel text, 1023. Quotations from the *Upaniṣad* below are taken from this text, with English translations by the author. Further references to the *Upaniṣad* will include only the title of the individual *Upaniṣad* and the number of the passage.

31. On this point Evan Thompson argues that "although dreamless sleep and anesthesia are not the same condition, the general point that retrospective oblivion does not prove a prior lack of consciousness must be kept in mind whenever we are tempted to infer that consciousness is absent in deep sleep because people report not being able to remember anything when they are woken up," Thompson, "Dreamless Sleep, the Embodied Mind, and Consciousness—The Relevance of a Classical Indian Debate to Cognitive Science," in *Open Mind*: 37(T), ed. T. Metzinger and J. M. Windt (Frankfurt am Main, 2015), 11. On deep sleep Georges Dreyfus notes: "Even deep sleep, often cited as the paradigm of a non-conscious state, has a certain phenomenological feel to it. It is part of the constantly changing flow of experiences that we undergo, and is retained as such. When we wake up from deep sleep, we do not feel that there was nothing before, but, rather, we feel that we are emerging from a particular mode of experience." See Georges Dreyfus, "Self and Subjectivity: A Middle Way Approach," in *Self, No Self? Perspectives From Analytical, Phenomenological, and Indian Traditions*, ed. Mark Siderits, Evan Thompson, and Dan Zahavi (Oxford: Oxford University Press, 2010), 147.

32. See Giulio Tononi, "Consciousness," 216–42. See also Marcello Massimini et al., "Breakdown of Cortical Effective Connectivity During Sleep," *Science* 309, no. 5744 (September 30, 2005): 2228–32, https://doi.org/10.1126/science.1117256. Giulio Tononi and Gerald M. Edelman, "Consciousness and Complexity," *Science* 282, no. 5395 (December 4, 1998): 1846–51, https://doi.org/10.1126/science.282.5395.1846.

33. Maciej Kamiński, Katarzyna Blinowska, and Waldemar Szelenberger, "Topographic Analysis of Coherence and Propagation of EEG Activity during Sleep and Wakefulness," *Electroencephalography and Clinical Neurophysiology* 102, no. 3 (March 1, 1997): 216–27, https://doi.org/10.1016/S0013-4694(96)95721-5.

34. Andrea Piarulli et al., "Ultra-Slow Mechanical Stimulation of Olfactory Epithelium Modulates Consciousness by Slowing Cerebral Rhythms in Humans," *Scientific Reports* 8, no. 1 (April 26, 2018): 6581, https://doi.org/10.1038/s41598-018-24924-9.

35. Sebastian Seung, *Connectome: How the Brain's Wiring Makes Us Who We Are* (Boston: Houghton Mifflin Harcourt, 2012).

36. *Bṛhadāraṇyaka Upaniṣad*, III. 2. 2, Raphael, *Upaniṣad*, 115. An interesting exploration of the connection between the dendrites of the olfactory bulb and the brain cortex and the effects of yogic breathing was carried out by yoga teacher André Van Lysebeth in *Pranayama: La dynamique du soufflé* (Paris, Flammarion, 1971), chapter 8.

37. Jacob Needleman used the term "inner empiricism" (Jacob Needleman, "Inner Empiricism as a Way to a Science of Consciousness," *Jacob Needleman Noetic Sciences Review*, Summer 1993).

38. "Yoga is the stilling of the changing states of the mind" Patañjali, I. 2, *The Yoga Sutras of Patañjali*, ed. E. F. Bryant (New York: North Point Press, 2009, 10). References to this edition of the *Yogasūtra* are made below without further detail. At the same time, a close examination will also be made of the Squarcini edition: Patañjali, *Yogasūtra*, ed. Federico Squarcini (Turin, Einaudi, 2019). Other classical editions of the *Yogasūtra* will be taken into account as appropriate.

39. It would be interesting to study in detail "off-periods" or "down-states," the electrical silences in the brain of 500 milliseconds found in non-REM sleep, and to situate them in relation to specific moments of yogic and meditative states of consciousness; see Thilo Hinterberger et al., "Decreased Electrophysiological Activity Represents the Conscious State of Emptiness in Meditation," *Frontiers in Psychology* 5 (2014), https://doi.org/10.3389/fpsyg.2014.00099.

40. The materialist view can be roughly sketched in the following terms: since brain stimulation is able to trigger an experience, consciousness

must be determined by the underlying neuronal level. However, this conclusion is too hasty; indeed, one could claim the opposite view by showing that training on the level of the mind, for example through yogic techniques, is able to trigger brain alterations. So, if there is reversibility and mutual influence, why are neural processes to be placed at the base? In other words, why should one not consider instead the anatomical changes to be reducible and determined by the mental level? Neural plasticity is confirmed in many articles: Sara W. Lazar et al., "Meditation Experience Is Associated with Increased Cortical Thickness," *Neuroreport* 16, no. 17 (November 28, 2005): 1893–97; Britta Holzel et al., "How Does Mindfulness Meditation Work? Proposing Mechanisms of Action from a Conceptual and Neural Perspective," *Perspectives on Psychological Science* 6 (November 1, 2011): 537–59, https://doi.org/10.1177/1745691611419671; Kieran Fox et al., "Is Meditation Associated with Altered Brain Structure? A Systematic Review and Meta-Analysis of Morphometric Neuroimaging in Meditation Practitioners," *Neuroscience & Biobehavioral Reviews* 43 (June 1, 2014), https://doi.org/10.1016/j.neubiorev.2014.03.016; Britta K. Hölzel et al., "Stress Reduction Correlates with Structural Changes in the Amygdala," *Social Cognitive and Affective Neuroscience* 5, no. 1 (March 2010): 11–17, https://doi.org/10.1093/scan/nsp034; Cyril R. Pernet et al., "Mindfulness Related Changes in Grey Matter: A Systematic Review and Meta-Analysis," *Brain Imaging and Behavior* 15, no. 5 (October 2021): 2720–30, https://doi.org/10.1007/s11682-021-00453-4; Michel Bitbol claims that "conscious experiences correlate with brain events, but the brain *qua object* is constituted out of a carefully selected set of conscious experiences"; see Bitbol, "The Tangled Dialectic of Body and Consciousness: A Metaphysical Counterpart of Radical Neurophenomenology," *Constructivist Foundations* 16, no. 2 (2021): 141–51.

41. In "Consciousness and its Place in Nature," Chalmers distinguishes between different types of non-reductionist views such as interactionism, epiphenomenalism, and panpsychism.

42. Evan Thompson, *Waking, Dreaming, Being: New Light on the Self and Consciousness from Neuroscience, Meditation, and Philosophy* (New York: Columbia University Press, 2015, 62–65).

43. Thompson, *Waking,* 105.

44. Ramakant Sinari argues that the "Husserlian path of bracketing would realize [the most advanced stages of absorption] only if it were stretched to a point at which some kind of pre-reflective, pre-conscious, inane stuff is 'touched'" Ramakant Sinari, "The Method of Phenomenological Reduction and Yoga," *Philosophy East and West,* 15, no. 3–4 (1965): 226. Also Pulighanda is of the opinion that since "for Husserl

phenomenological reductions, including the transcendental reduction, are logico-epistemological devices for establishing philosophy as a rigorous and presuppositionless science, He could never bring himself to abandon this goal in order to carry phenomenological reduction to a point where, with the collapse of the noesis and noema into a unity, the doctrine of the intentionality of consciousness itself breaks down" Ramakrishna Puligandla, "Phenomenological Reduction and Yoga Meditation," *Philosophy East and West* 20, no. 1 (1970): 30.

45. Consider for instance Jitendra Nat Mohanty's work. Note that Mohanty does not specifically concentrate his analysis on yoga but is more interested in bridging his interpretation of Vedanta toward Husserlian phenomenology: Jitendra Nat Mohanty, *Phenomenology and Indian Philosophy: The Concept of Rationality,* in *Phenomenology and Indian Philosophy,* edited by D. P. Chattopadhyaya, L. Embree, J. N. Mohanty (Albany: State University of New York Press, 1992, 8–19); and Jitendra Nat Mohanty, *Reason and Tradition in Indian Thought: An Essay on the Nature of Indian Philosophical Thinking* (Oxford, 1992). Also Jarava Lal Mehta's work can be included in a comparative framework, though interest in this case is centered more on hermeneutical issues.

46. Edmund Husserl, *The Crisis of European Sciences and Transcendental Phenomenology* (Evanston: Northwestern University Press, 1970).

47. I make an exception for certain Buddhist studies that have recently been taken into account thanks to Francisco Varela's groundbreaking work, although always in very restricted circles of discussion. See, for instance, Mark Siderits, Evan Thompson, and Dan Zahavi, *Self, No-Self? Perspectives from Analytical, Phenomenological and Indian Traditions* (New York: Oxford University Press, 2011).

48. "Everything in them [the Indians] is a fantasy and slavery. The annihilation [*Vernichtung*], the dumping [*Wegwerfung*] of any reason, morality and subjectivity, can reach a positive feeling and awareness only with a releasement into wild imagination. Unruled spirit, the Indian finds no peace and cannot grasp himself, but only in this way finds pleasure. Similar to a man completely ruined in his body and mind, he finds his existence dumped and painless and he creates, through opium, a world of dream and a joy of folly"; see Georg Wilhelm Friedrich Hegel, *Vorlesungen über der Philosophie del Geschichte*, Shurkamp-Taschenbuch Wissenschaft, nr 612, band 12, Frankfurt am Main, 207 (Engl. trans. by the author). In the essay on the Gita, Hegel's view is, however, more nuanced with regard to Indian thought. See Georg Wilhelm Friedrich Hegel, *Über die unter dem Namen Bhagavad-Gita bekannte Episode des Mahabharata von Wilhelm con Humboldt,* Akademie der Wissenshaften, Berlin, 1826 (Berliner Schriften, Humboldt-Rezension).

49. Wilhelm Halbfass, *India and Europe: An Essay in Understanding* (Albany: State University of New York Press, 1988); "The Exclusion of India from the History of Philosophy" is the title of the ninth chapter.

50. Historian Giuseppe Tucci speaks of a "pure consciousness, not obfuscated by any concrete thought, nonetheless the assumption of those concrete thoughts that make up the psychic reality of the human being," in Giuseppe Tucci, *Teoria e pratica del mandala* (Roma: Astrolabio, 1949, 12). English translation by the author.

51. "Gleichwohl ist das Sein seiender als jegliches Seiende. Weil das Nichten im Sein selbst west, deshalb können wir es nie als etwas Seiendes am Seienden gewahren"; see Martin Heidegger, *Über den Humanismus* (V. Klostermann Frankfurt am Main, 2000, Band 9 der Gesamtausgabe, 51).

52. *Bṛhadāraṇyaka Upaniṣad*, III, 7, 23, Raphael, *Upaniṣad*, 137. See also III, 4, 2, 123: "You cannot see the seer of seeing; you cannot hear the hearer of hearing; you cannot think of the thinker of thinking; you cannot know the knower of knowing."

53. Michel Bitbol, "Consciousness, Being and Life: Phenomenological Approaches to Mindfulness," *Journal of Phenomenological Psychology* 50, no. 2 (November 26, 2019): 139, https://doi.org/10.1163/15691624-12341360.

54. Jan Patočka, "Epoché and Reduktion—einige Bemerkungen" in *Bewusstsein. Gerhard Funke zu eigen*, ed. Bucher, Drüe and Seebohm (Bonn: Bouvier, 1975), 76–85). Translated from German by Matt Bower, Ivan Chvatík and Kenneth Maly, 48.

55. Maurice Merleau-Ponty, *The Visible and the Invisible*, trans. I. Lingis (Evanston: Northwestern University Press, 1968), 135. Here the original French has "making myself world" [*en me faisant monde*] and not "a world," as given in the English translation. See Maurice Merleau-Ponty, *Le visible et l'invisible*, ed. Claude Lefort (Paris: Gallimard, 1964), 176.

56. Maurice Merleau-Ponty, *Phenomenology of Perception*, trans. C. Smith (New York: Routledge, 1962) 493.

57. Lawrence Shapiro, *Embodied Cognition* (London: Routledge, 2010).

58. Andy Clark and David Chalmers, "The Extended Mind," *Analysis* 58, no. 1 (1998): 7–19.

59. "The fires of *prāṇa* alone awake in this city [of the body]," *Praśna Upaniṣad* IV. 3; Raphael, *Upaniṣad*, 935. English translation by the author.

60. An important exception are the forerunning articles on the topic by James Morley. See James Morley, "Inspiration and Expiration: Yoga Practice Through Merleau-Ponty's Phenomenology of the Body," *Philosophy East and West* 51, no. 1 (2001); and James Morley, "Embodied Consciousness in Tantric Yoga and the Phenomenology of Merleau-Ponty," *Religion and Arts* 12 (2008).

Chapter 2

1. Edmund Husserl, *Erste Philosophie. Zweiter Teil (1923–24)*, Husserliana VIII (Dordrecht: Kluwer Academic Publishers, 1996) 165.

2. Husserl, *The Crisis*, § 35, 137. Original text: Edmund Husserl, *Die Krisis der Europäischen Wissenschaften und die Transzendentale Phänomenologie*, Husserliana VI, ed. W. Biemel (The Hague: Martinus Nijhoff, 1954).

3. Husserl, *The Crisis*, § 35, 137.

4. Husserl, *The Crisis*, § 40, 151.

5. Phenomenology, which was founded by Edmund Husserl (1859–1938), remains a key trend in contemporary philosophy. Husserl's conversion to Lutheranism in 1886 appears not to have entailed major implications for his philosophical enquiry, as it occurred long before Husserl's engagement with the *Logical Investigations* (1901) and twenty-one years before the *Idea of Phenomenology* (1907) was published.

6. Edmund Husserl, "Über die Reden Gotamo Buddhos" (1925) in K. Schuhmann, "Husserl and Indian Thought," ed. C. Leijenhorst and P. Steenbakkers, *Selected Papers on Phenomenology* (Dordrecht: Kluwer Academic Publishers, 2004), 144. Fred Hanna emphasizes parallels between Buddhism and Husserl's transcendental phenomenology. See F. J. Hanna, "On the Teachings of the Buddha," *The Humanistic Psychologist*, September 1995, 365–72; F. J. Hanna, B. D. Wilkinson and J. Givens, "Recovering the Original Phenomenological Research Method: An Exploration of Husserl, Yoga, Buddhism and New Frontiers in Humanistic Counseling," *Journal of Humanistic Counseling* 56 (July): 144–62.

7. Husserl, *The Crisis*, § 6, 16; *Die Krisis*, 14.

8. Husserl, *The Crisis*, 275; *Die Krisis*, 320.

9. Schuhmann, "Husserl and Indian Thought," 160.

10. O. Stone, D. Zahavi, "Phenomenology and Mindfulness," *Journal of Consciousness Studies* 28, nos. 3–4 (2021): 158–85, *10.

11. Husserl, *Erste Philosophie*, 165.

12. Husserl, *The Crisis*, § 38, 146.

13. "The Phenomenological Judgment-Exclusions," E. Husserl, *Ideas Pertaining to a Pure Phenomenology and to a Phenomenological Philosophy*, First Book, trans. F. Kersten (The Hague: Martinus Nijhoff, 1983) § 33, [59], 65.

14. Phenomenologist Carmine Di Martino speaks about "questioning the obviousness of the world, seeing the givenness of the world as on day one, giving an account of its sense of being, without building it or deducing it" C. Di Martino, "Esperienza e intenzionalità nella fenomenologia di Husserl," *Memorandum* 13, no. 32 (2007): 51 (Eng. trans. by the author).

15. Husserl, *Erste Philosophie*, 166.

16. Husserl, *Ideas*, § 32, [56], 60.

17. Husserl, *Erste Philosophie*, § 33, 45.

18. Husserl, *Ideas I*, § 3, [10], 9.

19. Husserl, *Erste Philosophie*, § 33, 47.

20. See also Husserl, *The Crisis*, 158: "alteration of perspective [. . .] In the course of alteration they all [perspectives] play their role."

21. Husserl, *Erste Philosophie*, 51. Husserl points out that the course of ordinary perception [*Wahrnehmungsverlauf*] takes place only when prior-expectations [*Vorerwartungen*] are not disappointed [*enttäuschen*]. See Husserl, *Erste Philosophie*, 49.

22. Husserl, *Erste Philosophie*, 52.

23. Husserl, *Erste Philosophie*, 188.

24. Husserl, *Erste Philosophie*, 87.

25. Husserl, *Erste Philosophie*, 54.

26. Husserl, *Erste Philosophie*, 55.

27. Edmund Husserl, *The Idea of Phenomenology*, trans. W. P. Alston & J Nakhkikian (The Hague: Martinus Nijhoff, 1973, [44]) 34.

28. Max Wertheimer (1880–1943) was the founder of Gestalt psychology, together with his former students Kurt Koffka and Wolfgang Köhler.

29. According to the gestalt laws of perception in perception there is a tendency of animals and humans—called the "constancy phenomenon"—to see familiar objects as having standard shape, size, color, regardless of changes in the angle of perspective, distance, or lighting of the object itself; see William Woodward, *Gestalt Psychology*, in Vol. 7 of *Encyclopedia of Philosophy and the Social Sciences* (Sage, 2013), 383–87.

30. Husserl, *Erste Philosophie*, 186. This perception is, according to Husserl, the "most immediate form of experience [*unmittelbarste Erfahrungsform*]" Husserl, *Erste Philosophie*, 175.

31. Giovanni Piana, *Elementi di una dottrina dell'esperienza* (Milan: Cuem-Libreria Universitaria, 2003), 27. English translation by the author.

32. Husserl, *Ideas I*, 24, [44], 44—"dass jede originär gebende Anschauung eine Rechtsquelle der Erkenntnis sei, dass Alles, was sich uns in der "Intuition" originär, (sozusagen in seiner leibhaften Wirklichkeit) darbietet, einfach hinzunehmen sei, als was es sich gibt, aber auch nur in den Scharanken, in denen es sich da gibt" E. Husserl, *Ideen zu einer reinen Phenomenologie und phenomenologishen Philosophie*, Erstes Buch, Hrsg. von W. Biemel (The Hague: Martinus Nijhoff, 1950) § 24, [44], 52. The Italian translation of this passage better reflects Husserl's position that an originary vision is a deeply embodied one: "That every originary vision [*Anschauung*], offering itself, is a legitimizing source of *knowledge*, that everything that is given to us originarily (so to speak in its *living 'flesh and blood'* reality) in 'intuition' is to be accepted simply in the way

it gives itself out, but also only within the limits in which it gives itself out to be there" (English translation by the author, drawing from the Italian one): Edmund Husserl, *Idee per una fenomenologia pura e per una filosofia fenomenologica*, ed. Vincenzo Costa (Turin: Einaudi, 2002) 52–53.

33. Husserl makes an example of a simple perception of a house, Husserl, *Erste Philosophie*, 88.

34. Expression used by Michel Bitbol in "The Tangled Dialectic of Body and Consciousness: A Metaphysical Counterpart of Radical Neurophenomenology," *Constructivist Foundations* 16, no. 2 (2021): 141–51.*15.

35. Husserl, *Erste Philosophie*, 96.

36. Husserl, *Erste Philosophie*, 97.

37. "Because, now, the locutions, moments of consciousness, awarenesses, and similar constructions, and likewise because the locution, intentive moments, are made quite unusable by the many different equivocations which will be distinctly brought out in what follows, we introduce the term noetic moment or, in short, noesis" Husserl, *Ideas*, § 84, [174], 205. "Perception, for example, has its noema, most basically its perceptual sense, i.e., the perceived as perceived" Husserl, *Ideas*, § 88, [182], 214.

38. S. Gallagher, D. Zahavi, *The Phenomenological Mind* (New York: Routledge, 2008).

39. "Thus the particular object of our active consciousness and correlatively the active, conscious having of it, being directed toward it and dealing with it—all this is forever surrounded by an atmosphere of mute, concealed, but co-functioning validities, a vital horizon into which the active ego can also direct itself voluntarily, reactivating old acquisitions, consciously grasping new apperceptive ideas, transforming them into intuitions" Husserl, *The Crisis*, § 40, 149.

40. Jan Patočka, "Naturliche Welt und Phänomenologie. Phänomenologische Schriften II," in *Ausgewählte Schriftten* (Stuttgart: Klett-Cotta, 1991) 202.

41. See Jan Patočka, *Le monde naturel come problème philosophique* (The Hague: M. Nijhoff, 1976), 94.

42. A reference to J. Patočka will be made later when referring to an "a-subjective phenomenology."

43. Eugen Fink, *Sixth Cartesian Meditation*, trans. R. Bruzina (Indianapolis: Indiana University Press, 1995) [118–119], 108.

44. Husserl, *Erste Philosophie*, 98.

45. Husserl, *Erste Philosophie*, 108.

46. Sextus Empiricus defines the ancient Greek skeptical epoché introduced by Pyrrho of Elis (365–275 BCE), who did not leave written records, as follows: " 'Suspension of judgment' is a standstill of the intellect, owing to which we neither reject nor posit anything. Tranquillity [*Ataraxia*]

is freedom from disturbances or calmness of soul. We shall suggest in the chapter on the aim of scepticism how tranquility accompanies suspension of judgment" Sextus Empiricus, *Outlines of Pyrrhonism*, ed. J Annas and J. Barnes (Cambridge: Cambridge University Press, 2000), 5. Some fragments on Pyrrho's thought come from his disciple Timon of Phlius. Furthermore, Pyrrho's trip to the East in the entourage of Alexander the Great (327–26) and his encounter with the gymnosophists (naked sages) are reported by several authors, with major accounts in Diogenes Laërtius (180–240 CE), Sextus Empiricus (160–210 CE) and Plutarch. Diogenes Laërtius in the *Lives and Opinions of Eminent Philosophers* reports the following: "Pyrrho of Elis [. . .] was first a painter. He studied [. . .] with Anaxarchus, whom he accompanied everywhere, so that he even associated with the Naked Sages in India [Gymnosophists] and with the Magi. As a result, he seems to have adopted a profoundly noble philosophy, having introduced the notion of 'inability to attain conviction' [*akatalepsia*] and that of 'suspension of judgment' [*epoché*], as Ascanius of Abdera reports. For he said that nothing is beautiful or ugly, or just or unjust, and that likewise in all instances nothing exists in truth, but men do everything by custom and by habit; for each thing is no more this than that" Diogenes Laërtius, *Lives and Opinions of Eminent Philosophers*, XI, 61, trans. P. Mensch, ed. J. Miller (Oxford: Oxford University Press, 2018, 466). Sextus Empiricus in his *Adversos Mathematicos* (I. 282) adds some important piece of information about Pyrrho, as summarized by Christopher Beckwith in his *Greek Buddha*: "The story relates that while in India, 'Pyrrho heard an Indian reproach [his teacher] Anaxarchus, telling him that he would never be able to teach others what is good while he himself danced attendance on kings in their courts. Since Pyrrho himself had written a poem in praise of Alexander, for which he had been rewarded with ten thousand gold pieces, he withdrew from the world and lived in solitude, rarely showing himself to his relatives." Cristopher Beckwith, *Greek Buddha: Pyrrho's Encounter with Early Buddhism in Central Asia* (Princeton, NJ: Princeton University Press, 2017, 48). Beckwith adds: "The mentioning of 'withdrawing from the world' and family reflects the stereotypical Buddhist expression 'to leave the family' which means in practice 'to become a Buddhist ascetic practitioner' (in Pyrrho's days a Śramaṇa; later, a bhikṣu 'monk')" Beckwith, *Greek Buddha*, 94.

47. Husserl, *The Crisis*, § 40, 150—*Die Krisis*, 153: "eine ganz andere Weise der universalen Epoche möglich, nämlich die mit einem Schlage den durch die Gesamtheit des natürlichen Weltlebens und durch das gesamte (ob verborgene oder offene) Geflecht der Geltungen hindurchreichenden Gesamtvollzug außer Aktion setzt, eben den, der als einheitliche 'natürliche Einstellung' das 'schlicht' 'geradehin' Dahinleben ausmacht. Durch

die Vollzugsenthaltung, die diese ganze bisher ungebrochen verlaufene Lebensweise inhibiert, wird eine völlige Umstellung des gesamten Lebens gewonnen, eine durchaus neue Weise des Lebens."

48. Husserl, *Erste Philosophie,* 109.

49. Husserl, *Ideas,* § 32, [56], 61.

50. Husserl, *Erste Philosophie,* 108: "allen thematischen Objekten der jeweiligen Akte das Interesse der Geltung versagt. Und selbstverständlich das besagt phänomenologische Ausschaltung."

51. Husserl, *Erste Philosophie,* 111.

52. Husserl, *Erste Philosophie,* 111: "Wir bringen am Objekt gleichsam eine ausschaltende Klammer an, einen Index, der sagt: Hier will ich jedes Mitgelten-lassen, jedes Seinsinteresse, Wertinteresse usw. inhibieren, ich will das Objekt nur als intentionales seines Aktes, des Aktes, der ihm Geltung zumißt, gelten lassen."

53. The "reduction" in this context is not to be intended as a limitation; it might be useful to recall the etymology of the Latin *re-dùcere,* meant as a "leading" [*ducere*] "a new" [*re*]. The reduction is thus a reorientation of the field of attention.

54. Husserl, *Erste Philosophie,* 49.

55. Husserl, *Erste Philosophie,* 160.

56. Husserl, *Erste Philosophie,* 111.

57. Husser, *Ideas,* § 50, [94], 113.

58. Husserl, *Erste Philosophie,* 166.

59. Husserl, *Erste Philosophie,* 111.

60. Husserl, *Erste Philosophie,* 114: "Ich bin nicht das träumende und an Erträumtes mich hingebende Ich; sondern ich bin der Betrachter von Träumen und Erträumtem, von Phantasieren und Phantasiertem als solchen."

61. Husserl, *Erste Philosophie,* 120.

62. Husserl, *Erste Philosophie,* 121.

63. Husserl, *Erste Philosophie,* 121.

64. Husserl, *Erste Philosophie,* 167. The capacity of surprising oneself is at the heart of Eastern practices, as we shall see.

65. Husserl, *Erste Philosophie,* 122.

66. Also the term "refrain from" [*unterlassen*] is used.

67. Husserl, *Erste Philosophie,* 127.

68. Husserl, *Erste Philosophie,* 162.

69. Husserl, *Erste Philosophie,* 128, 163.

70. Husserl, *Erste Philosophie,* 129.

71. Husserl, *Ideas,* § 33, 59–60: "designating 'pure' consciousness, about which we shall have so much to say, as transcendental consciousness and the operation by which it is reached the transcendental epoché. As a

method this operation will be divided into different steps of 'excluding,' 'parenthesizing'; and thus our method will assume the characteristic of a step-by-step reduction. For this reason we shall, on most occasions, speak of *phenomenological reductions* (but also, with reference to their collective unity, we shall speak of the *phenomenological reduction*)." However some authors, in the wake of certain remarks by Patočka, have envisaged a distinction in Husserl between the phase of the epoché and that of the reduction, which is not relevant for the present endeavor: "Dans notre tentative d'établir une distinction aussi nette que possible entre la réduction et l'épochè (plus nette, à vrai dire, que dans bien des textes husserliens" Michel Bitbol, *La conscience a-t-elle une origine? Des neurosciences à la pleine conscience : une nouvelle approche de l'esprit* (Paris: Flammarion, 2014), 148.

72. Husserl, *Ideas,* § 50, 113; *Ideen,* 94.

73. The dream argument or the evil demon argument. Husserl admits that his phenomenology is in debt to the "cartesian method of the transcendental reduction" [*Cartesianische Methode der transzendentalen Reduktion*] Husserl, *Erste Philosophie,* 80.

74. Husserl, *Erste Philosophie,* 72–73.

75. Husserl, *Erste Philosophie,* 73. "If we retain a pure Ego as a residuum after our phenomenological exclusion of the world and of the empirical subjectivity included in it [. . .], then there is presented in the case of that Ego a transcendency of a peculiar kind—one which is not constituted—a *transcendency within immanency*" Husserl, *Ideas,* [110], 133.

76. Husserl, *Erste Philosophie,* 74.

77. Husserl, *Erste Philosophie,* 127.

78. Husserl, *Cartesian Meditations. An Introduction to Phenomenology,* trans. D. Cairns (New York: Springer, 1960) § 11, 26.

79. Husserl, *Erste Philosophie,* 76.

80. Husserl, *Erste Philosophie,* 74. [objektiven Geltung außer Spiel setze]

81. Husserl, *Erste Philosophie,* 78.

82. Husserl, *Erste Philosophie,* 76.

83. Husserl, *Erste Philosophie,* 92, 97.

84. Husserl, *Erste Philosophie,* 97.

85. Husserl, *Erste Philosophie,* 77: "Aber wie erlöst sich nun mein transzendentales Ich von dieser Selbstverhüllung?"

86. Sometimes Husserl referring to this same dimension speaks about the "*ego cogito*" but adds that with this expression he doesn't "intend a thought in the specific sense of the term" Husserl, *Erste Philosophie,* 83.

87. Husserl, *Erste Philosophie,* 123.

88. Husserl, *Ideas,* § 51, 114; *Ideen,* 95.

89. Husserl, *Ideas,* § 33, [59], 65.

90. Husserl, *Ideas,* § 33, [59], 66.

91. A reference to Jan Patočka's "a-subjective phenomenology" will be done again in the following.

92. Husserl, *Cartesian Meditations,* § 11, [65], 26.

93. This "transcendence" [to be bracketed] is part of the intrinsic sense of anything worldly, despite the fact that anything worldly necessarily acquires all the sense determining it, along with its existential status, exclusively from my experiencing, my objectivating, thinking, valuing, or doing, at particular times—notably the status of an evidently valid being is one it can acquire only from my own evidences, my grounding acts" Husserl, *Cartesian Meditations,* § 11, 26.

94. Husserl, *Ideas,* § 33, [59], 66.

95. Husserl, *Erste Philosophie,* 145.

96. "Die Rede von der 'Wendung' der Aufmerksamkeit ist bezeichnend; sie drückt aus, daß, worauf sie sich wendet, schon im Bewußtseinsfeld als Hintergrundgegen ständlichkeit daseiend war, nur eben nicht bemerkt, d.i. nicht thematische Gegenständlichkeit eines Aktes. [. . .] dasselbe, worauf ich jetzt speziell hin achte, war vordem schon in meinem Wahrnehmungsfelde, es stand schon da, ich hatte es nur nicht beachtet" Husserl, *Erste Philosophie,* 145. (Engl. trans by the author.)

97. Husserl, *Erste Philosophie,* 163.

98. Rubin's vase (known as the figure–ground vase) is a famous set of ambiguous or bi-stable two-dimensional forms developed around 1915 by Danish psychologist Edgar Rubin.

99. The duck-rabbit illusion is an image proposed in 1892 by American psychologist Joseph Jastrow to show a kind of optical illusion. On Gestalt images Maurice Merleau-Ponty remarks: "If we set ourselves to see as things the intervals between them, the appearance of the world would be just as strikingly altered" Merleau-Ponty, *Phenomenology of perception,* 18.

100. An anonymous German postcard from 1888 (right figure) depicts the image in its earliest known form.

101. Edmund Husserl, *Ideas Pertaining a Pure Phenomenology and a Phenomenological Philosophy,* Second Book, trans. R. Rojcewicz and A. Schuwer (Dordrecht: Kluwer Academic Publishers, 1989) § 5, [12], 13.

102. Husserl, *Cartesian Meditations,* § 38, 78. On the subject Didier Franck speaks of "passive pre-donation," D. Franck, *Chair e corps. Sur la phénomenologie de Husserl* (Paris: Les éditions de minuit, 1981), 75.

103. Edmund Husserl, *Analysen zur passiven Synthesis: Aus Vorlesungs- und Forschungsmanuskripten 1918–1926,* Husserliana XI (The Hague: Nijhoff, 1966). As Bruce Bégout and Natalie Depraz note in their introduction to the French version of the analysis concerning passive synthesis, Husserl

outlines a genesis of the transcendental through an exploration of the "sensory and ante-predicative." E. Husserl, *De la synthèse passive. Logique transcendantale et constitutions originaires*, ed. B. Bégout and J. Kessler (Grenoble: Jérôme Million, 1998) 10–12.

104. Husserl, *Erste Philosophie*, 145.

105. "das Klare immerfort seinen Leerhorizont der Unklarheit und Undeutlichkeit mit sich führt" Husserl, *Erste Philosophie*, 163.

106. "jedes so Wahrgenommene hat sozusagen in sich selbst seinen Hintergrund, jedes ist nur gegeben als sich darstellend durch eine sichtige Vorderseite mit unsichtigem Inneren und unsichtiger Rückseite" Husserl, *Erste Philosophie*, 146. Engl. Trans. by the author.

107. "haben wir [. . .] nie ein Wahrgenommenes ohne Horizontbewußtsein, wie immer wir auch das Wahrgenommene fassen und beschränken" Husserl, *Erste Philosophie*, 146. Engl. Trans. by the author.

108. Husserl, *Erste Philosophie*, 146.

109. Husserl, *Erste Philosophie*, 148.

110. Husserl, *Erste Philosophie*, 148.

111. Husserl, *Erste Philosophie*, 149.

112. Husserl, *Erste Philosophie*, 154.

113. Husserl, *Erste Philosophie*, 153, "Alleinheit eines endlosen Lebenszusammenhanges."

114. Husserl, *Erste Philosophie*, 159.

115. Husserl, *The idea of Phenomenology*, [62] 50; *L'idea della fenomenologia*, [62], 120.

116. Husserl, *Erste Philosophie*, 161.

117. On the dimensions of the passive synthesis and of the background-consciousness as opening fields to the transcendental, see L. Martelli, "Genesi passiva e hyle: la fondazione della coscienza trascendentale," *Philosophy Kitchen. Rivista di filosofia contemporanea*, 7, 2020, 115–31; S. Gonnella, "La sintesi passiva e le radici iletiche della sensibilità," *Philosophy Kitchen. Rivista di filosofia contemporanea*, 7, marzo 2020, 103–114. See also the already mentioned "Introduction" to the French version of Husserl's analysis concerning passive synthesis by Bruce Bégout and Natalie Depraz: Husserl, *De la synthèse passive.*

Chapter 3

1. Reiner Schürmann, "Heidegger and Meister Eckhart on Releasement," in *Research in Phenomenology* (Brill, 1973), 3:95–119.

2. Husserl, *Erste Philosophie*, 87.

3. Edmund Husserl, *Logical investigations*, J. N. Findlay (New York: Routledge, 2001), 168.

4. Husserl, *Erste Philosophie*, 109. Phenomenology is interested in the structure of evidence in its being a subjective act.

5. Husserl, *Erste Philosophie*, 110.

6. Husserl, *The Crisis*, 303.

7. Heidegger himself in 1925 in the book *History of the Concept of Time* claims pure consciousness to be an independent region of being and finally comes to state: "Consciousness is pure Being." Martin Heidegger, *History of the Concept of Time (Prolegomena)*, trans. T. Kisiel (Bloomington: Indiana University Press), 106.

8. Giulia Moiraghi, *In cammino verso la cosa. Heidegger dall'estetica all'ontologia* [*On the way to the thing. Heidegger from aesthetics to ontology*] (Milan: Mimesis, 2006).

9. Martin Heidegger, *Über den Humanismus* (Frankfurt am Main: V. Klostermann, 2000, Band 9 der Gesamtausgabe) 14. "[Die metaphysik] denkt nicht das Sein als soches, denkt nicht den Unterschied beider."

10. Husserl, *Erste Philosophie*, 78.

11. A decade later Husserl makes clear that: "Zunächst ist die Rede von phänomenologischem 'Residuum' besser zu meiden, wie auch die von der 'Ausschaltung der Welt.' Sie verführt leicht dazu, zu meinen, daß die Welt nunmehr aus dem phänomenologischen Thema herausfällt und stattdessen nur die 'subjektiven' Erscheinungsweisen etc., die sich auf die Welt beziehen, Thema wären" Husserl, *Erste Philosophie*, 432. English translation by the author: "It is better to avoid the term phenomenological 'Residuum,' as well as the one of 'switching off of the world.' These expressions induce a belief that the world would fall out of the phenomenological theme; instead, only subjective modes of appearance referring to the world [would be phenomenological themes]."

12. Husserl, *Erste Philosophie*, 81.

13. Husserl, *Erste Philosophie*, 83.

14. "The oblivion of Being makes itself known indirectly through the fact that the human being always observes and handles only beings" M. Heidegger, *Letter on Humanismus*, trans. F. A. Capuzzi, in *Pathmarks*, M. Heidegger, trans., ed. W. McNeil; and W. McNeil (Cambridge: Cambridge University Press, 1998), 258. "Die Seinsvergessenheit bekundet sich mittelbar darin, daß der Mensch immer nur das Seiende betrachtet und bearbeitet" Heidegger, *Über den Humanismus*, 31.

15. See M. Heidegger, "The Age of the World Picture," in *The Question Concerning Technology and Other Essays*, trans. W. Lovitt (London: Garland), 1977.

16. "'Being'—that is not God and not a cosmic ground" Heidegger, *Letter on Humanismus,* 252, "Das 'Sein'—das ist nicht Gott und nicht ein Weltgrund," Heidegger, *Über den Humanismus,* 23.

17. "Likewise, material truth always signifies the consonance of something at hand with the "rational" concept of its essence. The impression arises that this definition of the essence of truth is independent of the interpretation of the essence of the Being of all beings, which always includes a corresponding interpretation of the essence of the human being as the bearer and executor of intellect. Thus the formula for the essence of truth (*veritas est adaequatio intellectus et rei*) comes to have its general validity as something immediately evident to everyone. Under the domination of the obviousness that this concept of truth seems to have, but that is hardly attended to as regards its essential grounds, it is considered equally obvious that truth has an opposite, and that there is untruth. The untruth of the proposition (incorrectness) is the non accordance of the statement with the matter. The untruth of the matter (non genuineness) signifies nonagreement of a being with its essence" Martin Heidegger, *On the Essence of Truth* (1930), trans. J. Sallis, in *Pathmarks,* ed. W. McNeil and W. McNeil, trans. (Cambridge: Cambridge University, 1998), 139; Martin Heidegger, *Dell'essenza della verità,* Italian trans. F. Volpi, *Segnavia* (Milan: Adelphi, 2002) 137–38.

18. Martin Heidegger, *Gelassenheit* (Tübingen: Neske, 1959), 61; Martin Heidegger, *Discourse on Thinking,* English trans. J. M. Anderson and E. H. Freund (New York: Harper & Row Publishers, 1955) 81: "in accordance with Greek story and thought, we are aware of the nature of truth as a dis-closure and recovery [*Unverborgenheit und Entbergung*]."

19. "That which shows itself and at the same time withdraws is the essential trait of what we call the mystery. I call the comportment which enables us to keep open to the meaning hidden in technology, openness to the mystery" Heidegger, *Discourse on thinking,* 55. "Was auf solche Weise sich zeigt und zugleich sich entzieht, ist der Grundzug dessen, was wir das Geheimnis nennen. Ich nenne die Haltung, kraft deren wir uns fur den in der technischen Welt verborgenen Sinn offen halten: die Offenheit for das Geheimnis" Heidegger, *Gelassenheit,* 26.

20. Martin Heidegger, "The Origin of the Work of Art" in *Poetry, Language, Thought,* trans. Albert Hofstadter (New York: Harper Perennial, 1971), 51.

21. Heidegger, *Gelassenheit,* 44: "Das Offene selbst aber ist die Gegnet."

22. Heidegger, *Gelassenheit,* 40.

23. Heidegger, *Gelassenheit,* 40.

24. Heidegger, *Gelassenheit,* 109: "Die Gelassenheit ware dann nicht nur der Weg, sondern die Bewegung."

25. Heidegger, *Gelassenheit*, 34.

26. Heidegger, *Gelassenheit*, 34: "wenn unser Wesen zugelassen ist, sich auf das einzulassen, was nicht ein Wollen ist."

27. Heidegger, *Gelassenheit*, 35: "Vielleicht verbirgt sich in der Gelassenheit ein höheres Tun als in allen Taten der Welt und in den Machenschaften der Menschentümer."

28. M. Heidegger, "Zur Erörterung der Gelassenheit," in *Gelassenheit* (Tübingen: Neske, 1959). This discourse was taken from a conversation written down in 1944–45 between a scientist, a scholar, and a teacher.

29. Heidegger, "Zur Erörterung der Gelassenheit," 35.

30. Heidegger, "Zur Erörterung der Gelassenheit," 35.

31. Heidegger, "Zur Erörterung der Gelassenheit," 36: "Wir sollen nichts tun sondern warten."

32. Heidegger, *Discourse on Thinking*, 72. "And waiting means: to release oneself into the openness of that-which-regions," *Gelassenheit*, 50: "Und Warten heiBt: auf das Offene der Gegnet sich einlassen"—* Italian version 113–14.

33. "The region gathers, just as if nothing were happening, each to each and each to all into an abiding, while resting in itself" Heidegger, *Discourse on thinking*, 66. Heidegger, "Zur Erörterung der Gelassenheit," 41–42: "in das Verweilen beim Beruhen in sich selbst." (Italian translation: "La contrada raccoglie, sebbene nulla avvenga, ogni cosa nel suo rapporto ad ogni altra, facendola permanere nell'acquietarsi in se stessa").

34. "Regioning is a gathering and re-sheltering for an expanded resting in an abiding" Heidegger, *Discourse on thinking*, 66. Heidegger, "Zur Erörterung der Gelassenheit," 42: "Gegnen ist das versammelnde Zurückbergen zum weiten Beruhen in der Weile." (Italian translation: "Farsi-incontro è raccogliere e ricondurre al vasto acquietarsi nella permanenza").

35. Mediopassive form of the active φαίνω. M. Heidegger, *Being and Time* (New York: State University of New York Press, 2010), intro. II 28, 25.

36. See R. Calasso, *Le nozze di Cadmo e Armonia* (Milan: Adelphi, 1991), 225–30.

37. Husserl, *The Crisis*, § 42, 153.

38. Maitry *Upaniṣad*, VI, 30, 1179.

39. Heidegger, *Discourse on thinking*, 90.

40. Husserl, *Erste Philosophie*, 79.

41. Martin Heidegger, *Introduction to Metaphysics*, trans. G. Fried and R. Polt (New Haven and London: Yale University Press, 2014, [77] § The restriction of Being, III, "Being means appearing. Appearing does not mean something derivative, which from time to time meets up with Being. Being essentially unfolds as appearing."

42. On the topic Husserl's disciple E. Fink claims: "Mais en vérité c'est le problème le plus cardinal, par-dessus lequel la phénoménologie de Husserl saute, parce qu'elle recule devant la pensée spéculative. Elle décrète simplement que l'étant est identique au phénomène, identique à l'étant se montrant et s'exposant. Une chose an soi qui resterait fondamentalement soustraite à l'apparître, n'aurait aucun sens, serait un non-concept" E. Fink, *Proximité et distance* (Grenoble: Jérôme Millon, Grenoble, 1994), 120.

43. Husserl, *Ideas*, "Preface" to the English edition, 22.

44. Husserl, *The Idea of Phenomenology*, [12] 10.

Chapter 4

1. See first chapter on the doctrinal base of the mandala in Giuseppe Tucci, *Teoria e pratica del mandala* (Rome: Astrolabio, 1949), 22: "Knowledge to which action does not conform, is not good but bad, when knowledge does not change life and is not actualized in it, it is cause of disharmony" (English translation by the author).

2. See *Saṃyutta Nikāya*, 56. 11, *Dhammacakkappavattanasutta* "Rolling Forth the Wheel of Dhammacakkappavattanasutta," in *The Connected Discourses of the Buddha: A Translation from the Pāli of the Saṃyutta Nikāya*, ed. Bhikkhu Bodhi (Boston: Wisdom, 2000), 1843–47.

3. Patañjali, *Yogasūtra*, II. 15, 203. Furthermore, commentator Vyāsa argues for the existence of a modified version of the Buddhist "four noble truths" in Patañjali's aphorisms in II. 15, II. 17, and II. 25–26. Sanskrit phrases appear declined as found in the original text.

4. Svātmārāma, *Haṭhayogapradīpikā. Light on Hatha Yoga*, ed. Swami Muktibodhananda (Munger: Yoga Publications Trust, Bihar School of Yoga, 1985, 1998), online at https://archive.org/details/hatha-yoga-pradipika-swami-muktibodhananda_202206/page/34/mode/2up, I.10, 34. English translation modified by the author. Note that the word referring to suffering here is *tāpa* and not *tapas:* "Aśeṣatāpataptānāṁ samāśrayamaṭho haṭhaḥ | Aśeṣayogayuktānāmādhārakamaṭho haṭhaḥ." Though both *tāpa* and *tapas* derive from the same root, their meaning and usage differ widely.

5. *Śvetāśvatara Upaniṣad,* II, 14, in Raphael, *Upaniṣad,* 968.

6. *Śvetāśvatara Upaniṣad,* II, 12, in Raphael, *Upaniṣad,* 968.

7. Plato, *Republic*, book VII, in *Plato: Complete Works* (Indianapolis/Cambridge: Hackett, 1997), 1132–55.

8. A. Sander, "Phenomenological Reduction and Yogic Meditation: Commonalities and Divergencies," *Journal of East-West Thought* 5 (2015): 31.

9. Bitbol, *La conscience a-t-elle une origine?*, 158.

10. Puligandla had noted that "Whereas phenomenology merely talks of bracketing, ideating, and performing reduction, Patafijali's yoga provides a stepwise procedure for actually accomplishing them," R. Puligandla, "Phenomenological Reduction and Yoga Meditation," 33.

11. Western historiography has been imported to India in only a limited capacity and was unknown there before the nineteenth century.

12. There is both a broad and a narrower sense of the term prajñā, as we shall see.

13. *Māṇḍūkya Upaniṣad,* I. 1–2, in Raphael, *Upaniṣad,* 1022.

14. *Māṇḍūkya Upaniṣad,* I. 3, in Raphael, *Upaniṣad,* 1022.

15. *Māṇḍūkya Upaniṣad,* I. 4, in Raphael, *Upaniṣad,* 1022.

16. *Māṇḍūkya Upaniṣad,* I. 5, in Raphael, *Upaniṣad,* 1022.

17. See Chapter 1.

18. *Māṇḍūkya Upaniṣad,* I. 5, in Raphael, *Upaniṣad,* 1022.

19. See *Bṛhadāraṇyaka Upaniṣad,* II. 3. 6, in Raphael, *Upaniṣad,* 82.

20. *Māṇḍūkya Upaniṣad,* I. 7, 1026.

21. Other than the Vedic sage Yājñavalkya, credited with being the author of the oldest *Upaniṣad,* the *Bṛhadāraṇyaka* that is also the final part of the *Śatapatha Brāhmana.* Yājñavalkya is also traditionally considered the author of a much later text, the *Yoga* Yājñavalkya (see note 89).

22. *Māṇḍūkya Upaniṣad,* I. 13, in Raphael, *Upaniṣad,* 1026.

23. This is the comment of Gaudapada to the *Māṇḍūkya Upaniṣad* I. 11. Raphael, *Upaniṣad,* 1027.

24. Śaṅkarā, *Yoga Tarvali,* trans. Swami Narasimhananda, "Yoga-Taravali ofAcharya Shankara," *Traditional Wisdom* 124, no. 1 (2019): 7 n.21.

25. Śaṅkarā, *Yoga Tarvali,* 8 n.26.

26. The term "*Sat-citta-ananda*" occurs as a whole in the *Tejobindu Upaniṣad,* III. 1, in K. Nārāyaṇasvāmaiyar, *Thirty Minor Upanisahds* (Madras: Printed by Annie Besant at the Vasanta Press, 1914), 86. In Vedanta the term *citta* is frequently used as synonym of the seer or, in Śaṅkarā, of the "witness consciousness" [*Sākshin Caitanya*], see: S. K. Maharana, "Phenomenology of Consciousness in Ādi Śamkara and Edmund Husserl," *Indo-Pacific Journal of Phenomenology* 9, no. 1 (2009): 5. Since in Patañjali *citta* has just the ordinary meaning of "the space of the mind stuff," in this essay the term consciousness will be reserved to terms such as (*draṣṭṛ, puruṣa, prakāśa . . .*).

27. *Chāndogya Upaniṣad* III. 12.7–9, 390.

28. *Chāndogya Upaniṣad* III. 14.1, 396 [*sarvaṁ khalvidaṁ brahma*].

29. *Chāndogya Upaniṣad,* VI. II.1, 488 [*ekam evādvitīyam*].

30. *Isha Upaniṣad,* 16, 802 [*so'hamasmi*].

31. *Chāṇḍogya Upaniṣad,* VI. 8. 7, 502 [*tattvamasi*].

32. *Māṇḍūkya Upaniṣad,* I. 2, 1022 [*brahmāyamātmā*].

33. *Bṛhadāraṇyaka Upaniṣad,* I. IV. 10, 38 [*ahaṃ brahmāsmi*].

34. *Aitareya Upaniṣad,* III. 3, 698 [*prajñām brahman*].

35. *Maitry Upaniṣad,* VI. 19, 1168.

36. *Maitry Upaniṣad,* VI, 19 "rests without forming concepts . . ."

37. *Muṇḍaka Upaniṣad,* III, 2, 6, 900.

38. See *Śvetāśvatara Upaniṣad,* 1.15, 960.

39. *Bṛhadāraṇyaka Upaniṣad,* I. II. 6, 16. *Taitttirīya Upaniṣad* I. IX. 1, 623, *Muṇḍaka Upaniṣad* III, I, 5, 895, *Kena Upaniṣad* IV, 8, 791, *Śvetāśvatara Upaniṣad,* I. 15, 960 (just to mention a few).

40. See A. L. Murdoch, *Tapas in the Rigveda* (MA thesis, York University, 1983).

41. For example, in the *Bṛhadāraṇyaka Upaniṣad* it is said that Prajapati toiled and heated "śrāmyatsa tapo 'tapyata" emanating splendor, *Bṛhadāraṇyaka Upaniṣad,* I. II. 6, 16.

42. S. N. Dasgupta claims that "*tapas* does not mean any such thing as asceticism, expiatory penances or the like, but devoted meditation upon the particular objects which would have to be created." S. N. Dasgupta, *Yoga Philosophy. In Relation to Other Systems of Indian thought* (Delhi: Motilal Banarsidass, 1930), 43.

43. See Walter O. Kaelber, *Tapta Marga: Asceticism and Initiation in Vedic India* (Albany: State University of New York Press, 1989), 143.

44. Experiencing *tapas* means experiencing "magical heat" or "psychic heat," which in its essence corresponds to the burning sensation of a "creative exudation." Mircea Eliade, *Yoga: Immortality and Freedom,* trans. W. R. Trask (Princeton: Princeton University Press, 2009), 331–32.

45. A contradiction? Yes and no: it is the circularity that characterizes myths in general, and Indian literature in particular. Roberto Calasso defines it as "mutual procreation," according to which he who generates is, in turn, often generated by his own descendants. See Roberto Calasso, *Ardor,* trans. by R. Dixon (New York: Farrar, Straus and Giroux, 2014), 70.

46. *Rigveda* Hymn 1.1, "Agni do I invoke [Oṁ a̱gnimīḻe]—the one placed to the fore [. . .]" in S. W. Jamison and J. P. Brereton, ed., *The Rigveda: The Earliest Religious Poetry of India* (Oxford: Oxford University Press, 2014), 89.

47. These recall, respectively, the earthly dimension that is linked to the churning of the sticks that kindle the flame and symbolize the sexual union, the atmospheric dimension of lightning that in the myth is created by the water held in the clouds, and the sky, where Agni appears as Sūrya, the sun.

48. *Rigveda* III, 18 in Kaelber, *Tapta Marga,* 45.

49. Kaelber, *Tapta Marga,* 46.

50. See Kaelber, *Tapta Mārga,* 45–60.

51. See *Rigveda* X.68, I.32, 55 in R. Panikkar: *I veda,* ed. M. Carrara Pavan (Milan: Bur, 2012), 198.

52. One of the faces of Agni, Sūrya, is also a *tapasvin* which can make it rain, nourish the earth and ripen the harvest: *". . . for from fire springs smoke, from smoke the cloud, from the cloud rain, it is from fire that these are produced: hence he says 'born of heat.'" Satapatha Brahmana* 5.3.5.17. In the *Chāndogya Upaniṣad* the sun, named Aditi, is said to be the Brahman, *Chāndogya Upaniṣad,* III, XIX, 1, 409.

53. Calasso, *Ardor,* 25.

54. See *Tattirīya-Samhitā,* 5, 1.8.2, in W. O. Kaelber, "Tapas, Birth and Spiritual Rebirth in the Veda," *History of Religions* 15, no. 4 (May 1976): 348.

55. See *Rigveda* X.129.4, in Kaelber, "Tapas, Birth and Spiritual Rebirth in the Veda," 348.

56. *Jāiminīya Upanisad Brāhmana,* 1.47.7, in Kaelber, "Tapas, Birth and Spiritual Rebirth in the Veda," 349.

57. See Stefano Castelli, "Editoriale," *Percorsi Yoga,* No. 70, luglio 2016, 6.

58. *Chāndogya Upaniṣad,* 2.23.2–3 in Kaelber, "Tapas, Birth and Spiritual Rebirth in the Veda," 373.

59. Also the Ṛṣi, the primordial winds, "sat down with Tapas" and "brooded upon" "abhi- √tap" the world. See Kaelber, "Tapas, Birth and Spiritual Rebirth in the Veda," 374. Also in the *Brahmana* XI–IX: *abhi-tap.*

60. See Hume, Radhakrishnan and Nikhilananda cited in Kaelber, "Tapas, Birth and Spiritual Rebirth in the Veda," 372.

61. *Maitry Upaniṣad,* VI, 27, 1176.

62. Calasso, *Ardor,* 175.

63. With derivatives that mean: "reins," "ropes."

64. Literally: yoking a pair of bulls/horses under the weight of a plough/chariot. See, for example, *Rigveda* I.5.4: "Whose pair of tawny horses yoked in battles foemen challenge not: To him, to Indra sing your song" trans. by Ralph T. H. Griffith. See also "Thus to thee, Indra, yoker of Bay Coursers, the Gotamas have brought their prayers to please thee" *Rigveda* I.61.16.

65. Rigveda X.61.10. *"ṛtaṃ vadanta ṛtayuktimaghman."*

66. *Śvetāśvatara Upaniṣad,* II.9, 968.

67. *Śvetāśvatara Upaniṣad,* II.11, 968.

68. *Śvetāśvatara Upaniṣad,* II.10, 968. "In a level, clean place, free from gravel, fire and sand. With soundless water, a dwelling and so on. Pleasing to the mind and not harsh on the eye, secret and sheltered from the wind, one should practise yoga."

69. *Kaṭha Upanishad,* II. III. 11, 854.

70. See *Kaṭha Upanishad* II. III. 11, 854. *"Yadā pañcāvatisthante jñānāni manasā saha | buddhiśka na vicestati tāmāhuh paramāṃ gatim."*

71. *Maitry Upaniṣad,* VI, 17, 1166.

72. *Maitry Upaniṣad,* VI, 18, 1166.

73. *Maitry Upaniṣad,* VI. 25, 1174.

74. "The means to liberation is uninterrupted discriminative discernment" Patañjali, *The Yoga Sutras of Patañjali,* ed. E. F. Bryant Patañjali, II.26, 234.

75. "By the removal of ignorance [*avidyā*], conjunction [*saṃyoga*] is removed. This is the absolute freedom of the seer" Patañjali, *The Yoga Sutras of Patañjali,* II, 25, 234. Another expression partially related to *saṃyoga* is *yogakṣema,* safety from the ordinary bondage on (is this "on" correct) conjunction, recurring in Vedanta (see, for instance, *Kaṭha Upanishad* I.2.2) but also in Buddhism in which the process of "rest/liberation from bondage" [*yogakkhema*] refers to the *nirvana*. See C. Neri, T. Pontillo, "On the Boundary between Yogakkhema in the Suttapiṭaka and Yogakṣema in the Upaniṣads and Bhagavadgītā," *Cracow Indological Studies* XXI, no. 2 (2019): 139–57, 151.

76. Karen O' Brien-Kop in *Rethinking 'Classical Yoga' and Buddhism* acknowledges that "the discourse of yoga was employed by various communities in a shared religio-cultural environment." She also claims that her book "has challenged the idea that the Pātañjalayogaśaśtra is only Hindu—it certainly is Hindu (and the text clearly addresses Brahmins) but not only, since Buddhist soteriology is also integral to understanding this text"; K. O' Brien-Kop, *Rethinking 'Classical Yoga' and Buddhism* (London: Bloomsbury Academic, 2022), 6, 152.

77. *Milinda Pañha,* [Questions of Milinda], in *La rivelazione del Buddha,* ed. R. Gnoli (Milan: Mondadori, 2001), 115. In the text (c. 2nd–3rd century CE), the Buddhist sage Nāgasena, of the early Buddhist school of the Sarvāstivāda, answers the questions posed by Greek king Milinda (Menander I).

78. In the Vedic world carrying out the sacrifice reproduced Prajāpati's creation and therefore had largely worldly, ontic ends, understood from the point of view of singularity.

79. *Rigveda* X.136, Panikkar, *I Veda,* 536–37.

80. Calasso, *Ardor,* 217.

81. *Atharvaveda,* XV.15 in R.T.H. Griffith, *The Hymns of the Atharva Veda* (Benares: E. J. Lazarus and Co., 1895), 197–98.

82. M. Eliade, *Yoga. Immortality and Freedom,* 108–9.

83. *Bhagavadgītā* 4.25, 28–29, in *The Bhagavad Gita,* ed. Sri Swami Sivananda (The Divine Life Society, 2000) 43–44.

84. See Eliade, *Yoga. Immortality and Freedom,* 114.

85. Calasso, *Ardor,* 217.

86. Traditionally six schools are listed within Hinduism: Sāṃkhya, Nyāya, Vaiśeṣika, Yoga, Mīmāṃsā, Vedānta.

87. Patañjali, *The Yoga Sutras of Patañjali,* II.29, 241; *aṣṭāṅga* inevitably recalls the Buddhist Eightfold Path, probably testifying for mutual connections and more specifically for a Buddhist influence on the exposition of the *Yogasūtra,* although the steps of the path are fairly different in the two traditions.

88. The five *yamāḥ* are: (1) nonviolence [*ahiṁsā*], (2) being-truth [*satyā*], (3) abstaining from stealing [*asteya*], (4) controlling sexual energy [*brahmacarya*], (5) refraining from greediness [*aparigrahāḥ*]. Patañjali, *The Yoga Sutras of* Patañjali, II. 30, 242.

89. *Tapas* appears listed also as one of the five *nyamāḥ,* which are (1) cleanliness [*śauca]* (2) contentment *[śantośa]* (3) power of heat [*tapas*], (4) study [*svādhyāya*], (5) releasement [*Īshvara-praṇidhāna*]. Patañjali, *The Yoga Sutras of Patañjali,* II.32, 252.

90. Patañjali's indication on the *āsana* is analyzed in the paragraph about *āsanas.*

91. A text most likely later, as the *Yoga Yājñavalkya,* attributed to the mythical figure of Yājñavalkya, provides a description of the *Pratyāhāra* as an internal focus on eighteen vital points called Marma-sthāna. See *Yoga Yājñavalkya,* J. Ely, ed., trans. A. G. Mohan (Madras: Ganesh & Co, 2013), n. 8–11, 93.

92. The term "zen" as in Zen Buddhism is etymologically linked to *dhyāna,* meditation. When Bodhidharma brought Buddhism to China, *dhyāna* underwent these transformations, as Red Pine notes in his commentary on Hui-Neng's zen teachings: "When Buddhist meditation was introduced to the Chinese, the Sanskrit term dhyana was rendered zenna and later shortened to zen. In the beginning, this word simply meant 'meditation.' But it was used by the heirs of Bodhidharma to refer to the practice of pointing directly to the mind, and it became the name of their school as well. Nowadays, this term is pronounced ch'an in Mandarin Chinese"; see R. Pine, ed. and trans., *The Platform Sutra: The Zen Teaching of Hui-Neng* (Berkeley: Counterpoint, 2006), 146. In Buddhism, the notion of "meditation" or "contemplation" is generally rendered with the term

bhāvana, which literally means "cultivating" (*bhava* meaning: becoming) and thus refers to a specific calling into existence.

93. De La Valleé Poussin was one of the first scholars who drew comparisons between Buddhist terminology and the one of the *Yogasūtra.* See L. de La Valleé Poussin, "Le Bouddhisme et le yoga de Patañjali," *Mélanges Chinois et Bouddhiques* 5 (1936): 223–41. Recently O' Brien-Kop has claimed that "Patañjali was certainly familiar with the concepts of the Buddhist Sarvāstivāda and yogācāra milieux—and we must assume that his audience was too" (O'Brien-Kop, *Rethinking 'Classical Yoga' and Buddhism,* 19).

94. The Yogācāra tradition is to be traced back to authors such as Asaṅga (c. 330–405 CE), author of the *Yogācārabhūmiśāstra*) and Vasubandhu. "The two centuries prior to the composition of the Pātañjalayogaśāstra saw the beginnings of the Buddhist Yogācāra school, whose identifying feature was the practice of yoga"; J. Mallinson and M. Singleton, *Roots of Yoga* (Penguin Classics, 2017) (digital edition), § on Yogācāra Buddhism; See also Squarcini, ed., *Yogasūtra,* "Introduzione," LIX, LXIV, and D. Lusthaus, *Buddhist Phenomenology. A Philosophical Investigation of Yogācāra Buddhism and the Ch'eng Wei-shih lun* (New York: Routledge, 2002), § "What Is and Isn't Yogacara?."

95. Squarcini, *Yogasūtra,* "Introduction," XCVII.

96. Patañjali, *The Yoga Sutras of Patañjali,* IV.29, 450. Also the term *vāsanā,* the subliminal impressions, used by Pātañjali in IV. 8 e IV. 24 is to be found also in Vasubandhu *Abhidharmakośa.*

97. This is the title of the second section or *pādaḥ.*

98. Patañjali, *The Yoga Sutras of* Patañjali, II.1, 169 "*tapaḥ-svādhyāyeśvara-Praṇidhānāni kriya-yogaḥ.*" In this sutra Patañjali connects his *kriyāyoga* to *tapas,* the power of heat, *svādhyāya,* the study of the self, and *Īśhvara-Praṇidhāna,* the capacity of releasement to a wider dimension (*Īśhvara* is a deity and intended as the master or guru of the yogis). These latter can be intended as the two aspects that comprise *tapas* itself.

99. Patañjali, *The Yoga Sutras of* Patañjali, II.43, 272.

100. Same root of the term detrimental [*kliṣṭa*].

101. Patañjali, *The Yoga Sutras of* Patañjali, II.2, 173. Here we will not delve into the very elaborate structure of the different grades of *samādhi* envisaged by Patañjali, in which the earlier stages still entail the presence of mental seeds [*sambīja*] and of discrimintive knowledge [*samprajñata*] [I. 17–21] while the deeper [*a-samprajñta samādhi*] don't. Finally, the seedless *samadhi* [*nirbīja*] is beyond any trace or seed [1.51].

102. The term *Kaivalya* is the title of the fourth *pādaḥ.*

103. Ignorance, the breeding ground for all the other afflictions.

104. Patañjali, *The Yoga Sutras of Patañjali,* II. 3, 175. The attachment to life as an object [*abhiniveśāḥ*] is considered the hardest affliction to overcome, also by the wise one.

105. Patañjali, *The Yoga Sutras of Patañjali,* II.10, 192.

106. Ganganatha Jha, ed., *Yoga-Darshana. Sūtra of Patañjali with Bhāṣya of Vyāsa* (Fremont, CA: Asian Humanities Press, 2002), 88.

107. See the gloss by commentator *Vāchapati Miśra* to the sutra II.10, R. Prasāda, *Patañjali's Yoga Sutras with the commentary of Vyāsa and the gloss of Vāchaspati Miśra* (Munshiram: Manoharlal, 1998), 103. On the subject O' Brien-Kop argues: "Thus *Patañjjali*'s discourse appears to be aware not only of the core seed metaphor of the Abhidharmakośabhāṣya but also of the predominant trace (vāsanā) metaphor of the Yogācārabhūmiśāstra and with the anuśaya-āśaya-āśraya semantic continuum of both Buddhist texts" K. O' Brien-Kop, *Rethinking 'Classical Yoga' and Buddhism,* 70.

108. Patañjali, *The Yoga Sutras of Patañjali,* III.9, 315. At the origin of the afflictions are *saṃskāra* directed outward, toward external objects [*Vyutthāna-saṃskāra*]. They can be specifically counteracted by restraining and neutralizing *saṃskāra* [*Nirodha-saṃskāra*].

109. "Everything transcendent (that which is not given to me immanently) is to be assigned the index zero" Husserl, *The Idea of Phenomenology,* 6.

110. Patañjali, *The Yoga Sutras of Patañjali,* III.11, 318.

111. Patañjali, *The Yoga Sutras of Patañjali,* III.11, 318.

112. Patañjali, *The Yoga Sutras of Patañjali,* I.2, 10.

113. Patañjali, *The Yoga Sutras of Patañjali,* I.2, 10.

114. Indologist Larson notes that the different dimensions of the mind that in *Sāṃkhya* were distinguished are conflated in Patañjali's notion of *citta.* For this reason the term *citta* might be rendered with the collective term of "mind-stuff": "Where classical *Sāṃkhya speaks of buddhi, ahaṃkāra* and *manas* as three distinct faculties that make up the *anthaḥkaraṇa* or 'internal organ,' classical Yoga philosophy reduces the three to one all-pervasive *citta* or 'mind-stuff' "; G. J. Larson, "Classical Yoga as Neo-Sāṃkhya: A Chapter in the History of Indian Philosophy," in *Asian Studies* 53, no. 3 (1999): 728. In Buddhist Yogācāra tradition (strongly connected to Patañjali's yoga *darśana*) the term *citta* is one of the names of the "store-consciousness" [*ālayavijñāna*]: "In Asaṅga's school *citta* is one of the names of the *ālayavijñāna* ('store-consciousness') and there is no more important term in Asaṅga's system than the latter term"; A. Wayman, *Analysis of the Śrāvakabhūmi Manuscript* (Berkeley: University of California Press, 1961), 49.

115. Patañjali lists five kinds of fluctuations [*vṛitti*]. Patañjali, *The Yoga Sutras of Patañjali,* I.6 "right knowledge [*pramāṇa*], error [*viparyaya*], imagination [*vikalpa*], sleep [*nidrā*] and memory [*smṛtayaḥ*]": It is interesting to notice that in Patañjali's view also sleep is a modification of the space of mind somehow comparable to the other *vṛttis,* and is separated from the condition of consciousness (prajñā), which belongs only to the stages of contemplative absorption. This marks a difference with the Vedanta in which deep sleep and the fourth state had a lot in common.

116. Patañjali, *The Yoga Sutras of Patañjali,* I.7 "Direct perception [*pratyakṣa*], inference [*anumāna*] and revealed authority [*āgamāḥ*]" Patañjali, *Yoga-Sutras of Patañjali with the exposition of Vyāsa,* trans. Usharbudh Arya, D. Litt (Honesdale, PA: The Himalayan International Institute of Yoga Science and Philosophy of the USA, 1986), 149.

117. See for example the supernatural perception referred to by Patañjali with the term *viṣayavati* (Patañjali, *The Yoga Sutras of Patañjali,* I. 35). See also sutra I. 43. "Nirvitarka, 'absorption without conceptualization,' occurs when memory [*smṛiti*] has been purged and the mind is empty [*śūnyā*], as it were, of its own [reflective] nature. Now only the object [of meditation] shines forth" Patañjali, *The Yoga Sutras of Patañjali,* 147.

118. Patañjali, *The Yoga Sutras of Patañjali,* I. 5, 27.

119. Eliade adds that the worldly man "opposes his static posture, the immobility of *āsana,* to agitated, unrhythmical, changing respiration, he opposes the *prāṇāyāma.*" Eliade, *Yoga. Immortality and Freedom,* 95. See also this other passage: "The orientation is the same: reacting against the 'habitual,' 'profane,' 'human' inclination," Mircea Eliade, *Tecniche dello yoga* (Turin: Bollati Boringhieri, 2013), 85.

120. Interesting are the connections that Peter Sloterdijk envisages between his notion of "anthropotechnics" and Eastern transformative techniques. See P. Sloterdijk, *You Must Change Your Life: On Anthropotechnics* (Malden, MA: Polity, 2013).

121. Husserl, *Erste Philosophie,* [121], 122: "Es handelt sich also in der Tat um eine ganz 'unnatürliche' Einstellung und eine ganz unnatürliche Selbst- und Weltbetrachtung. Das natürliche Leben vollzieht sich als eine ursprüngliche, als eine anfangs durchaus notwendige Welthingabe, Weltverlorenheit. Das Unnatürliche ist das der radikalen und reinen Selbstbesinnung, der Selbst besinnung auf das reine."

122. Husserl, *The Crisis,* § 39, 148 (Italian translation, 176)." Michel Bitbol expresses this point referring to both phenomenology and mindfulness meditation, which unlike Western epistemology do not entail "disentangling knowledge from the existential transformation of the knower" Bitbol, *Consciousness, Being and Life,* 127–61, * 4.

123. Patañjali, *The Yoga Sutras of Patañjali,* II.20, 222.

124. Patañjali, *The Yoga Sutras of Patañjali*, I.3, 22, *"tadā draṣṭuḥ svarūpe 'vasthānam,"* "when that is accomplished, the seer abides in its own true nature."

125. Husserl, *Erste Philosophie*, 111. As already mentioned, the very root of the word "phenomenon" comes from the Greek term *Phanes*, "light."

126. *"Sama"* has a similar meaning to the word "same" in English.

127. Patañjali, *Yogasūtra*, ed. by Squarcini, I.41. English trans. by the author: "reaching concordance [*samāmpatti*], that is to the condition in which the effects of the vortices are nearly extinguished (kṣ*īṇa*). Thus the gem is completely transparent, [finally] able to take the colour of any object it is placed before her, [revealing the conjunction] between the seizer *[grahītṛ]* the seizing [*grahaṇa*] and the seized [*grāhya*]," 10.

128. "Otherwise, at other times, [the seer] is absorbed in the changing state [of the mind]" *"vṛtti-sārūpyam itaratra"* Patañjali, *The Yoga Sutras of Patañjali*, I.4, 24.

129. Patañjali, *The Yoga Sutras of Patañjali*, II.17, 213.

130. Advaita Vedānta is a tradition within Vedānta that emphasize the nondual nature of reality. Ramanuja (founder of Vishishtadvaita Vedānta), accused Śaṅkarācārya of being a hidden or "crypto-Buddhist" [*Prachanna Bauddha*]; see S. Biderman, "Śankara and the Buddhists," *Journal of Indian Philosophy* 6 no. 4 (1978): 405–13. Also Bhattacharya Saxena argues that "Adi Śhankaracharya, erroneously known as *prachanna Bouddha* or a hidden Buddhist, attempted to assimilate Buddha's wisdom into his Brahmanical fold"; see N. Bhattacharya Saxena, *Absent Mother God of The West* (London: Lexington Books, 2016), 19.

131. Swami Nikhilananda, ed., *Drgdriśyaviveka. An Inquiry into the Nature of the 'Seer' and the 'Seen,'* trans. Swami Nikhilananda (Mysore: Sri Ramanakrishna Asrama, 1931), 1.

132. Husserl, *Erste Philosophie*, 121.

133. Ian Whicher suggests translating nirodha as "cessation," referring to this "'undoing' or dissolution of the conjunction [*saṁyoga*] between *puruṣa*—the 'seer' [*draṣṭṛ*]—and *prakṛti*—the 'seeable.'" I. Whicher, "Nirodha, Yoga Praxis and the Transformation of the Mind," *Journal of Indian Philosophy* 25 (1997): 4.

134. "[the *vṛtti* states of mind] are stilled by practice and dispassion" *"abhyāsa-vairāgyābhyāṁ tan-nirodhaḥ"* Patañjali, *The Yoga Sutras of Patañjali*, I.12. 47.

135. Husserl, *The Crisis*, § 40, 150.

136. Husserl, *Ideas*, Introduction [3], XIX.

137. Husserl, *Ideas*, Introduction, [3] XIX.

138. Husserl, *Ideas*, Introduction [1] XVII.

139. See Patañjali, *The Yoga Sutras of Patañjali*, I. 13, 48.

140. Patañjali, *The Yoga Sutras of Patañjali,* I. 14, 49.

141. Patañjali, *The Yoga Sutras of Patañjali,* I. 15, 49 ("Dispassion is the controlled consciousness of one who is without craving for sense objects, whether these are actually perceived, or described"). Having taken a closer look at the phenomenological concept of placing out of validity everyday objectivities gives us important insights in how to understand from a different perspective the detachment involved in *vairagya,* which is often misleadingly translated as "renunciation." It is not a question of penance intended as a pious renunciation; rather, it is a question of gaining a distance from the relation that usually takes place with the world, characterized by the belief in an independent external existence of objects. Preparing this *vairagya* as a first step, the abstentions [yamas] are to be found in the eight-step path of yoga explored by Patañjali.

142. Patañjali, *The Yoga Sutras of Patañjali,* II. 17, 213.

143. Husserl, *The Crisis,* part III B, 259.

144. Husserl, *The Crisis,* cit., 249.

145. Husserl, Ideas, § 59, 111.

146. Husserl, *The Crisis,* Appendix 1, *The Vienna Lectures,* 297.

147. Husserl, *The Crisis,* 303.

148. Husserl, *The Crisis,* 329.

149. Patañjali, *The Yoga Sutras of Patañjali,* I. 36, 133.

150. Patañjali, *The Yoga Sutras of Patañjali,* III. 3, 306.

151. Patañjali, *The Yoga Sutras of Patañjali,* III. 5, 311.

152. Patañjali, *The Yoga Sutras of Patañjali,* I. 48, 158.

153. Patañjali, *The Yoga Sutras of Patañjali,* III. 1, 301.

154. Patañjali, *The Yoga Sutras of Patañjali,* III. 3, 306.

Chapter 5

1. D. R. Komito, *Nāgārjuna's Seventy Stanzas: A Buddhist Psychology of Emptiness* [*Shūnvatāsaptatikārikānāma*] (New York: Snow Lion Publications, 1987).

2. This approach relies only on the alleged dualist *Sāṃkhya* influences on the *Yogasūtra.*

3. Vidhushekhara Bhattacharya stresses the fact that Gaudapāda, commentator of the *Māṇḍūkya Upaniṣad,* is influenced and draws from Buddhist traditions. More specifically Bhattacharya considers the striking similarties between Gaudapada's comment to the *Māṇḍūkya Upaniṣad* and Nāgārjuna's *Mūla-madyamaka-kārikā.* Vidhushekhara Bhattacharya, ed., *The ĀgamaŚāstṛa of Gaudapāda* (Calcutta: University of Calcutta, 1943), 120–27.

4. *Maitry Upaniṣad* VI. 20, 1169.

5. See for instance the already mentioned passages from the *Bṛhadāraṇyaka Upaniṣad* II. 3. 6. and the *Māṇḍūkya Upaniṣad,* I.7.

6. Taishō Tripiṭaka, ed., *Prajñāpāramitā Hṛdaya Sūtra,* Lapis Lazuli Texts, vol. 8, no. 251, online resource:apislazulitexts.com/tripitaka/T0253-LL-prajnaparamita-hrdaya/

7. Nāgārjuna, *Fundamental Wisdom of the Middle Way. Nāgārjuna's Mūla-madyamaka-kārikā,* trans., ed. J. L. Garfield (Oxford: Oxford University Press, 1995, XVIII.18), 248. See also: M. Siderits and S. Katsura, eds., *Nāgārjuna's Middle Way* (Somerville, MA: Wisdom Publications, 2013), 197.

8. It might be worth noting that in India the term *śūnyatā* before indicating the grade zero of the enumeration was used in grammar and music to indicate the empty measure. On the subject see: C. Bartocci, P. Martin, and A. Tagliapietra, *Zerologia. Sullo zero, il vuoto e il nulla* (Milan: Il Mulino, 2016).

9. The sense of having an individual "self" is an illusion that masks the fact that, under this virtual self, there are the aggregates [*pancha-skandha*] that are ever-changing and impermanent: *rūpa* (form, environment), *vedanā* (sensation), *saṃjñā* (conceptuality), *saṃskāra* (power of formation), *vijñāna* (ordinary consciousness).

10. See section of this text on the *Māṇḍūkya Upaniṣad.*

11. Geographically connected to the Vulture Peak Mountain, Gṛdhrakūṭaparvata. The "first turning" are the early teachings of the Buddha that were pronounced at the Gazelle Park of Sarnath.

12. Tenzin Gyatso, *The World of Tibetan Buddhism,* trans. Geshe Thupten Jinpa (Boston: Wisdom Publications, 1995, 10): "The Individual Vehicle expounds the view of selflessness only in relation to person or personal identity but not in relation to things and events in general, whereas in the Universal Vehicle, the principle of selflessness is not confined to the limited scope of the person but encompasses the entire spectrum of existence, all phenomena."

13. Nāgārjuna, *The Dispeller of Disputes. Nāgārjuna's Vigrahavyāvartanī,* ed. and trans., J. Westerhoff (Oxford: Oxford University Press, 2010; kārikā no. 22), 27.

14. Nāgārjuna, *The Dispeller of Disputes,* n. 70, 41.

15. Nāgārjuna, *Fundamental Wisdom of the Middle Way,* XXIV, 19, 69.

16. E. Husserl, *Ideas I,* § 50, [94] 113.

17. The *tetralemma, Catuṣkoṭi* is present in Early Buddhism and also in the *Māṇḍūkya Upaniṣad* IV.83, IV.84. Eastern influences on skeptic philosopher Pyrrho of Elis could exist because of his journey to India (when joining the expedition led by Alexander the Great—fourth century BCE)

and his encounter with the Indian gymnosophists. However, according to Beckwith, claiming that Pyrrho learned the *tetralemma* in India can be problematic. See Beckwith, *Greek Buddha,* 219.

18. J. Westerhoff, "Nāgārjuna's Catuṣkoṭi," *Journal of Indian Philosophy* (2006) 34, 391. Westerhoff also adds that "there is, however, one notorious exception in Nāgārjuna's writings, in verse 18:8 of the *Mūla-madyamaka-kārikā*. There Nāgārjuna seems to affirm all four alternatives by claiming that 'all is real, all is not real, both real and not real, neither real nor not real. This is Buddha's teaching.'"

19. Nāgārjuna, *The Dispeller of Disputes,* kārikā, 24, 63, p. 28, 38.

20. Nāgārjuna, *The Dispeller of Disputes,* kārikā n° 28, 29.

21. Nāgārjuna, *Fundamental Wisdom of the Middle Way,* XXIV.8, 68.

22. Nāgārjuna, *Fundamental Wisdom of the Middle Way,* XXIV.11, 68.

23. Nāgārjuna, *Fundamental Wisdom of the Middle Way,* XXIV, 20.

24. Nāgārjuna, *Fundamental Wisdom of the Middle Way,* XXIV, 21.

25. Nāgārjuna, *Fundamental Wisdom of the Middle Way,* XXIV, 38.

26. The image of Indra's net which in the *Atharva Veda* is only mentioned as a net to imprison enemies [8.8.6 | 8.8.8] finds fortune in Buddhism (developed in the *Avatamsaka Sutra* of *Mahayana* school) and especially in Chinese and Japanese *Huayan* Buddhism. H. Cook, *Hua-Yen Buddhism: The Jewel Net of Indra* (Penn State Press, 1977), 2.

27. Nāgārjuna, *Fundamental Wisdom of the Middle Way,* 1995, XXIV.40.

28. Nāgārjuna, *The Dispeller of Disputes,* 70, 41.

29. Heidegger, *Über den Humanismus,* 52.

30. In his dialogue with Thai Buddhist monk Bikkhu Maha Mani, Heidegger confirms "to be often in tune with Lao-tzu, but to know him only through German translators" H. W. Petzt, *Auf einen Stern zugehen. Begegnungen mit Martin Heidegger 1929 bis 1976* (Frankfurt am Main: Societäts-Verlag, 1983) 179–91.

31. "Count Kuki has a lasting place in my memory" M. Heidegger, *On the Way to Language,* trans. P. D. Hertz (New York: Perennial Library, 1971) 1.

32. Heidegger, *On the Way to Language,* 3.

33. Heidegger, *On the Way to Language,* 3.

34. Heidegger, *On the Way to Language,* 19.

35. Heidegger, *On the Way to Language,* 5.

36. "that emptiness then is the same as nothingness, that essential Being"; Heidegger, *On the Way to Language,* 19.

37. Heidegger, *On the Way to Language,* 19.

38. *Ni-ente,* in Italian, literally no-entity.

39. Petzt, *Auf einen Stern zugehen. Begegnungen mit Martin Heidegger 1929 bis 1976,* 179–91. English translation by the author.

40. Giuseppe Tucci, "The Rātnāvali of Nāgārjuna," *The Journal of the Royal Asiatic Society of Great Britain and Ireland* (1936) 95–96, 434.

41. These teachings can be traced back to the master-disciple lineage of Tilopa (988–1069) Nāropā-Marpa-Milarepa (1051–1135) from which the Kaghyupa school of Tibetan Buddhist originated and are at the base of the Gelug school founded by Lama Tsong Khapa (to which Tenzin Gyatso, the XIVth Dalai Lama, belongs).

42. *Dharmakāya*: literally the body [*kaya*] of *Dharma*. The Mahayana doctrine of the *Trikaya* includes: 1. *Nirmāṇakāya*, the body of creation (gross); 2. *Saṃbhogakāya*, the body of enjoyment (subtle); 3. *Dharmakāya*, the body of emptiness (very subtle).

43. Milarepa, *The Hundred Thousand Songs of Milarepa*, trans., ed. Qarma C. C. Chang (New York: Shambhala Publications, 1962), 684.

44. Milarepa, *The Hundred Thousand Songs of Milarepa*, "The Conversion of the Goddess Tserinma," 325.

45. Milarepa, *The Hundred Thousand Songs of Milarepa*, 679.

46. Also known as "The Mad Yogi from gTsan"—"who was a disciple of Phag.Mo.Gru.Pa. (1110–1170 CE), the celebrated pupil of Gambopa (1079–1161 CE), Milarepa's chief disciple" in Milarepa, *The Hundred Thousand Songs of Milarepa*, 688.

47. Geographically connected to the Dhanyakataka sanctuary of Amaravati.

48. The kind of nondual interpretation here explored is only one of the ways that the early Madhyamaka evolved in India and later Tibet. Speaking about Nāgārjuna, Giuseppe Tucci claims: "His thought has permeated, as it were, not only the Abhidharma of Māhāyana, but also the mystical experiences of Tantric systems" (Giuseppe Tucci, "The Rātnāvali of Nāgārjuna," *Journal of the Royal Asiatic Society of Great Britain and Ireland*, 1934, 307).

49. Milarepa, *The Hundred Thousand Songs of Milarepa*, "Milarepa and the Pigeon," 88–89.

50. Milarepa, *The Hundred Thousand Songs of Milarepa*, "The Song of Yogi's Joy," 79.

51. Milarepa, *The Hundred Thousand Songs of Milarepa*, "The Song of Yogi's Joy," 512.

52. Milarepa, *The Hundred Thousand Songs of Milarepa*, "The Grey Rock *Vajra* Enclosure," 99.

53. Nāgārjuna, *Fundamental Wisdom of the Middle Way*, XXV.19.

54. Milarepa, *The Hundred Thousand Songs of Milarepa*, "Heartfelt Advice to Rechungpa," 582.

55. Milarepa, *The Hundred Thousand Songs of Milarepa*, "Heartfelt Advice to Rechungpa," 578.

56. See D. Duckworth, "From Yogācāra to Philosophical Tantra in Kashmir and Tibet," *Sophia* (2018): 57, 611–23.

57. A. Padoux, "Tantrism," in *Encyclopedia of Religions,* vol. 14, ed. Mircea Eliade (New York: Macmillan, 1986), 273.

58. Abhinavagupta, *Tantrāloka. Luce dei Tantra,* ed. R. Gnoli (Milan: Adelphi, 2017, 106–109, 92.); English translation by the author. In the belief that everything has the potential to be a door through which to access the supreme consciousness, the more radical left hand lineage tantric schools used specific secret rituals to explore forbidden practices like meditating in cremation grounds, eating meat, and including yogic sexual practices.

59. Vasgupta, *Śivasūtra* of Vasgupta, ed. R. Torella (Milan: Adelphi, 2013) 139 n. 18; Why did you put here the page number before the aphorism? English translation by the author.

60. A. Sironi, ed. *Vijñānabhairava Tantra* (Milan: Adelphi, 1989, no. 73); English translation by the author.

61. Sironi, ed. *Vijñānabhairava Tantra,* n. 62.

62. Milarepa, *The Hundred Thousand Songs of Milarepa,* "The Song at the Inn," 154.

63. Milarepa, *The Hundred Thousand Songs of Milarepa,* "The Song of the Eight Wondrous Joys," 508.

64. Clear Light is referred to also with the term *prakāśa*. The term *prakāśa* (often in relation to *Vimarśa*) is also used in the Tantric Śiva-Śakti tradition of Śrīvidyā: "May the Great Lord who is ever wakeful in the blissful play of the repeated acts of Creation, Maintenance, and Dissolution of all the worlds that issue from Him, protect you. He is mere illumination (*Prakāśa*). Merged in him is *Vimarśa(-śakti)*" Puṇyānandanātha, *Kāma-Kalā-Vilāsa* (fourteenth century CE), trans. by A. Avalon. Madras: Ganesh and co. 1953, verse 1, 1.

65. Milarepa, *The Hundred Thousand Songs of Milarepa,* "The Shepherd's Search for Mind," 128.

66. Milarepa, *The Hundred Thousand Songs of Milarepa,* 128.

67. Milarepa, *The Hundred Thousand Songs of Milarepa,* "In the Dread Bardo Path," 345.

68. Padmasambhava (approximately 755–797 CE) is the author of the *Bardo Tödöl Chenmo* and brought Buddhism to Tibet.

69. *Ba* meaning "between," *Do*: "suspended," *Thos*: "listening," *Grol*: "liberation."

70. Padmasambhava, *The Tibetan Book of the Dead: The Great Liberation through Hearing in the Bardo,* ed. Guru Rinpoche according to Karma Lingpa, trans. by Francesca Fremantle and Chogyam Trungpa (Boston and London: Shambala, 1987), 43: "At that moment do not be afraid of the sharp, brilliant, luminous and clear white light, but recognise it as

wisdom." Padmasambhava, *Il libro tibetano dei morti*, ed. Giuseppe Tucci (Milan: Bur, 2019) 107.

71. In the *Bardo Tödöl Chenmo* six intermediate states are described: 1) matrix, 2) dream state, 3) concentration, 4) moment of death, 5) existential plane, 6) transmigration. The last three are described more at length. Padmasambhava, *Il libro tibetano dei morti*, 112.

72. Padmasambhava, *The Tibetan Book of the Dead*, 64: "Do not be afraid of him, do not be terrified, do not be bewildered. Recognise him as the form of your own mind. . . . Recognition and liberation are simultaneous." Within the Tibetan tradition, once the signs of death have emerged, the practitioners can choose to begin a final meditation from which they will not come back: "Thukdam is an honorific term meaning 'to be engaged in meditation practice,' but it's usually reserved specifically for the meditation practice of abiding in the clear light of pure awareness or the ground luminosity at death." Thompson, *Waking, Dreaming, Being*, 294.

73. Padmasambhava, *The Tibetan Book of the Dead*, 78. Padmasambhava, *Il libro tibetano dei morti*, 171: "Until yesterday you were distracted, so although so much of the bardo state has appeared you have not recognised, and you have so much fear. If you are distracted now, the rope of compassion will be cut off and you will go to a place where there is no liberation, so be careful" Padmasambhava, *The Tibetan Book of the Dead*, 78.

74. Tilopa-Nāropā-Marpa-Milarepa lineage, from which the Kagyu school originates.

75. Tenzin Gyatso, *The World of Tibetan Buddhism*, 95–96. "The reference here is to the experience of entering into union with a consort of the opposite sex, through which the vital elements located at the crown are melted, and then, through the power of meditation, their flow is reversed upward. One of the prerequisites for engaging in such an advanced practice of sexual union is that the practitioner should have the ability to abstain from the fault of emission. Emission of sexual fluids is said to be damaging to one's practice, particularly according to the explanations found in the Kālacakra Tantra."

76. Sironi, ed., *Vijñānabhairava Tantra*, n. 113, n. 116, 51. English translation by the author.

77. See paragraph on Husserl's distinction between body as object [*Koerper*] and lived-body [*Leib*].

78. *Chāndogya Upaniṣad*, VIII. 12. 3, 594.

79. *Kaṭha Upanishad*, I. 3. 5, 834.

80. *Māṇḍūkya Upaniṣad*, II. 17, 1048.

81. *Māṇḍūkya Upaniṣad*, III. 39, in Raphael, *Upaniṣad*, 1071.

82. *Vaiśeṣikasūtra*, 28 5.2.15–16, cited in Mallinson and Singleton, *Roots of Yoga*, chap. 1, "Yoga," 1.1.7.

83. A. David-Néel, *The Secret Oral Teachings in Tibetan Buddhist Sects* (San Francisco: City Lights, 1972) 17–18.

84. Patañjali, *Yogasūtra*, II. 43, 272.

85. Tenzin Gyatso, *The World of Tibetan Buddhism*, "The Distinctive Features of Tantra," 80 and following.

86. Nāgārjuna, *Fundamental Wisdom of the Middle Way*, XXIV. 11, 68.

87. Kālacakra literally means the wheel [*cakra*] of time [*Kāla*]. Kālacakra is also the primal Buddha, liberator of creatures, the one who destroys the wheel of time.

88. Tenzin Gyatso, *The World of Tibetan Buddhism*, 24.

89. It is the surviving part of the *Mulachakratantra;* mentioned in the *Laghuchakratantra* and in the comment to the *Vimalaprabha,*"The Radiance of Purity" by Puṇḍarīka (King Kalkin, ninth century CE—succesor of Sucandra as king of Śambala). In this latter text the first occurrences of the term *haṭha* are to be found.

90. The bliss sensation is described as a thousand times greater than the one arising from ordinary intercourse, that is from one who has not yet realized emptiness and is still a victim of the objects of the mind.

91. Nāropā, *Iniziazione. Kālacakra,* [*Sekoddesa*], ed., R. Gnoli (Milan: Adelphi, 1994), 344. Nāropā's comment to this verse reads as follows: "Sin is born from the destruction of desire, because from it the aversion towards the beloved woman is born, from aversion come obfuscation, and from this, with a fallen vajra, a state of mental confusion, and activity directed only towards other mean objects, as food and drinks, ecc. The from-all-this-deluded mind becomes without pleasure and wanders through the six births [. . .] Compassion is linked with the silent gaze, benevolence with the embrace, joy with the contact of the woman, equanimity with the motionless pleasure that takes place within union. In this way the one who is united with such a yoga how can he be bond to desire [vulgar]."

92. V. A. Wallace, ed., *The Kālacakra Tantra*. The Chapter on Sadhana. Together with the Vimalaprabha commentary, trans. V. A. Wallace (New York: Columbia University's Center for Buddhist Studies, 2010), 130.

93. *Samyutta Nikāya*, 12. 61. Also Sutta Nipata 4.4: "Having left a former (object) they attach themselves to another, dominated by craving they do not go beyond attachment. They reject and seize, like a monkey letting go of a branch to take hold of another."

94. Nāropā, *Kālacakra*, 341–43. It is also added: "just so the stain of the mind is destructed thanks to its conjunction with emptiness," n. 133, 342.

95. The initiation can include a ritual of adoration of the deity embracing his consort, the so called Prajña.

96. The list of six stages is: *Pratyāhāra, Dhyāna, Prāṇāyāma, Dhāraṇā* [rintention of the bindu], *Anusmṛti* [recollection], *Samādhi*. Comparing these

six limbs to Patañjali's one, what is noticeable is the absence of the first three limbs of the *aṣṭāṅga-yoga*. However, within the Kālacakra tradition great emphasis is placed on the preliminary practices that, together with the *bodhicitta* resolution, hold the place of the prescriptions that must be fulfilled (*Yamā* and *Nyamā*). The place of the *āsana* [seat, posture] is covered within this tradition by physical practices performed with a partner [*mudrā*], called *yogini-tantra* or *karma-mudrā*; in more advanced stages these are replaced with figured meditations [*jñana-mudrā*]. It is important to highlight the presence of a number of female practitioners and *yogini* masters within Tibetan traditions. Marpa's wife was considered to be a yogini herself. Another example is Machig Labdrön [1055–1149 CE) a female Tibetan Buddhist monk, a tantric master and yogini who originated several Tibetan lineages of the Vajrayana practice of Chöd.

97. Nāropā, *Kālacakra*, n. 147, 355.

98. Here it is worth noting that not all tantric traditions prescribe practices with no emission of sexual fluid.

99. Nāropā, *Kālacakra*, n. 141, 346–47.

100. Wallace, *The Kālacakra Tantra*, 141.

101. Wallace, *The Kālacakra Tantra*, chapter II, 27.

102. Tzong Kapha (1357–1419).

103. A commentary to the *Bodhi-patha-pradipa* by Atiśa.

104. G. H. Mullin, *The Six Yogas of Naropa*, Snowlion, Colorado, 1996, 117. Tzong Kapha is not for the subtle when speaking of the risks faced by the one who doesn't undergo initiation.

105. The six yogas, literally called *dhammas* [*dharmas*] within the text, are: 1. yoga of Internal heat, 2. yoga of the illusionary body, 3. yoga of the clear light, 4. yoga of the *bardo*, 5. yoga of the consciousness transference, towards paradises, 6. yoga of the forceful projection, in a new residence (mentioned already by Patañjali III. 38).

106. Tzongkapha, *The Six Yogas of Naropa: Tsongkhapa's commentary entitled A Book of Three Inspirations*, ed. and trans. G. H. Mullin (New York: Snow Lion Publications, 1996) 134–35.

107. Tzongkapha, *The Six Yogas of Naropa*, 122–26.

108. Tzongkapha, *The Six Yogas of Naropa*, 134, 150–53.

109. Tzongkapha, *The Six Yogas of Naropa*, 156.

110. Tzongkapha, *The Six Yogas of Naropa*, 139.

111. Tzongkapha, *The Six Yogas of Naropa*, 161.

112. Tzongkapha, *The Six Yogas of Naropa*, 172–73.

113. Tzongkapha, *The Six Yogas of Naropa*, 207.

114. Tzongkapha, *The Six Yogas of Naropa*, 183.

115. Tzongkapha, *The Six Yogas of Naropa*, 205–6.

116. Tzongkapha, *The Six Yogas of Naropa*, 206.

117. Tzongkapha, *The Six Yogas of Naropa,* 209.

118. Lama Yeshe, *The Bliss of the Inner Fire. Heart Practice of the Six Yogas of Naropa* (Somerville, MA: Wisdom Publications, 1998) 181 [Lama Yeshe, *La beatitudine del fuoco interiore.* Pomaia: Chiara Luce edizioni, 2003].

119. Lama Yeshe, *The Bliss of the Inner Fire,* 211.

120. Lama Yeshe, *The bliss of the inner fire,* 99 [*La beatitudine del fuoco interiore,* 116].

121. Lama Yeshe, *The bliss of the inner fire,* 126, 166 [*La beatitudine del fuoco interiore,* 145, 191]

122. It is a purifying exercise in which the practitioner is asked to visualize "every negative energy" and "your internal garbage, is forced out through the openings of your lower body in the form of snakes, scorpions, worms, ants, or whatever else you find effective"; Lama Yeshe, *The Bliss of the Inner Fire,* 55 [*La beatitudine del fuoco interiore,* 61].

123. Lama Yeshe, *The Bliss of the Inner Fire,* 139 [*La beatitudine del fuoco interiore,* 159]

124. The connection between the inner flames of the chandali and the kundalini will become evident in the paragraph on *haṭha* yoga.

125. Nāropā, *Kālacakra,* 238, 246.

126. A. David-Néel, *My Journey to Lhasa: The Personal Story of the Only White Woman Who Succeeded in Entering the Forbidden City* (New York: Harper and Brothers, 1927), 132.

127. David-Néel, *My Journey to Lhasa,* 132.

128. David-Néel, *My Journey to Lhasa,* 134.

129. The union of emptiness and compassion is often depicted as taking the shape of the Buddha Vajrasattva, the union of feminine and masculine.

130. Nāgārjuna, *Fundamental Wisdom of the Middle Way,* VII.16, 20.

131. Nāgārjuna, *Fundamental Wisdom of the Middle Way,* 152.

Chapter 6

1. Heisenberg summarizes the situation as follows: "Classical physics can be considered as that idealization according to which we speak of the world as something entirely separable from us [. . .] the world appears [in quantum physics] as a complex tissue of events, in which different relations take turn, overlap and combine." See W. Heisenberg, *Fisica e filosofia* (Milan: Feltrinelli, 2021, 127, 128) English translation by the author.

2. Rovelli speaking about entanglement in physics: "knotting, imbrication, involvement, intertwin, tangling, sentimental relation [. . .] two particles that have met on the past, maintain a sort of strange bond,

as if they continued talking to each other [. . .] Schrödinger's wave of two objects is not the whole of the two waves: it is a more complex wave that contains other information" Carlo Rovelli, *Helgoland* (Milan: Adelphi, 2020, 100, 103). This and the following quotes by Rovelli are translated in English by the author. Rovelli adds that "a correlation between two objects is a property of both objects: as all properties it exists only in relation to a further, third object. Entanglement is not dancing in two: it is a dance between three," 106.

3. Rovelli, *Helgoland,* 142.

4. Rovelli, *Helgoland,* 153–55.

5. Rovelli, *Helgoland,* 24.

6. "We cannot describe any elementary entity, unless within the context with which it interacts [. . .] Quantum theory is the theory of how things influence each other [. . .] properties of things are relative to other things and are realized within interactions" Rovelli, *Helgoland,* 148, 86, 99. Merleau-Ponty on the topic states: "The function ψ (x, y, z.) represents a maximum description of the composed 'object;' consisting in the object properly called (x), the apparatus (y), and the observer (z); nevertheless we do not know in what state the object x is found." Maurice Merleau-Ponty, *Nature. Course Notes from the Collège de France,* trans. R. Vallier (Evanston: Northwestern University Press, 2003), 92.

7. "Niels Bohr writes: 'there is no quantic world. There is only an abstract quantic description. It is wrong to think that the task of physics is to describe how nature is'" Rovelli, *Helgoland,* 49.

8. Merleau-Ponty, *Nature. Course Notes from the Collège de France,* 100.

9. Maurice Merleau-Ponty, *Résumés de Cours. Collège de France 1952–1960,* [Écrits 1957–58] (Paris: Gallimard, 1968), 129; Merleau-Ponty, *La nature. Notes cours du Collège de France,* ed. D. Seglard (Paris: Éditions de Seuil, 1995), 372. This and the following quotes are translated to English by the author; Merleau-Ponty, *Linguaggio, Storia, Natura. Corsi al Collège de France, 1952–1961,* ed. M. Carbone (Milan: Bompiani, 1995), 99.

10. Merleau-Ponty, *Nature. Course Notes from the Collège de France,* 91.

11. Merleau-Ponty, *Résumés de Cours,* 132 / Merleau-Ponty, *La nature. Notes cours du Collège de France,* 373 / Merleau-Ponty, *Linguaggio, storia, natura,* 100.

12. Merleau-Ponty, *Résumés de Cours,* 120/ Merleau-Ponty *Linguaggio, storia, natura,* 92.

13. According to philosopher of science Michel Bitbol, quantum theories are "a general procedure for anticipating probabilistically the replies to context-dependent experimental solicitations." Bitbol refers to Anton Zeilinger (pioneer of quantum computer science and recently awarded the Nobel Prize) as "the forerunner of this new trend" in that "according

to this interpretation, the information made available by experiments exhausts 'reality' " M. Bitbol, "A Phenomenological Ontology for Physics. Merleau-Ponty and QBism," in *Phenomenological Approaches to Physics*, ed. H. Wiltsche and P. Berghofer (Springer, 2020), *3, 4*. Bitbol argues that "the most consistent phenomenological approach of quantum mechanics is presumably QBism. QBism is an acronym for "Quantum Bayesianism." According to QBism, "state" vectors are just probabilistic valuations, in a Bayesian sense. They are not statements about what is the case, but statements about what each agent can reasonably expect to be the case. [. . .] According to QBism, the quantum "state" has no direct representational bearing on physical processes; it is a symbolic tool within 'a calculus for gambling on each agent's own experience.' [. . .] Quantum entangled states *predict* that a correlation *will* be observed in the *future* with a high *probability*"; M. Bitbol, "Is the Life-World Reduction Sufficient in Quantum Physics?" *Continental Philosophy Review* (2020): 20–21.

14. "By now, even for science, the objective-being cannot be any longer being-itself: objective' and 'subjective' are domains hastily constructed out of a totalizing experience" Merleau-Ponty, *The Visible and the Invisible*, 37.

15. See Giulia Moiraghi, *In cammino verso la cosa* (Milan: Mimesis, 2006), 29–31.

16. Heidegger, *Being and Time*, 69, 66.

17. Heidegger, *Being and Time*, 69, 66.

18. "Objectification is a matter of method, founded upon prescientific data of experience. Mathematical method "constructs," out of intuitive representation, ideal objects and teaches how to deal with them operatively and systematically"; Husserl, *The Crisis*, 348.

19. Heidegger, "The Age of the World Picture," 115.

20. According to Heidegger the means refers to the one who employs it; it is shaped on the body of the one who will make use of it. See the connections with Gibson's concept of affordance in James J. Gibson, *The Senses Considered as Perceptual Systems* (Boston: Houghton Mifflin, 1966).

21. See Heidegger, *Being and Time*, § 22 [102 and following], *94. From a genealogical point of view "handiness" [*Zuhandenheit*], the distinctive character of the equipment [*Zeug*], comes before simple presence [*Vor-handenheit*].

22. Heidegger, *Being and Time*, [63], 68–69.

23. "Thus in whatever way we may be conscious of the world as universal horizon, as coherent universe of existing objects, we, each 'I-the-man' and all of us together, belong to the world as living with one another in the world; and the world is our world, valid for our consciousness as existing precisely through this 'living together.' We, as living in wakeful world-consciousness, are constantly active on the basis

of our passive having of the world [. . .] we, in living together, have the world pregiven in this 'together,' as the world valid as existing for us and to which we, together, belong, the world as world for all, pregiven with this ontic meaning. Constantly functioning in wakeful life, we also function together" Husserl, *The Crisis*, 108–9.

24. Varela et al., *The Embodied Mind*, 3–4.

25. Varela et al., *The Embodied Mind*, 217.

26. Varela et al., *The Embodied Mind*, 202.

27. F. J. Varela, "Neurophenomenology. A Methodological Remedy for the Hard Problem," *Journal of Consciousness Studies* 3, no. 4 (1996): 339.

28. Merleau-Ponty, *Phenomenology of Perception*, 159.

29. Merleau-Ponty, *Phenomenology of Perception*, 499–500.

30. F. J. Varela, *Ethical Know-how* (Stanford, CA: Stanford University Press, 1999), 17.

31. Varela, *The Embodied Mind*, 9.

32. One should imagine another "*homunculus*" existing within the brain of the previous *homunculus* and so on.

33. Dennett, *Consciousness Explained*, 107.

34. F. Crick, *The Astonishing Hypothesis* (New York: Charles Scribner's Sons, 1994).

35. Examples include Jackendoff's projective mechanism, Baars's global workspace theory, Dennett's multiple drafts model of consciousness, Calvin's Darwin machines, and Edelman's neural Darwinism.

36. Varela speaks of "mysterians" referring for example T. Nagel (1986) and C. McGinn (1991) Varela, "Neurophenomenology," 333.

37. Varela, "Neurophenomenology," 333. More recent theories such as the Integrated Information Theory by Giulio Tononi or Roger Penrose and Stuart Hameroff debate on the microtubules are obviously not considered in Varela's overview.

38. Varela, "Neurophenomenology," 345–46.

39. Varela, "Neurophenomenology," 347.

40. Varela, "Neurophenomenology," 337.

41. Husserl, *The Crisis*, § 38, 144 [*La Crisi*, 172].

42. Varela, "Neurophenomenology," 337.

43. Husserl, *The idea of Phenomenology*, [8], 5 [Husserl, *L'idea della fenomenologia*, 46].

44. Husserl, *Erste Philosophie*, 142.

45. Husserl, *Ideas*, XIX, [3].

46. Varela, "Neurophenomenology," 33.

47. Varela, "Neurophenomenology," 338–39.

48. Varela, "Neurophenomenology," 337.

49. Varela, "Neurophenomenology," 341.

50. Varela, "Neurophenomenology," 343.

51. "Phenomenological accounts of the structure of experience and their counterparts in cognitive science relate to each other through reciprocal constraints"; Varela, "Neurophenomenology," 343.

52. Varela, "Neurophenomenology," 344.

53. F. J. Varela, "The Specious Present: A Neurophenomenology of Time Consciousness," to appear in: J. Petitot, F. J. Varela, J.-M. Roy, B. Pachoud and (Eds.), *Naturalizing Phenomenology: Issues in Contemporary Phenomenology and Cognitive Science*. Stanford University Press, 1997.

54. Husserl, *Analysen zur passiven synthesis*.

55. Varela, "Neurophenomenology," 342. See also N. Depraz, F. Varela, and P. Vermersch, *On Becoming Aware* (Amsterdam: John Benjamins, 2002), 123.

56. Varela et al., *On Becoming Aware* (Amsterdam: John Benjamins, 2002), 342.

57. Varela, "Neurophenomenology," 346.

58. Varela, "Neurophenomenology," 133.

59. Varela et al., *The Embodied Mind*, 144.

60. Tsongkhapa, *The Great Treatise on the stages of the Path to Enlightenment*, ed. J. Cutler, G. Newland (New York: Snow Lion Publications, 2002, [660]) 211.

61. Tsongkhapa, *The Great Treatise on the stages of the Path to Enlightenment*, [575], 120.

62. Tsongkhapa, *The Great Treatise on the Stages of the Path to Enlightenment*, [575], 120.

Chapter 7

1. See Dasgupta, *Obscure Religious Cults*, cited in M. Eliade, *Immortality and Freedom*, 228.

2. *Yogabija*, 170, 187, in Mallinson and Singleton, *The Roots of Yoga*, [170], [187], 365, 389.

3. The first meaning of *dharma/dhamma* is: "cosmic law and order."

4. There are many meanings orbiting around the term "phenomenon." It is commonly used as the object of observation and study in the hard sciences and especially the human sciences. Consequently, "phenomenology" in this framework comes to indicate an empirically based investigation and description. The use of the term to describe an extraordinary event, common among journalists, is indebted to this first meaning of the word. In psychology, some authors use the terms "phenomenology" or "phenomenological" to refer to psychological theories of introspection,

while others intend the branch of psychology that has developed under the name "phenomenological psychology," which is more closely connected to Husserl's views. Giorgi and Ashworth distinguish this form of phenomenological psychology from other branches of psychology that are more loosely classified as phenomenological. See A. Giorgi, "Concerning the Possibility of Phenomenological Psychological Research," *Journal of Phenomenological Psychology* 14, no. 1–2 (1983), 129–69; and P. Ashworth, "Some Notes on Phenomenological Approaches in Psychology," *Bulletin of the British Psychological Society* 29 (1976): 363–68.

5. This is the kind of depth to which the Greeks, according to Nietzsche, were devoted to: "Those Greeks were superficial—out of profundity"; F. Nietzsche, *The Gay Science*, ed. B. Williams (Cambridge: Cambridge University Press, 2001), 9.

6. *Māṇḍūkya Upaniṣad,* IV 99, 1099.

7. *Chāndogya Upaniṣad* VI. VIII. 7, 502.

8. A. Schopenhauer, *Die Welt als Wille und Forstellung,* Zweiter Tailband (Diogenes, 2017) 480: "die schon erwähnte Formel des Veda: 'Tat twam asi!' (Dieses bist du!)." This problem of translation is not recognizable in the English version of the text, in which the phrase is generally rendered in the philologically correct form: "you are that."

9. Schopenhauer, *Die Welt als Wille und Forstellung II,* 280 "Tat twam asi, das heißt: Dieses Lebende bist du."

10. On the theme see P. Deussen, *Outlines of Indian Philosophy: with an appendix on the philosophy of the Vedanta in its Relation to Occidental Metaphysics* (K. Curtious, 1907) 58–63.

11. *Yogabīja* 51, in Mallinson and Singleton, *The Roots of Yoga,* 5.6.2.

12. Husserl, *Erste Philosophie,* 167.

13. Iris, the messenger of the gods, is the rainbow which passes between earth and heaven.

14. *Theaetetus,* 155 d, Plato, *Complete works,* edited by J. M. Cooper (Hackett, 1997), 173.

15. Śivasūtra no. 12 [*vismayo yogabhūmikāḥ*], Vasugupta, *Śivasūtra,* 126. English translation by the author.

16. Vasugupta, *Śivasūtra,* 126.

17. David-Néel, *The Secret Oral Teachings in Tibetan Buddhist Sects,* 15–16.

18. Calasso, *Ardor,* 25.

19. Bitbol, *La conscience a-t-elle une origine?,* 12 English translation by the author.

20. It is the seventh consciousness after the five sense-consciousness, and the analytical consciousness, the sixth. And comes before the Ālaya-vijñāna (store house/foundation consciousness). On the relations between

Madhyamaka and Yogācāra see J. L. Garfield J. Westerhoff, *Madhyamaka and Yogācāra—Allies or Rivals?* (Oxford: Oxford University Press, 2015).

21. Mircea Eliade, *Lo sciamanismo e le tecniche dell'estasi* (Rome: Mediterranee, 1974), 456, 321; see also Eliade, *Yoga. Immortality and Freedom*, 322.

22. Eliade, *Yoga. Immortality and Freedom*, 442, 453; Padoux describes this relationship as "a particular attitude on the part of the Tantric adept toward the cosmos, whereby he feels integrated within an all-embracing system of micro-macrocosmic correlations" A. Padoux, "Tantrism," in *Encyclopedia of Religions* 14, ed. Mircea Eliade (New York: Macmillan, 1986), 273.

23. Swami Lakshmanjoo, *Śiva Sutras* (Universal Shaiva Fellowship, 2007), 57.

24. An ithyphallic Śivapaśupati seated in a position similar to *Baddhakoṇāsana* and surrounded by all sorts of animals appears on the Mohenjo-Daro seal. This theory was promoted by archaeologist John Marshall and though controversial today is still credited by many: J. H. Marshall, *Mohenjo-Daro and the Indus Civilization* (London: Probsthain, 1931).

25. Gorakṣanātha lived between the IXth and the XIIth century and is traditionally considered the founder of the Nāth Haṭha Yoga and of the Śaiva order.

26. "The *Amṛtasiddhi* was directly drawn upon in the production of several subsequent *haṭha* texts, none of which was Buddhist and the earliest of which was probably the Nāth Śaiva Amaraughaprabodha" J. Mallinson, "Kālavañcana in the Konkan: How a Vajrayāna Haṭhayoga Tradition Cheated Buddhism's Death in India," *Religions* (2019): 10, 273, 2.

27. Mallinson, "Kālavañcana in the Konkan," 2.

28. Mallinson, "Kālavañcana in the Konkan," 2.

29. Dating to roughly the fifteenth century CE. A settled system comparable to the one of *Haṭhayogapradīpikā* is anticipated by a Vaishnava text of the thirteenth century, a system that also considers the presence of the yogini. Mallinson and Singleton, *The Roots of Yoga*, 240.

30. Svātmārāma, *Haṭhayogapradīpikā*, IV. 18, in *Light on Hatha Yoga*, ed. Swami Muktibodhananda (Munger: Yoga Publications Trust, Bihar School of Yoga, 1985), 493.

31. (c. 1000 BCE) *Atharvaveda*, XV.15–18 in R. T. H. Griffith, *The Hymns of the Atharva Veda*, 197–98.

32. *Praśna Upaniṣad*, IV.3.4, Raphael, *Upaniṣad*, 935–37.

33. In the *Śiva Saṃhitā* it is said that "One should work hard at it" I. 18; "If he energetically practices thus every day for three months, then his *nāḍī*-s are sure to be purified forthwith" II. 26; "with uninterrupted exercise" V. 73. J. Mallinson, ed., *The Shiva Samhita* (Yoga Vidya, 2007).

34. The central channel is flanked by two other important *nāḍī*-s: Iḍā (the moon channel) and Piṅgalā (the sun channel).

35. *Bṛhadāraṇyaka Upaniṣad*, II. 1. 19, in Raphael, *Upaniṣad*, 73.

36. Svātmārāma, *Haṭhayogapradīpikā*, II. 5, 160.

37. *prānavāyu, apānavāyu, samānavāyu, udānavāyu* and *vyānavāyu.*

38. Svātmārāma, *Haṭhayogapradīpikā*, II. 47, 236.

39. T.K.V. Desikachar (1938—2016), the son of Tirumalai Krishnamacharya, belongs to the Krishnamacharya lineage.

40. T.K.V. Desikachar, *The Heart of Yoga* (Rochester, VT: Inner Traditions, 1999) 116.

41. Svātmārāma, *Haṭhayogapradīpikā*, II. 20, 183; Also specific *prāṇāyāma* rapid breathing patterns, such as the *bhastrika* are described in connection with the metaphor of the fire: "with the same motion as a pair of bellows [*bhastrā*] being pumped" II. 62, 205.

42. See *The serpent power* by the British orientalist John Woodroffe, alias, A. Avalon (1865–1936), (sixth chapter of the *Sri Tattva Chintamani*, XVI CE) by Swami Purnananda: A. Avalon, *The Serpent Power: Being the Sat-Cakra-Nirupana and Paduka-Pancaka* [1919] (New York: Dover Publications, 1958).

43. Root √*tap* of *tapas.*

44. Svātmārāma, *Haṭhayogapradīpikā*, III. 66, 67, 68, 69, 349–351.

45. "At the end of inhalation, *jālandhara* bandha is done. At the end of *kumbhaka* and beginning of exhalation, *uḍḍīyāna* bandha is done" Svātmārāma, *Haṭhayogapradīpikā*, II. 45, 234; III. 55, 332; III. 61, 340; the *Mahābandha* is the conjunction of the three locks, II. 46, 234; *uḍḍīyāna* literally means "flying up," whereas *jālandhara* literally means the "net bearer," referring to the net of *nāḍī*-s.

46. In haṭhayoga, the centrality of tapas and the purifying fire is such that Mallinson and Singleton claim that the "Tamil *Tirumandiram*, whose teachings on yoga are perhaps contemporaneous with or a little later than those of the *Dattātreyayogaśāstra*, *haṭhayoga* is called *tavayoga*, *tava* being the Tamil form of the Sanskrit *tapas*" Mallinson Singleton, *The Roots of Yoga*, "Introduction," chapter on *Haṭhayoga*.

47. Svātmārāma, *Haṭhayogapradīpikā*, II. 22, 186 "*Dhautī, basti, netī, trāṭaka, naulī* and kapālabhāti; these are known as *shatkarma* or the six cleansing processes."

48. Such as the hands or the tongue, as for example the *khecarī mudrā*: "Having turned, the tongue back, the three channels of Iḍā, Piṅgalā and Suṣumnā are controlled. This is *khecarī mudrā* and it is called the center [*cakra*] of ether" Svātmārāma, *Haṭhayogapradīpikā*, III.37, 312.

49. Also *āsana* means seat.

50. Svātmārāma, *Haṭhayogapradīpikā,* I.39, 110.

51. Svātmārāma, *Haṭhayogapradīpikā,* III.10, 291.

52. Literally indicating the male sexual fluid.

53. Svātmārāma, *Haṭhayogapradīpikā,* "The knower of yoga, perfect in the practice, conserves his *bindu* and the woman's rajas by drawing it up through the generative organ" III. 91, 389; III. 64, 344.

54. *Yogabīja,* 148, 149, ed. Rām Lāl Śrīvāstav (Gorakhpur: Śrī Gorakhnāth Mandir, 1982).

55. J. Birch, "The Meaning of Haṭha in Early Haṭhayoga," *Journal of the American Oriental Society* 131, no. 4 (October–December 2011): 527–58.

56. Svātmārāma, *Haṭhayogapradīpikā,* III.77, 78, 363.

57. Svātmārāma, *Haṭhayogapradīpikā,* III. 79, 363.

58. This explains the cryptic nature of the text, intended to be used just as a support for the one who has already learned the techniques by his own teacher: "Yoga should be practiced in the way instructed by the guru" Svātmārāma, *Haṭhayogapradīpikā,* I.14, II.1, 47, 149.

59. However in later versions of the *Haṭhayogapradīpikā, Yamāḥ* and *Nyamāḥ* are restored to the text for the sake of ecumenism.

60. Svātmārāma, *Haṭhayogapradīpikā* I. 15, 50.

61. Husserl, *Erste Philosophie,* 11.

62. Svātmārāma, *Haṭhayogapradīpikā* I.11, 37.

63. "When mind attains *unmanī,* duality [*a-dvaita*] is lost" Svātmārāma, *Haṭhayogapradīpikā,* IV. 61, 553.

64. Svātmārāma, *Haṭhayogapradīpikā,* IV. 58, 549.

65. Svātmārāma, *Haṭhayogapradīpikā,* IV. 3–4, 472: "*Rājayogah samādhiścha unmanī cha manonmanī Amaratvam layastattvam śūnyāśūnyam param padam Amanaskam tathādvaitam nirālambam nirañjanam Jīvanmuktiścha sahajā turyā chetyekavāchakāh.*"

66. Svātmārāma, *Haṭhayogapradīpikā,* IV. 10, 480. See also IV. 37, 522: "the state of *śūnyā-aśūnyā* arises"

67. Patañjali, *The Yoga Sutras of* Patañjali, III. 26, 353.

68. Patañjali, *The Yoga Sutras of* Patañjali, III. 27, 356. As Bryant notes: "Hariharānanda relates this sutra, too, to tantric physiology," 356.

69. Patañjali, *The Yoga Sutras of* Patañjali, III. 29, 357.

70. Patañjali, *The Yoga Sutras of* Patañjali, III. 36–37, 366–67.

71. Bitbol, *La conscience a-t-elle une origine?* 180; "un rélévateur de l'ici comme on ne savait plus le rencontrer à force de trops savoir"). English translation by the author.

72. Patañjali, *Yogasūtra of Patañjali,* 330.

73. This how contemporary tantric teacher Eric Baret refers to this deconditioning role: "The practice of exploring the subtle body gradually

leads to the brain becoming deconditioned. Notions of time and space are called into question when these openings take place. [. . .] The sites of a sacred geography are then clearly disclosed" (E. Baret, *Yoga Tantrico* (Rome: Mediterranee, Roma, 2005), 35. English Translation by the author.

74. Needleman, "Inner Empiricism as a Way to a Science of Consciousness."

75. Ludwig Wittgenstein, *Tractatus Logico-Philosophicus,* trans. D. F. Pears and B. F. McGuinness (London: Routledge, 2001), 54, 89.

76. Husserl, *The Crisis,* 298.

77. Merleau-Ponty argues against what he calls a high-altitude thinking [*pensée de survol*] and claims that "depth cannot be understood as belonging to the thought of an acosmic subject, but as a possibility of a subject involved in the world," Merleau-Ponty, *Phenomenology of Perception,* 311.

78. "Thus the particular object of our active consciousness, and correlatively the active, conscious having of it, being directed toward it, and dealing with it—all this is forever surrounded by an atmosphere of mute, concealed, but co-functioning validities, a vital horizon" Husserl, *The Crisis,* § 40, 149.

79. Literally a "constantly flowing horizonal character" Husserl, *The Crisis,* § 40, 149.

80. Husserl, *The Crisis,* § 47, 188.

81. Husserl, *Ideas,* § 40, [157] 164.

82. Husserl, *The Crisis,* § 47, 88.

83. Husserl, *Ideas,* § 41, [158], 165–66.

84. Husserl, *Ideas,* § 41, [158], 166.

85. "Between appearing of things and the kinesthetic system (the whole of the movement possibilities) there is a coordination, the lived body takes over a transcendental function, from this a belief in the world is established and the hypothesis of a brain in a vat is excluded" (V. Costa, E. Franzini, P. Spinicci, *La fenomenologia.* Milan: Einaudi, 2002), 182.

86. Husserl, *Ideas,* § 41, [158], 166.

87. Husserl, *Ideas,* § 41 [159], 166.

88. Husserl, *Ideas,* § 37 [150], 157.

89. See the topic tackled in T. Metzinger, *The Ego Tunnel: The Science of the Mind and the Myth of the Self* (New York: Basic Books, 2010).

90. Y. Ataria, "Where Do We End, and Where Does the World Begin? The Case of Insight Meditation," *Philosophical Psychology* 28, no. 8 (2014): 1128–46, 1128–46; Evan Thompson also reports of cases of electrical induced out-of-body experiences: Thompson, *Waking, Dreaming, Being,*

207–13. On the topic neuroscientist Thomas Metzinger argues as follows: "It is interesting to note how OBEs [out-of-body experiences], phenomenologically, are not states of disembodiment" T. Metzinger, "Out-of-Body Experiences as the Origin of the Concept of a 'Soul,'" *Mind & Matter* 3 (2005): 57–84, 68.

91. Husserl, *Ideas,* § 36 [145], 153.

92. Husserl, *Ideas,* § 36 [146], 153.

93. Husserl, *Ideas,* § 37, [148], 155.

94. Husserl, *Ideas,* [146], 154.

95. Husserl, *Ideas,* [146–47] 154.

96. Husserl, *Ideas,* [147] 154.

97. The view of the author here differs from the one summarized by O'Brien-Kop in her introduction to Patañjali: "What I hope to have conveyed in this book is that the method proposed by Patanjali is not physical practice, since sitting (āsana) is a preparation for meditation, which is rational reflection" (K. O'Brien-Kop, *The Philosophy of the Yogasūtra. An Introduction* (London, Bloomsbury Academic, 2023), 156.

98. The paucity of indications by Vyāsa is explained by *Śankara* as again being due to requiring from the specific teacher a detailed instruction on the execution of the *āsanas*.

99. *Vāchaspati Miśra*'s comment to II. 47, in R. Prasāda, *Patañjali's Yoga Sutras with the commentary of Vyāsa and the gloss of Vāchaspati Miśra* (Munshiram: Manoharlal Publishers, 1998), 170.

100. Vijñānabhikṣu, *Yogabhasyavārtika,* 2.46, in P. A. Maas, "Sthirasukham *āsanam:* Posture and Performance in Classical Yoga and Beyond," in Baier, K., Maas, P. A. and Preisendanz K. (Eds.), *Yoga in Transformation.* Göttingen: Vienna University Press, 49–100 accessed Nov 9, 2018, 80. Sanskritist Philip Mass comments on this by noting that "in the final part of his explanation, Vijñānabhikṣu apparently refers to the fact that the number of postures that have their names derived from animals, of which the *Patañjalayogaśāstra* lists three, i.e., Sitting Like a Sarus Crane, Sitting Like an Elephant and Sitting Like a Camel, can easily be manifolded by taking the sitting poses of other species as a model for specific modes of positioning the body." Maas, "Sthirasukham āsanam," 80.

101. Śankara, *Yogasūtrabhasyavivaraṇa* II. 46, in Maas, "Sthirasukham āsanam," 71, note 75.

102. "The description of the yoga hermitage as prescribed by the siddhas for the *haṭha* yoga practitioners. The room of sadhana should have a small door, without aperture (window), holes or cracks, being neither too high nor too low. It should be spotlessly clean, wiped with cow manure and free from animals or insects. Outside, there should be an open platform with a thatched roof, a well and a surrounding wall (fence). The appearance

of the hermitage should be pleasant" Svātmārāma, *Haṭhayogapradīpikā*, I. 13, 43. This recalls the famous Upanishadic passage: "In a level, clean place, free from gravel, fire and sand. With soundless water, a dwelling and so on. Pleasing to the mind and not harsh on the eye, secret and sheltered from the wind, one should practise yoga" *Śvetāśvatara Upaniṣad*, II, 10.

103. Svātmārāma, *Haṭhayogapradīpikā*, II. 16, 180.

104. Whereas "the *Gheraṇḍa Saṃhitā* teaches the most *āsanas*, namely, thirty-two"; J. Birch, "The Proliferation of āsana-s in Late-Medieval Yoga Texts," in *Yoga in Transformation Historical and Contemporary Perspectives*, ed. K. Baier, P. A. Maas, and K. Preisendanz (Gottingen: Vienne University Press, 2018), 101.

105. Svātmārāma, *Haṭhayogapradīpikā*, I. 25, 82.

106. Svātmārāma, *Haṭhayogapradīpikā*, I. 28, 90.

107. Svātmārāma, *Haṭhayogapradīpikā*, I. 23, 78; I. 30, 94.

108. Svātmārāma, *Haṭhayogapradīpikā*, I. 32, 98.

109. Svātmārāma, *Haṭhayogapradīpikā*, III, 78, 363.

110. According to Mark Singleton, postural *haṭha* yoga owed a large debt to Western gymnastics, bodybuilding, and callisthenic techniques imported into India during the British Raj. Mark Singleton, *Yoga Body. The Origins of Modern Posture Practice* (Oxford University Press, 2010).

111. Birch, "The Proliferation of āsana-s in Late-Medieval Yoga Texts," 104.

112. See V. Sarde, "Yoga on Stone': Sculptural Representation of Yoga on Mahuḍī Gate at Dabhoī in Gujarāt," *Journal of Multidisciplinary Studies in Archaeology*, 5 (2017), 659. See also Mallinson, "Kālavañcana in the Konkan," 3.

113. See Sarde, "Yoga on Stone," 659–75.

114. Sarde, "Yoga on Stone," 659.

115. V. Sarde, "A Medieval Religious Center of Natha and Mahanubhava Sect in Maharashtra," online resource on *Tattva mag*., 2021 https://tattvamag.org/a-medieval-religious-center-of-natha-and-mahanubhava-sect-in-maharashtra. In the online conference "Early images of Nāth yogis in Maharashtra" (2020) Vijay Sarde shows the pillars of the hall of the Ballālāi Devī temple, Brahmani, curved with Nāth yogis and yoginis: https://www.youtube.com/watch?v=wsGB3CKb7zg.

116. Vijay Sarde also confirmed this quite obvious reconstruction at the end of the online conference noted above.

117. Birch, "The Proliferation of āsana-s in Late-Medieval Yoga Texts," 104.

118. Seth Powell, "Etched in Stone: Sixteenth-Century Visual and Material Evidence of Śaiva Ascetics and Yogis in Complex Non-Seated āsana-s at Vijayangara," *Journal of Yoga Studies* 1, no. 48 (2018).

Chapter 8

1. Patañjali, *Yogasūtra,* II. 46, 283 *"Sthira-sukham āsanam"*

2. Patañjali, *Yogasūtra,* II. 47, 287. Within this relaxation, a consonance/concordance [*samapatti*] with the infinite [*ananta*] takes place.

3. Typical of when the moment when the body releases the posture and takes the corpse pose.

4. According to *Vachaspati Misra* the kind of effort at stake is very special and different from the ordinary one, as recalled by Maas: "According to him, the yogi has to replace natural effort with a special yogic effort that finally leads to the perfection of postures: 'After all, a natural effort to hold up the body does not bring about the ancillary of yoga, that is, the posture which is to be taught here; if it did bring about that posture, instruction would be pointless, because it could be achieved all by itself. Therefore, this natural effort does not bring about the posture that is to be taught. And natural effort is counter-productive, because it impedes restraint in posture inasmuch as it is the cause of spontaneous postures. Therefore, a person who is practising the posture that has been taught should make an effort to slacken natural effort. The posture that has been taught cannot be achieved any other way. And so it is that slackening natural effort causes the achievement of the posture.' "; P. A. Maas, "Sthirasukham āsanam," 82.

5. See Vyāsa's comment to *Yogasūtra* II. 47, in R. Prasāda, *Patañjali's Yoga Sutras with the commentary of Vyāsa and the gloss of Vāchaspati Miśra* (Munshiram: Manoharlal, 1998), 170.

6. Vijñānabhikṣu, *Yogabhasyavārtika,* 2.47, in Maas, "Sthirasukham āsanam," 82.

7. Patañjali, *Yogasūtra,* I. 2, I. 3, 10, 22.

8. See Vyāsa's comment to *Yogasūtra* II. 47, in Prasāda, *Patañjali's Yoga Sutras with the Commentary of Vyāsa and the Gloss of Vachaspati Misra,* 170.

9. Both the "study of the self" [*Svādhyāya*] and the "surrendering to Ishvara" [*ĪshvaraPranidhāna*] mentioned in the first aphorism of the second *pada* can be taken as two phases of *tapas*: *Svādhyāya* matches the scorching of the conventional attitude toward reality and the deepening of the field of observation between consciousness and world, while *ĪshvaraPranidhāna* corresponds to the release before the dimension of Being. From a certain perspective, these are parts of *tapas* itself and are expressions of the two moments of the burning flame and the welcoming care.

10. Patañjali, *Yogasūtra,* I. 12, 47.

11. Varela, Depraz, and Vermersch in their book *On Becoming Aware* single out a threefold structure in developing a method inspired by Husserl's phenomenology, to be applied to a meditative setting; it basically

entails a phase of "suspension," a phase of "redirection" and a one of "intuitive completion" (Depraz, Varela, Vermersch, *On Becoming Aware*, 60). The model I offer here takes into account how phenomenology has also unfolded among Husserl's heirs and suggests simplifying the pattern into two main stages: the suspensive one, which includes the reorientation of the attention and draws mainly from Husserl, and the phase of welcoming or letting happen, which draws more from the inputs of Heidegger and Merleau-Ponty. From my point of view, a two-phase dynamic enables the understanding as seen thus far as the two moments of *tapas* and thus to grasp from a phenomenological perspective the central yogic meaning of purification.

12. This very "stage" ultimately is not different from the singular forms themselves.

13. Here a reference to the "I" in terms of *asmitā* or of *ahaṁkāra* is made and not to the "I-consciousness" referred to in Kashmir Śivaism that, on the contrary, somewhat corresponds to the "Transcendental-Ego" in Husserl. On the topic scholar Dyczkowsky says: "Somananda and Utpaladeva enjoy the distinction of having introduced a number of fundamental concepts previously unknown or poorly understood. Certainly the most important of these new ideas was the concept of the Superego. According to these philosophers ultimate reality is Siva Who is the identity of all beings as pure 'I' consciousness. This entirely original idea had important repercussions in the later monistic philosophies through which the Tantras were interpreted"; M. S. G. Dyczkowsky, *Doctrine of Vibration: An Analysis of the Doctrines and Practices of Kashmir Shivaism* (Delhi: Motilal Banarsidass, 1987), 19.

14. "Then from the intellect emerges the egoity principle, by means of which an erroneous notion of non-self as Self is conceived [. . .] This is the erroneous notion, just like mistaking mother-of-pearl for silver. Therefore the word *ahaṃ* is suffixed with *kāra*, the active agent. This suffix also indicates that something has been created' "; Abhinavagupta, *Tantrasāra*, ed. H. N. Chakravarty (Portland: Rudra Press, 2012), chapter 8, 119. Also Patañjali speaks of a similar kind of projection in terms of superimposition [*adhyāsa*], *Yogasūtra*, III.17, 339.

15. J. Patočka, "Weltganzes and Menschenwelt. Bemerkungen zu einem zeitgenössischen kosmologischen Ansatz. Phänomenologische Schriften II," in *Ausgewählte Schriftten* (Stuttgart: Klett-Cotta, 1991), 259.

16. "la problematique fondamentale de la phénoménologie" J. Patočka, *Qu'est-ce que la phénoménologie?*, trans. E. Abrams (Grenoble: Millon, 1988) 264.

17. J. Patočka, *Essais hérétiques sur la philosophie de l'histoire*, trad. E. Abrams (Lagrasse: Verdier, 1999) 25.

18. J. Patočka, *Il mondo naturale e la fenomenologia,* a cura di A. Pantano, Mimesis, Milano, 2003, p. 148. English trans. by the author.

19. J. Patočka, *Il mondo naturale e la fenomenologia,* 94.

20. J. Patočka, *Papiers phénoménologiques,* 122.

21. J. Patočka, *Il mondo naturale e la fenomenologia,* 90–91.

22. J. Patočka, "Le subjectivisme de la phénoménologie husserlienne et la possibilité d'une phénoménologie 'asubjective,'" in *Qu'est-ce que la phénoménologie?,* 211.

23. J. Patočka, *Papiers phénoménologiques,* trans. E. Abrams (Grenoble: Millon, 1995), 27.

24. Patočka, *Papiers phénoménologiques,* 166.

25. Patočka, *Papiers phénoménologiques,* 127. English translation by the author.

26. See J. Patočka, *Introduction à la phénoménologie de Husserl* (Grenoble: Millon, 1992), 260.

27. Merleau-Ponty, *The Visible and the Invisible,* 257.

28. *Viñānabhairava tantra,* n. 115, 43. English translation by the author.

29. T. Metzinger, *The No-Self Alternative* in *The Oxford Handbook of the Self,* ed. S. Gallagher (New York: Oxford University Press, 2011), 279–80. Metzinger acknowledges that "relations do not hold between objects with intrinsic properties, but even the *relata* themselves can be decomposed into sets of relations."

30. Svātmārāma, *Haṭhayogapradīpikā,* II. 76, 270.

31. The union of concentration, meditation and absorption, Patañjali, *Yogasūtra,* III. 4.

32. Patañjali describes three kinds of transformation [*pariṇāma*]: 1) concerning the outgoing [*vyutthāna*] *saṃskāra*: *nirodha-pariṇāma;* 2) concerning *samādhi*: *samādhi-pariṇāma;* 3) concerning one-pointedness: *ekagrata-pariṇāma.* Patañjali, *Yogasūtra,* III. 9–III. 12, 315–19.

33. G. Bachelard, *The Psychoanalysis of Fire* (Boston: Beacon, 1977), 16.

34. Traditionally this posture is known with the already mentioned term of *viparīta-karaṇī* that means "inverted action."

35. This often leads to hidden contraction and long-term tensions in the body.

36. Merleau-Ponty, *Phenomenology of Perception,* 493.

37. Patañjali, *Yogasūtra,* II. 48, 288.

38. Patañjali, *Yogasūtra,* II. 49, 289.

39. Patañjali, *Yogasūtra,* II. 50, 290.

40. Svātmārāma, *Haṭhayogapradīpikā,* II. 2, 150: "Cale vāte calaṁ cittaṁ niścale niścalaṁ bhavet."

41. See Svātmārāma, *Haṭhayogapradīpikā,* II. 2.

42. See for example: Crawford et al., *Self-Regulation of Breathing as a Primary Treatment for Anxiety.* "Appl Psychophysiol Biofeedback," 40, 107–15 (2015).

43. See the already mentioned Piarulli et al., "Ultra-slow Mechanical Stimulation of Olfactory Epithelium Modulates Consciousness." See also A. Zaccaro et al., "How Breath-Control Can Change Your Life: A Systematic Review on Psycho-Physiological Correlates of Slow Breathing," *Frontiers in Human Neuroscience* (September 7, 2018): 12, 353.

44. *Chāndogya Upaniṣad,* VI. 8.2, 501.

45. *Śvetāśvatara Upaniṣad,* II. 9, 968.

46. Svātmārāma, *Haṭhayogapradīpikā,* II. 71, 268.

47. "Sitting in the *Padmāsana* posture the yogi should fill in the air through the left nostril (closing the right one); and, keeping it confined according to one's ability, it should be expelled slowly through the *sūrya* (right nostril). Then, drawing in the air through the *sūrya* slowly, the belly should be filled, and after performing *kumbhaka* (the retention) as before, it should be expelled slowly through the *candra* (left nostril)" Svātmārāma, *Haṭhayogapradīpikā,* II. 8, 54.

48. Patañjali, *Yogasūtra,* II. 50.

49. "by systematically restraining the *prāṇa* (breath) the *nāḍī*-s and *cakras* are purified. Thus the *prāṇa* bursts open the doorway to *suṣumnā* and easily enters it" Svātmārāma, *Haṭhayogapradīpikā,* II. 41, 230.

50. Svātmārāma, *Haṭhayogapradīpikā,* II. 65, 253.

51. In the *Haṭhayogapradīpikā* the term *kumbhaka* takes over a more general meaning and becomes synonymous with different kinds of *prāṇāyāma* (*Haṭhayogapradīpikā,* II. 43–44, 232).

52. In the *Haṭhayogapradīpikā* it is referred to in terms of the *kevala kumbhaka.* Svātmārāma, *Haṭhayogapradīpikā,* II. 71, 268.

53. Surpassing "both the limits of the external and the internal" Patañjali, *Yogasūtra,* II. 51, 292.

54. Patañjali, *Yogasūtra,* II. 52, 295.

55. On the topic of the eidetic variation in Husserl see Depraz, Varela, and Vermersch, *On Becoming Aware,* 21, 58.

56. It must be noted that according to one scholarly classification, Patañjali's yoga *darśana* is considered a dualist school because of its alleged borrowing of the dualist Sāṃkhya ontology of the Puruṣa and Prakṛti. However, *the Yogasūtra* contains an essential overturning of the Sāṃkhya realist and hypostatizing tendencies, which instead appear to have something in common with nonsubstantializing Buddhist views. In addition, the use of terms like ātman in the *Yogasūtra* is usually from a

methodological or provisional perspective rather than a metaphysical or ultimate perspective.

57. Merleau-Ponty, *The Visible and the Invisible,* 102.

58. Merleau-Ponty, *Phenomenology of Perception,* VII.

Chapter 9

1. Merleau-Ponty, *Phenomenology of Perception,* 71.

2. "Consciousness must be faced with its own unreflective life in things and awakened to its own history which it was forgetting: such is the true part that philosophical reflection has to play, and thus do we arrive at a true theory of attention." Merleau-Ponty, *Phenomenology of Perception,* 36.

3. Merleau-Ponty, *Phenomenology of Perception,* 34.

4. Svātmārāma, *Haṭhayogapradīpikā,* III. 127, 456.

5. Svātmārāma, *Haṭhayogapradīpikā,* IV. 52, 545. [*vāyurmanastatraiva līyate*]

6. Merleau-Ponty, *Phenomenology of Perception,* 33.

7. Merleau-Ponty, *Phenomenology of Perception,* 500.

8. Merleau-Ponty, *Phenomenology of Perception,* 33.

9. Rovelli, *Helgoland,* 37, 42, 49.

10. *Mataṅgapārameśvara Yogapāda* 2.10c–11d [c. 6th–10th century CE—Tantra] in J. Mallinson M. Singleton, *The Roots of Yoga.*

11. Kaelber, "Tapas, Birth, and spiritual rebirth in the Veda," 375.

12. Merleau-Ponty, *Phenomenology of Perception,* 35.

13. Merleau-Ponty, *The Visible and the Invisible,* 36.

14. Merleau-Ponty, *Phenomenology of Perception,* 35.

15. Merleau-Ponty, *Phenomenology of Perception,* 40.

16. Merleau-Ponty, *Phenomenology of Perception,* 70. This idea will be maintained throughout his life: "Gestalt is original" (Merleau-Ponty, *The Visible and the Invisible,* 106).

17. Merleau-Ponty, *Phenomenology of Perception,* 35.

18. Merleau-Ponty, *Phenomenology of Perception,* 302.

19. "My perception is not a sum of data, I perceive in an undivided way with my whole being, I catch one structure of the thing, one way of existing that speaks directly to all my senses," Merleau-Ponty, *The Visible and the Invisible,* 78.

20. Merleau-Ponty, *Phenomenology of Perception,* 474.

21. Merleau-Ponty, *The Visible and the Invisible,* 345.

22. Merleau-Ponty, *Phenomenology of Perception,* "Working Notes," 197.

23. Madyamaka's perspective is a middle way between absolute existence and inexistence.

24. Merleau-Ponty, *Phenomenology of Perception,* Preface, XI–XII.

25. Merleau-Ponty, *Phenomenology of Perception*, 297.
26. Merleau-Ponty, *The Visible and the Invisible*, 157.
27. Merleau-Ponty, *Phenomenology of Perception*, XVII.
28. Merleau-Ponty, *Phenomenology of Perception*, 68.
29. "The Kantian subject posits a world, but, in order to be able to assert a truth, the actual subject must in the first place have a world or be in the world" Merleau-Ponty, *Phenomenology of Perception*, 149.
30. Merleau-Ponty, *Phenomenology of Perception*, 159. Merleau-Ponty calls for the following reintegration to take place: "I think is reintegrated in I am, and consciousness in existence," 493.
31. Merleau-Ponty, *The Visible and the Invisible*, 130. "To be a consciousness or rather to be an experience," Merleau-Ponty, *Phenomenology of Perception*, 111.
32. Merleau-Ponty, *Phenomenology of Perception*, XVIII–XIX.
33. Merleau-Ponty, *Phenomenology of Perception*, 169.
34. Merleau-Ponty, *Phenomenology of Perception*, 191.
35. Merleau-Ponty, *Phenomenology of Perception*, 193.
36. Merleau-Ponty, *Phenomenology of Perception*, 193.
37. On the relations between Merleau-Ponty and Tantra see J. Morley, "Embodied Consciousness in Tantric Yoga," 144–63.
38. Husserl, *Erste Philosophie*, 163.
39. Husserl, *Erste Philosophie*, 163.
40. Maurice Merleau-Ponty, *Les Philosophes de l`Antiquité au XXe siècle: Histoire & Portraits* (Paris: Le Livre de Poche, 2006) cited in *Merleau-Ponty and Buddhism*, 1.
41. Jin Y. Park and Gereon Kopf, "Philosophy, Nonphilosophy and Comparative Philosophy," in *Merleau-Ponty and Buddhism*, 1.
42. Merleau-Ponty, *Phenomenology of Perception*, 273.
43. Abhinavagupta, *Tantrāloka* (11th century), in Gioia Lussana, *La dea che scorre. La matrice femminile dello yoga tantrico* (Bologna: Om Edizioni, 2017), 171. English translation by the author.
44. *Jayadrathayamala* Tantra, 68, Lussana, *La dea che scorre*, 171–72.
45. Merleau-Ponty, *Phenomenology of Perception*, 161.
46. Merleau-Ponty, *Phenomenology of Perception*, 278–79.
47. Merleau-Ponty, *Phenomenology of Perception*, 162.
48. Husserl, *Erste Philosophie*, 135: "Leib in seiner Verflechtung mit meinem Seelenleben."
49. Merleau-Ponty, *Phenomenology of Perception*, 257.
50. Merleau-Ponty, *Phenomenology of Perception*, Preface, XI.
51. Merleau-Ponty, *Phenomenology of Perception*, 44.
52. Merleau-Ponty, *Phenomenology of Perception*, 250–51; emphasis in original.
53. Merleau-Ponty, *Phenomenology of Perception*, 255.

54. Merleau-Ponty, *Phenomenology of Perception*, 255.

55. Merleau-Ponty, *Phenomenology of Perception*, 12.

56. Copper statue *The Supreme Goddess as a void*, 18th–19th century, Andhra Pradesh, India, Accession No. 2017-00058, Collection of Asian Civilisations Museum.

57. Merleau-Ponty, *Phenomenology of Perception*, 281.

58. Merleau-Ponty, *Phenomenology of Perception*, 191.

59. "Neither by wearing the garb of a siddha, nor by talking about it (is perfection attained). Only through practical application does one become a siddha. This is the truth without a doubt" Svātmārāma, *Haṭha-yogapradīpikā* I, 66, 143.

60. *Vijñānabhairava*, n. 102.

61. K. Wilber, *No Boundary* (Boston: Shambala, 2001), 54.

62. Merleau-Ponty, *The Visible and the Invisible*, 123.

63. Śamatha or "calm abiding meditation" is the first stage and focuses the mind on a single object in order to allow it to be present to itself long enough and thus penetrate its own nature and functioning.

64. Vipaśyanā, "insight or clear vision meditation," is the second stage, where the spaciousness of mind is explored. The capacity to be aware [*sati*] is extended to embrace all arising and changing mental events. Most contemporary Buddhist schools combine the two stages into a single meditative practice.

65. *Satipaṭṭhāna Sutta*, Bhikkhu Anālayo ed. (Poggio Nativo: Santa Cittarama Edizioni, 2018), 3–14.

66. In this "mode" the mind tends to drift around like a drunken monkey, clinging to thoughts, feelings, judgment, opinions, and phantasies in an endless stream of disconnected mental events.

67. J. Kabat-Zinn, "Mindfulness-Based Interventions in Context: Past, Present, and Future," *Clinical Psychology* 10, no. 2 (2003): 144–56.

68. In the revised edition of *The Embodied Mind* published in 2016 there is a foreword by Kabat-Zinn in which, however, no specific link between mindfulness and phenomenology is drawn. Only recent articles are starting to think the relationship between the two. See Michel Bitbol, "Consciousness, Being and Life: Phenomenological Approaches to Mindfulness," 127–61.

69. John Dunne in his article "Toward an Understanding of Non-Dual Mindfulness" addresses the problem of the sources of contemporary mindfulness teachings: "Indeed, it seems highly problematic to use any Buddhist sources prior to the seventh century (C.E.) to explicate the cognitive details of non-dual practices, inasmuch as these sources lack the theoretical tools and terminology to address non-dual meditations, including their features such as non-dual Mindfulness" John Dunne,

"Toward an Understanding of Non-Dual Mindfulness," *Contemporary Buddhism* 12, no. 1 (2011): 74.

70. See M. E. Kemeny et al., "Contemplative/Emotion Training Reduces Negative Emotional Behavior and Promotes Prosocial Responses, Emotion," *American Psychological Association* 12, no. 2 (2012): 338–50; Ekman, et al., "Buddhist and Psychological Perspectives on Emotions and Well-Being," *Current Directions in Psychological Science* 14 (2005): 59.

71. Merleau-Ponty, *Phenomenology of Perception*, 409.

72. Merleau-Ponty, *Résumés de cours. Collège de France 1952–1960* (Écrits 1957–58), 121 "Nature et la conscience ne peuvent communiquer vraiment qu'en nous et par notre être charnel" (English translation by the author).

73. Varela, Thompson, and Rosch, *The Embodied Mind*, XV–XVI.

74. Varela, Thompson, and Rosch, *The Embodied Mind*, 217.

75. Merleau-Ponty, *Phenomenology of Perception*, X.

76. Merleau-Ponty, *Phenomenology of Perception*, 493.

77. Merleau-Ponty, *Phenomenology of Perception*, 263–64.

78. Merleau-Ponty, *Phenomenology of Perception*, 264.

79. Merleau-Ponty, *Phenomenology of Perception*, 380. Merleau-Ponty also speaks of a synesthetic perception.

80. Merleau-Ponty, *Phenomenology of Perception*, 248.

81. Merleau-Ponty, *Phenomenology of Perception*, 257.

82. Merleau-Ponty, *Phenomenology of Perception*, 104.

83. Merleau-Ponty, *Phenomenology of Perception*, 107.

84. Maurice Merleau-Ponty, "The Eye and the Mind," in *Basic Writings*, T. Baldwin ed. (London: Routledge, 2003), 295.

85. Merleau-Ponty, *The Visible and the Invisible*, 138.

86. André Van Lysebeth, *Tantra. El culto de lo femenino* (Barcelona: Urano, 1990), 73. English translation by the author.

87. See Tucci, *Teoria e pratica della mandala*, 35.

88. 5.2.2 *Amṛtasiddhi* 1.15–21, 2.1–8, in Mallinson and Singleton, *The Roots of Yoga*, 203. Also following Nath *haṭha* yoga texts, as the *Śiva Samhita*, offer very similar descriptions: "In this body there is the Mount Meru surrounded by seven islands; here, too, are rivers, seas, mountains, fields and guardians of the fields. Herein are sages, all the stars and planets, sacred pilgrimage, temples (*pithani*) and presiding deities of the temple. Agents of emanation and contraction, sun and moon; here indeed are mist, air, fire, water and earth. All objects of the three worlds [*trialoka*] [are in] the body, performing their various functions around Meru. The yogi alone knows all this, there is no doubt" *Śivasamhitā*, 2.1–5, cited in M. Burley, *Haṭha Yoga* (Delhi: Motilal Banarsidass, 2000) 145.

89. Merleau-Ponty, *The Visible and the Invisible*, 136.

90. Merleau-Ponty, *Phenomenology of Perception*, 249.

91. "I can at each moment absorb myself almost wholly into the sense of touch or sight, and even that I can never see or touch without my consciousness becoming thereby in some measure saturated, and losing something of its availability," Merleau-Ponty, *Phenomenology of Perception*, 257.

92. 5.6.2 Yogabīja 53, in Mallinson and Singleton, *The Roots of Yoga*.

93. Merleau-Ponty, *Phenomenology of Perception*, 250.

94. Merleau-Ponty, *Phenomenology of Perception*, 373.

95. See Morley, "Inspiration and Expiration," 73–82.

96. "Others offer as sacrifice the outgoing breath in the incoming, and the incoming in the outgoing, restraining the courses of the outgoing and the incoming breaths" *Bhagavadgītā* 4.25, 28–29, Sri Swami Sivananda, ed., *The Bhagavad Gita* (Rishikesh: The Divine Life Society, 2000), 43–44.

97. Merleau-Ponty, *Phenomenology of Perception*, 474.

98. This is a *leitmotiv* in yoga, when it comes to the powers [*siddhi*] that the practitioner develops on the path and that entail, among others the capacity of changing size. See the third section of the *Yogasūtra*, the *vibhūti pādaḥ*.

99. Merleau-Ponty *The Visible and the Invisible*, 38.

100. Merleau-Ponty, *Phenomenology of Perception*, XV. Bitbol elaborates on the topic when writing: "Whereas phenomenologists impose nearly always a factual halt to the categorial deconstruction induced by the *epoché*, assigning a domain of reduction, practitioners of meditative states have as an ideal horizon the integral a-categorial of a limitless *epoché*" M. Bitbol, *La conscience a-t-elle une origine?* 168.

101. Merleau-Ponty, *Phenomenology of Perception*, 503.

102. And not as "in Hegel's phrase, a 'hole in being' " Merleau-Ponty, *Phenomenology of Perception*, 250.

103. Merleau-Ponty, *Phenomenology of Perception*, 198.

104. See Leonardo Colletti and Pablo Pellegrini, "Merleau-Ponty's Phenomenology as a Hermeneutic Framework for Quantum Mechanics," *Axiomathes* 30, no. 1 (2020): 49–68.

105. Merleau-Ponty, *Phenomenology of Perception*, Preface, XXIII. Here the original French has "knot" [*noeud*] and not "network" as given in the English translation.

106. Merleau-Ponty *The Visible and the Invisible*, 84.

107. "The other can be evident to me because I am not transparent for myself, and because my subjectivity draws its body in its wake" Merleau-Ponty, *Phenomenology of Perception*, 410.

108. Merleau-Ponty *The Visible and the Invisible*, 136.

109. Merleau-Ponty *The Visible and the Invisible*, 136.

110. Merleau-Ponty *The Visible and the Invisible*, 137.

111. Merleau-Ponty, *Phenomenology of Perception*, 109.

112. Merleau-Ponty *The Visible and the Invisible*, 135. Here the original French has "making myself world" [*en me faisant monde*] and not "a world," as given in the English translation. See note on *Le visible et invisible* in chapter 1.

113. "When we speak of the flesh of the visible, we do not mean to do anthropology" Merleau-Ponty, *The Visible and the Invisible*, 136. Some authors have however developed phenomenological premises along with Christian interpretations, as for example phenomenologist Jean-Luc Marion.

114. Merleau-Ponty, *The Visible and the Invisible*, 138.

115. Merleau-Ponty, *The Visible and the Invisible*, 139.

116. Merleau-Ponty, *The Visible and the Invisible*, 138.

117. Merleau-Ponty, *The Visible and the Invisible*, 139–40.

118. Merleau-Ponty, *The Visible and the Invisible*, 179.

119. G. A. Mazis, "The Flesh of the World is Emptiness and Emptiness is the Flesh of the World, and their Ethical Implications," in *Merleau-Ponty and Buddhism*, 183–208.

120. Merleau-Ponty, *Phenomenology of Perception*, 298.

121. M. Berman, "Merleau-Ponty and Nagarjuna: Relational Social Ontology and the Ground of Ethics," *Asian Philosophy* 14, no. 2 (July 2004): 131–45.

122. M. Iofrida, *Per un paradigma del corpo: una rifondazione filosofica dell'ecologia* (Macerata: Quodlibet, 2019).

123. Merleau-Ponty, *Phenomenology of Perception*, 528.

124. Merleau-Ponty, *The Visible and the Invisible*, "Working notes," 226, 229.

125. Michel Bitbol, "A Phenomenological Ontology for Physics. Merleau-Ponty and QBism," in *Phenomenological Approaches to Physics*, ed. H. Wiltsche and P. Berghofer (Springer, 2020), 9.

126. See Merleau-Ponty, *Nature. Course Notes from the Collège de France*, 97–98. Merleau-Ponty refers to philosopher of physics of Paulette Destouches Février and her concept of "participatory realism." On the subject Michel Bitbol argues: "Intra-ontology considers the phenomenon as a self-revelation of Being, or as an effect of the selfsplitting of the "flesh" out of which appearing appears (according to the scheme of intentionality), rather than the superficial manifestation of beings that supposedly exist beyond appearance" Bitbol, "The Tangled Dialectic of Body and Consciousness," 7. According to Bitbol, Chris Fuchs, one of the other actors of the QBist adventure, refers to an ontology which is akin to Merleau-Ponty's one in that it "was inspired by John Wheeler's post-Bohrian idea that quantum mechanics involves 'observer-participancy'" Bitbol, "A Phenomenological Ontology for Physics," 10.

127. Merleau-Ponty, *The Visible and the Invisible,* "Working notes," 38.

128. Jonathan Shear and Francisco J. Varela, *The View From Within: First-Person Approaches to the Study of Consciousness* (Imprint Academic, 1999).

129. Merleau-Ponty, *Phenomenology of Perception,* 493.

130. Husserl, *Cartesian Meditations,* § 11, [65], 2.

131. In *First Philosophy,* Husserl explains that it is better to avoid the expression "phenomenological residuum" because it could lead to believing that only subjective acts are of interest for phenomenology, to the detriment of the other correlate of the relation: namely, the world. See *Erste Philosophie* (Zur 46. Vorlesung), 432.

132. Merleau-Ponty, *Résumés de cours. Collège de France 1952–1960* (Écrits 1956–57), 95–96. English Translation by the author; Merleau-Ponty, *Linguaggio, storia, natura,* ed. by M. Carbone (Milano: Bompiani, 1995) 79.

133. As it has been done until now.

134. Z. Josipovic, "Nondual Awareness: Consciousness-as-such as non-representational reflexivity," 292.

135. Z. Josipovic, "Neural Correlates of Nondual Awareness in Meditation," 5.

136. Z. Josipovic, "Neural Correlates of Nondual Awareness in Meditation," 6.

137. Z. Josipovic, "Nondual Awareness: Consciousness-as-such as non-representational reflexivity," 291.

138. Z. Josipovic, "Nondual Awareness: Consciousness-as-such as non-representational reflexivity," 288.

139. Z. Josipovic, "Neural Correlates of Nondual Awareness in Meditation," *Annals of the New York Academy of Sciences,* September 2013, 2.

140. Z. Josipovic, "Nondual Awareness: Consciousness-as-such as non-representational reflexivity," 279.

141. See A. Lutz et al., "Meditation and the Neuroscience of Consciousness: An Introduction," in *The Cambridge Handbook of Consciousness,* ed. Philip David Zelazo et al. (Cambridge: Cambridge University Press, 2007), 499–553; J. Fell et al., "From Alpha to Gamma: Electrophysiological Correlates of Meditation-Related States of Consciousness," *Medical Hypotheses* 75 (2010): 218–24; B. R. Cahn et al., "Occipital Gamma Activation During Vipassana Meditation," *Cognitive Processing* 11 (2010): 39–56; A. Lutz et al., "Changes in the Tonic High-Amplitude Gamma Oscillations During Meditation Correlate with Long-Term Practitioners' Verbal Reports," Association for the Scientific Study of Consciousness Annual Meeting, Poster Presentation, 2006; Zaccaro, et al., "The Consciousness State of Traditional Nidrâ Yoga / Modern Yoga Nidra: Phenomenological Characterization and Preliminary Insights from an EEG Study," *International Journal*

of Yoga Therapy 31, no. 1 (January 2021): 14. An agreement between the Tibetan University, the Monastery of Sera Jay, and the University of Pisa has seen the research group (led by Bruno Neri and Angelo Gemignani) of the University of Pisa carrying out studies on the effects of meditation on brain activity in skilled meditators.

142. See, for example, A. Dutta et al., "A Comprehensive Review of Yoga Research in 2020," *The Journal of Integrative and Complementary Medicine* 28, no. 2 (2022), 115; A. Kumar et al., "Effect of Yoga as Add-on Therapy in Migraine: A Randomized Clinical Trial," *Neurology* (May 2020); S. Parker, "Training Attention for Conscious non-REM Sleep: The Yogic Practice of Yoga-Nidrā and its Implications for Neuroscience Research," *Progress in Brain Research* 244 (2019); C. C. Streeter, "Treatment of Major Depressive Disorder with Iyengar Yoga and Coherent Breathing: A Randomized Controlled Dosing Study," *The Journal of Integrative and complementary medicine* 23, no. 3 (2017); C. C. Streeter et al., "Effects of Yoga versus Walking on Mood, Anxiety, and Brain GABA Levels: A Randomized Controlled MRS Study," *The Journal of Alternative and Complementary Medicine* 16, no. 11 (November 2010); C. Villemure et al., "Insular Cortex Mediates Increased Pain Tolerance in Yoga Practitioners," *Cerebral Cortex* 24, no. 10 (October 2014).

143. This can happen in combination with a precise reference to the style of yoga considered in terms of the lineage: information that in itself is not enough to understand the involved dimensions.

144. Dutta et al., "A Comprehensive Review of Yoga Research in 2020," 115.

145. Undergoing solely the experience of being stressed out and pulled from all sides, as often happens to researchers beset by deadlines and demands for scientific productivity and academic performance, is quite paradoxical in the case of a scientist working on the domain of consciousness.

146. Heidegger, *Being and Time*, § 7, 38, 34.

147. Q. Lauer, *Phenomenology: its Genesis and Prospect* (New York: Harper & Row, 1965), 60.

148. Legget, *The Complete Commentary by Śaṅkara on the Yoga Sūtra-s*, III. 6, 479.

Bibliography

Abhinavagupta, *Tantrasāra*, edited by H. N. Chakravarty. Portland: Rudra Press, 2012.

Abhinavagupta, *Tantrāloka. Luce dei Tantra*, edited by R. Gnoli. Milan: Adelphi, 2017.

P. Ashworth, "Some Notes on Phenomenological Approaches in Psychology." *Bulletin of the British Psychological Society* 29 (1976): 363–68.

Y. Ataria, "Where Do We End, and Where Does the World Begin? The Case of Insight Meditation." *Philosophical Psychology* 28, no. 8 (2014): 1128–46.

A. Avalon, *The Serpent Power: Being the Sat-Cakra-Nirupana and Paduka-Pancaka*. [1919] New York: Dover Publications, 1958.

B. J. Baars, *A Cognitive Theory of Consciousness*. Cambridge: Cambridge University Press, 1988.

B. J. Baars, "A Scientific Approach to Silent Consciousness." *Frontiers in Psychology*, October 2013.

G. Bachelard, *The Psychoanalysis of Fire*. Boston: Beacon Press, 1977.

E. Baret, *Yoga Tantrico*. Rome: Mediterranee, 2005.

C. Beckwith, *Greek Buddha: Pyrrho's Encounter with Early Buddhism in Central Asia*. Princeton, NJ: Princeton University Press, 2017.

M. Berman, "Merleau-Ponty and Nagarjuna: Relational Social Ontology and the Ground of Ethics." *Asian Philosophy* 14, no. 2 (July 2004).

C. Bartocci, P. Martin, and A. Tagliapietra, *Zerologia. Sullo zero, il vuoto e il nulla*. Milan: Il Mulino, 2016.

N. Bhattacharya Saxena, *Absent Mother God of The West*. London: Lexington Books, 2016.

V. Bhattacharya, ed. *The Āgamaśāstṛa of Gaudapāda*. Calcutta: University of Calcutta, 1943.

S. Biderman, "Śankara and the Buddhists." *Journal of Indian Philosophy*, 6, no. 4 (1978): 405–413.

J. Birch, "The Meaning of Haṭha in Early Haṭhayoga." *Journal of the American Oriental Society* 131, no. 4 (October–December 2011).

J. Birch, "The Proliferation of āsana-s in Late-Medieval Yoga Texts." In *Yoga in Transformation Historical and Contemporary Perspectives*, edited by K. Baier, P. A. Maas, K. Preisendanz. Gottingen: Vienne University Press, 2018.

M. Bitbol, *La conscience a-t-elle une origine?Des neurosciences à la pleine conscience: une nouvelle approche de l'esprit.* Paris: Flammarion, 2014.

M. Bitbol, "Beyond Panpsychism: The Radicality of Phenomenology." In *Self, Culture and Consciousness*, edited by S. Menon, N. Nagaraj, and V.V. Binoy. Berlin: Springer, 2018.

M. Bitbol, "Consciousness, Being and Life: Phenomenological Approaches to Mindfulness." *Journal of Phenomenological Psychology* 50 (2019): 127–61.

M. Bitbol, "The Tangled Dialectic of Body and Consciousness: A Metaphysical Counterpart of Radical Neurophenomenology." *Constructivist Foundations* 16, no. 2 (2021): 141–51.

M. Bitbol, "Is the Life-World Reduction Sufficient in Quantum Physics?" *Continental Philosophy Review.* Berlin: Springer, 2020.

M. Bitbol, "A Phenomenological Ontology for Physics: Merleau-Ponty and QBism." In *Phenomenological Approaches to Physics*, edited by H. Wiltsche and P. Berghofer. Berlin: Springer, 2020.

N. Block, "On a Confusion about a Function of Consciousness." *Behavioral and Brain Sciences* 18, no. 2 (June 1995): 230.

N. Block, "Comparing the Major Theories of Consciousness." In *The Cognitive Neurosciences IV*, edited by M. Gazzaniga (2009): 1111–22.

B. Bodhi, ed., *The Connected Discourses of the Buddha. A Translation from the Pāli of the Saṃyutta Nikāya*. Boston: Wisdom Publications, 2000.

M. Burley, *Haṭha Yoga.* Delhi: Motilal Banarsidass, 2000.

B. R. Cahn et al., "Occipital Gamma Activation During Vipassana Meditation." *Cognitive Processing* 11 (2010): 39–56.

R. Calasso, *Le nozze di Cadmo e Armonia*. Milan: Adelphi, 1991.

R. Calasso, *Ardor*, trans. R. Dixon. New York: Farrar, Straus and Giroux, 2014.

S. Castelli, "Editoriale," *Percorsi Yoga*, no. 70, luglio 2016, Milan.

D. J. Chalmers, "Facing Up to the Problem of Consciousness." *Journal of Consciousness Studies* 2, no. 3 (1995): 200–19.

D. J. Chalmers, "Consciousness and its Place in Nature." In *Blackwell Guide to Philosophy of Mind*, edited by S. Stich and T. Warfield. Malden, MA: Blackwell, 2003.

A. Clark and D. Chalmers, "The Extended Mind." *Analysis* 58, no. 1 (1998): 7–19.

M. A. Cohen and D. C. Dennett, "Consciousness Cannot Be Separated from Function." *Trends in Cognitive Sciences* 15, no. 8 (August 2011): 361.

L. Colletti and P. Pellegrini, "Merleau-Ponty's Phenomenology as a Hermeneutic Framework for Quantum Mechanics." *Axiomathes* 30, no. 1 (2020): 49–68.

H. Cook, *Hua-Yen Buddhism: The Jewel Net of Indra*. University Park: Pennsylvania State University Press, 1977.

J. M. Cooper and D. S. Hutchinson, ed., *Plato. Complete Works*. Indianapolis/Cambridge: Hackett Publishing, 1997.

V. Costa, E. Franzini, and P. Spinicci, *La fenomenologia*. Milan: Einaudi, 2002.

R. Crawford and M.W. Barnes et al., "Self-Regulation of Breathing as a Primary Treatment for Anxiety." *Appl Psychophysiol Biofeedback* 40 (2015): 107–15.

F. Crick, *The Astonishing Hypothesis*. New York: Charles Scribner's Sons, 1994.

A. Damasio, "Thinking about Brain and Consciousness." In *Characterizing Consciousness: From Cognition to the Clinic?*, edited by S. Dehaene and T. Christen. Berlin: Springer, 2011.

S. N. Dasgupta, *Yoga philosophy. In Relation to Other Systems of Indian Thought*. Delhi: Motilal Banarsidass, 1930.

S. N. Dasgupta, *Philosophical Essays*. Calcutta: University of Calcutta, 1941.

A. David-Néel, *The Secret Oral Teachings in Tibetan Buddhist Sects*. San Francisco: City Lights, 1972.

A. David-Néel, *My Journey to Lhasa: The Personal Story of the Only White Woman who Succeeded in Entering the Forbidden City*. New York: Harper and Brothers, 1927.

S. Dehaene, J. Changeux, and L. Naccache, "The Global Neuronal Workspace Model of Conscious Access: From Neuronal Architectures to Clinical Applications." In *Characterizing Consciousness: From Cognition to the Clinic?*, edited by Stanislas Dehaene and Yves Christen, 55–85. Berlin and Heidelberg: Springer Berlin Heidelberg, 2011.

S. Dehaene, H. Lau, and S. Kouider, "What Is Consciousness, and Could Machines Have It?" *Science* (New York) 358, no. 6362 (October 27, 2017): 486–92.

D. C. Dennett, *Consciousness Explained*. New York: Little, Brown, 2017.

N. Depraz, F. Varela, and P. Vermersch, *On Becoming Aware*. Amsterdam: John Benjamins Publishing, 2002.

T. K. V. Desikachar, *The Heart of Yoga*. Rochester: Inner Traditions, 1999.

P. Deussen, *Outlines of Indian Philosophy: with an Appendix on the Philosophy of the Vedanta in its Relation to Occidental Metaphysics*. K. Curtious, 1907.

Diogenes Laërtius, *Lives and Opinions of Eminent Philosophers*, XI, 61, translated by P. Mensch, edited by J. Miller. Oxford: Oxford University Press, 2018.

C. Di Martino, "Esperienza e intenzionalità nella fenomenologia di Husserl." *Memorandum* 13, no. 32 (2007).

G. Dreyfus, "Self and Subjectivity: A Middle Way Approach." In *Self, No-Self? Perspectives from Analytical, Phenomenological and Indian Traditions*, edited by Mark Siderits, Evan Thompson, and Dan Zahavi. New York: Oxford University Press, 2011.

D. Duckworth, "From Yogācāra to Philosophical Tantra in Kashmir and Tibet." *Sophia* 57 (2018): 611–23.

J. Dunne, "Toward an Understanding of Non-Dual Mindfulness." *Contemporary Buddhism*, 12:01 (2011): 71–88.

A. Dutta et al., "A Comprehensive Review of Yoga Research in 2020." *The Journal of Integrative and Complementary Medicine* 28, no. 2 (2022).

M. S. G. Dyczkowsky, *Doctrine of Vibration. An Analysis of the Doctrines and Practices of Kashmir Shivaism*. Delhi: Motilal Banarsidass, 1987.

P. Ekman, R. J. Davidson, M. Ricard, and B. A. Wallace, "Buddhist and Psychological Perspectives on Emotions and Well-Being." *Current Directions in Psychological Science* 14 (2005): 59.

M. Eliade, *Yoga. Immortality and Freedom*, translated by W. R. Trask. Princeton, NJ: Princeton University Press, 2009.

M. Eliade, *Tecniche dello yoga*. Turin: Bollati Boringhieri, 2013.

M. Eliade, *Lo sciamanismo e le tecniche dell'estasi*. Rome: Mediterranee, 1974.

J. Fell et al., "From Alpha to Gamma: Electrophysiological Correlates of Meditation-Related States of Consciousness." *Medical Hypotheses* 75 (2010): 218–24.

E. Fink, *Proximité et distance*. Grenoble: Jérôme Millon, 1994.

E. Fink, *Sixth Cartesian Meditation*, trans. R. Bruzina. Indianapolis: Indiana University Press, 1995.

K. Fox et al., "Is Meditation Associated with Altered Brain Structure? A Systematic Review and Meta-Analysis of Morphometric Neuroimaging in Meditation Practitioners." *Neuroscience & Biobehavioral Reviews* 43 (June 1, 2014).

D. Franck, *Chair et corps. Sur la phénomenologie de Husserl*. Paris: Les éditions de Minuit, 1981.

S. Gallagher and D. Zahavi, *The Phenomenological Mind*. New York: Routledge, 2008.

G. Jha, ed., *Yoga-Darshana. Sūtra of Patañjali with Bhāṣya of Vyāsa*. Fremont: Asian Humanities Press, 2002.

J. L. Garfield and J. Westerhoff, *Madhyamaka and Yogācāra — Allies or Rivals?* Oxford: Oxford University Press, 2015.

J. J. Gibson, *The Senses Considered as Perceptual Systems*. Boston: Houghton Mifflin, 1966.

A. Giorgi, "Concerning the Possibility of Phenomenological Psychological Research." *Journal of Phenomenological Psychology* 14 (1–2) (1983).

R. Gnoli, ed., *La rivelazione del Buddha*. Milan: Mondadori, 2001.

S. Gonnella, "La sintesi passiva e le radici iletiche della sensibilità." *Philosophy Kitchen. Rivista di filosofia contemporanea* 7 (March 2020): 103–14.

R. T. H. Griffith, *The Hymns of the Atharva Veda*. Benares: E.J. Lazarus and Co., 1895.

T. Gyatso, *The World of Tibetan Buddhism*, trans. Geshe Thupten Jinpa. Boston: Wisdom Publications, 1995.

W. Halbfass, *India and Europe: An Essay in Understanding*. Albany: State University of New York Press, 1988.

F. J. Hanna, "On the Teachings of the Buddha." *The Humanistic Psychologist*, September 1995.

F. J. Hanna, B. D. Wilkinson, and J. Givens, "Recovering the Original Phenomenological Research Method: An Exploration of Husserl, Yoga, Buddhism, and New Frontiers in Humanistic Counseling." *Journal of Humanistic Counseling* 56 (July 2017): 144–62.

G. W. F. Hegel, *Vorlesungen über der Philosophie del Geschichte*. Frankfurt am Main: Shurkamp-Taschenbuch Wissenschaft, No. 612, Band 12.

G. W. F. Hegel, *Über die unter dem Namen Bhagavad-Gita bekannte Episode des Mahabharata von Wilhelm con Humboldt*. Berlin: Akademie der Wissenshaften, 1826. Berliner Schriften, Humboldt-Rezension.

M. Heidegger, *Being and Time*. Albany: State University of New York Press, 2010.

M. Heidegger, *Vom Wesen der Wahrheit*, in F.-W. von Herrmann, ed., *Wegmarken*. Frankfurt a. M.: Klostermann, 1976.

M. Heidegger, *On the Essence of Truth* (1930), trans. J. Sallis, in *Pathmarks*, edited by M. Heidegger, W. McNeil, translated by W. McNeil. Cambridge: Cambridge University Press, 1998.

M. Heidegger, *Über den Humanismus*. Frankfurt am Main: V. Klostermann, 2000 (Band 9 der Gesamtausgabe).

M. Heidegger, *Letter on Humanismus*. In *Pathmarks*, edited by M. Heidegger, W. McNeil, translated by W. McNeil. Cambridge: Cambridge University Press, 1998.

M. Heidegger, "The Origin of the Work of Art" in *Poetry, Language, Thought*, trans. Albert Hofstadter. New York: Harper Perennial, 1971.

M. Heidegger, *The Age of the World Picture*, in *The Question Concerning Technology and Other Essays*, translated by W. Lovitt. London: Garland Publishing, 1977.

M. Heidegger, *On the Way to Language*, translated by P. D. Hertz. New York: Perennial Library, 1971.

M. Heidegger, *Gelassenheit*. Tübingen: Neske, 1959.

M. Heidegger, "Zur Erörterung der Gelassenheit." In *Gelassenheit*. Tübingen: Neske, 1959.

M. Heidegger, *Discourse on Thinking*, translated by J. M. Anderson, E. H. Freund. New York: Harper & Row, 1955.

M. Heidegger, *History of the Concept of Time (Prolegomena)*, translated by T. Kisiel. Bloomington: Indiana University Press, 1985.

M. Heidegger, *Introduction to Metaphysics*, translated by G. Fried and R. Polt. New Haven, CT, and London: Yale University Press, 2014.

W. Heisenberg, *Fisica e filosofia*. Milan: Feltrinelli, 2021.

T. Hinterberger et al., "Decreased Electrophysiological Activity Represents the Conscious State of Emptiness in Meditation." *Frontiers in Psychology* 5 (2014).

B. K. Hölzel et al., "Stress Reduction Correlates with Structural Changes in the Amygdala." *Social Cognitive and Affective Neuroscience* 5, no. 1 (March 2010): 11–17.

B. Holzel et al., "How Does Mindfulness Meditation Work? Proposing Mechanisms of Action From a Conceptual and Neural Perspective." *Perspectives on Psychological Science* 6 (November 1, 2011): 537–59.

E. Husserl, *Logical Investigations*, J. N. Findlay. New York: Routledge, 2001.

E. Husserl, *The Idea of Phenomenology*, translated by W. P. Alston and J Nakhkikian. The Hague: Martinus Nijhoff, 1973.

E. Husserl, *Ideas Pertaining to a Pure Phenomenology and to a Phenomenological Philosophy*, First Book, translated by F. Kersten. The Hague: Martinus Nijhoff, 1983.

E. Husserl, *Ideas Pertaining a Pure Phenomenology and a Phenomenological Philosophy*, Second Book, translated by R. Rojcewicz and A. Schuwer. Dordrecht: Kluwer Academic Publishers, 1989.

E. Husserl, *Ideen zu einer reinen Phenomenologie und phenomenologishen Philosophie*, edited by Erstes Buch, Hrsg. von W. Biemel. The Hague: Martinus Nijhoff, 1950.

E. Husserl, *Idee per una fenomenologia pura e per una filosofia fenomenologica*, edited by Vincenzo Costa. Turin: Einaudi, 2002.

E. Husserl, *Erste Philosophie. Zweiter Teil (1923–24)*. Husserliana VIII. Dordrecht: Kluwer Academic Publishers, 1996.

E. Husserl, *Analysen zur passiven Synthesis: Aus Vorlesungs- und Forschungsmanuskripten 1918–1926*, Husserliana XI. The Hague: Nijhoff, 1966.

E. Husserl, *De la synthèse passive. Logique transcendantale et constitutions originaires*, edited by B. Bégout and J. Kessler. Grenoble: Jérôme Million, 1998.

E. Husserl, *Cartesian Meditations. An Introduction to Phenomenology*, translated by D. Cairns. New York: Springer, 1960.

E. Husserl, *Die Krisis der Europischen Wissenschaften und die Transzendentale Phenomenologie*, Husserliana VI, W. Biemel. The Hague: Nijhoff, 1954.

E. Husserl, "Über di Reden Gotamo Buddhos" (1925) in K. Schuhmann, "Husserl and Indian Thought," edited by C. Leijenhorst and P. Steenbakkers. *Selected Papers on Phenomenology*. Dordrecht: Kluwer Academic Publishers, 2004.

E. Husserl, *The Crisis of European Sciences and Transcendental Phenomenology*. Evanston: Northwestern University Press, 1970.

M. Iofrida, *Per un paradigma del corpo: una rifondazione filosofica dell'ecologia*. Macerata: Quodlibet, 2019.

W. James, *The Principles of Psychology, Vol. I*. New York: Henry Holt and Co., 1890.

W. James, "Does 'Consciousness' Exist?" *The Journal of Philosophy, Psychology and Scientific Methods* 1, no. 18 (1904).

W. James, *The Varieties of Religious Experience: A Study in Human Nature*. London and New York: Routledge, 2008.

S. W. Jamison and J. P. Brereton, ed., *The Rigveda. The Earliest Religious Poetry of India*. Oxford: Oxford University Press, 2014.

Z. Josipovic, "Neural Correlates of Nondual Awareness in Meditation." *Annals of the New York Academy of Sciences*, September 2013.

Z. Josipovic, "Nondual Awareness: Consciousness-as-such as Non-representational Reflexivity," edited by Narayanan Srinivasa. *Progress in Brain Research* 244, ch. 12, Elsevier, 2019, 273–98.

J. Kabat-Zinn, "Mindfulness-Based Interventions in Context: Past, Present, and Future." *Clinical Psychology* 10, no. 2 (2003).

W. O. Kaelber, "Tapas, Birth and Spiritual Rebirth in the Veda." *History of Religions* 15, no. 4 (May 1976).

W. O. Kaelber, *Tapta Marga: Asceticism and Initiation in Vedic India*. Albany: State University of New York Press, 1989.

M. Kamiński, K. Blinowska, and W. Szelenberger, "Topographic Analysis of Coherence and Propagation of EEG Activity during Sleep and Wakefulness." *Electroencephalography and Clinical Neurophysiology* 102, no. 3 (March 1, 1997): 216–27.

M. E. Kemeny et al., "Contemplative/Emotion Training Reduces Negative Emotional Behavior and Promotes Prosocial Responses, Emotion." *American Psychological Association* 12, no. 2 (2012): 338–50.

D. R. Komito, *Nāgārjuna's Seventy Stanzas: A Buddhist Psychology of Emptiness* [*Shūnvatāsaptatikārikānāma*]. New York: Snow Lion Publications, 1987.

A. Kumar et al, "Effect of Yoga as Add-on Therapy in Migraine: A Randomized Clinical Trial." *Neurology*, May 2020.

L. de La Valleé Poussin, "Le Bouddhisme et le yoga de Patañjali." *Mélanges Chinois et Bouddhiques* 5 (1936) 232–420.

Swami Lakshmanjoo, *Śiva Sutras*. Universal Shaiva Fellowship, 2007.

G. J. Larson, "Classical Yoga as Neo-Sāṃkhya. A Chapter in the History of Indian Philosophy." *Asian Studies* 53, no. 3 (1999).

Q. Lauer, *Phenomenology: its Genesis and Prospect*. New York: Harper & Row, 1965.

S. W. Lazar et al., "Meditation Experience Is Associated with Increased Cortical Thickness." *Neuroreport* 16, no. 17 (November 28, 2005): 1893–97.

T. Legget, *The Complete Commentary by Śaṅkara on the Yoga Sūtra-s*. Adhyatma Yoga Trust, 2016.

J. Levine, "Materialism and Qualia: The Explanatory Gap." *Pacific Philosophical Quarterly* 64, no. 4 (1983): 354–61.

G. Lussana, *La dea che scorre. La matrice femminile dello yoga tantrico.* Bologna: Om Edizioni, 2017.

D. Lusthaus, *Buddhist Phenomenology. A Philosophical Investigation of Yogācāra Buddhism and the Ch'eng Wei-shih lun*. New York: Routledge, 2002.

A. Lutz et al., "Changes in the Tonic High-Amplitude Gamma Oscillations During Meditation Correlate with Long-Term Practitioners' Verbal Reports." Association for the Scientific Study of Consciousness Annual Meeting, Poster Presentation, 2006.

A. Lutz et al., "Meditation and the Neuroscience of Consciousness: An Introduction." In *The Cambridge Handbook of Consciousness*, edited by Philip David Zelazo, et al. Cambridge: Cambridge University Press, 2007.

J.-F. Lyotard, *The Postmodern Condition. A Report on Knowledge*, translated by Geoff Bennington and Brian Massumi. Manchester: Manchester University Press, 1984.

P. A. Maas, "Sthirasukham *āsanam:* Posture and Performance in Classical Yoga and Beyond." In *Yoga in Transformation,* edited by K. Baier, P. A. Maas, and K. Preisendanz, 49–100. Göttingen: Vienna University Press.

R. Mcintyre, "Husserl and the Representational Theory of Mind." In *Historical Foundations of Cognitive Science,* edited by J C. Smith. Philosophical Studies Series, vol. 46. Dordrecht: Springer, 1991.

S. K. Maharana, "Phenomenology of Consciousness in Ādi Śamkara and Edmund Husserl." *Indo-Pacific Journal of Phenomenology* 9 (2009).

J. Mallinson, ed., *The Shiva Samhita*. Yoga Vidya, 2007.

J. Mallinson, "Haṭhayoga's Philosophy: A Fortuitous Union of Non-Dualities." *Journal of Indian Philosophy* 42, no. 1 (2014).

J. Mallinson and M. Singleton, *Roots of Yoga*. New York: Penguin Classics, 2017 (digital edition).

J. Mallinson, "Kāḷavañcana in the Konkan: How a Vajrayāna Haṭhayoga Tradition Cheated Buddhism's Death in India." *Religions* 10 (2019): 273.

M. Massimini et al., "Breakdown of Cortical Effective Connectivity During Sleep." *Science* 309, no. 5744 (September 30, 2005): 2228–32.

J. H. Marshall, *Mohenjo-Daro and the Indus Civilization*. London: Probsthain, 1931.

L. Martelli, "Genesi passiva e hyle: la fondazione della coscienza trascendentale." *Philosophy Kitchen. Rivista di filosofia contemporanea* 7 (2020): 115–31.

G. A. Mazis, "The Flesh of the World is Emptiness and Emptiness is the Flesh of the World, and their Ethical Implications." In *Merleau-Ponty and Buddhism*, edited by Y. Park and G. Kopf. Lanham, MD: Lexington Books, 2009.

M. Merleau-Ponty, *Phenomenology of Perception*, trans. C. Smith. New York: Routledge, 1962.

M. Merleau-Ponty, *The Visible and the Invisible*, trans. I. Lingis. Evanston: Northwestern University Press, 1968.

M. Merleau-Ponty, *Le visible et l'invisible*, edited by Claude Lefort. Paris: Gallimard, 1964.

M. Merleau-Ponty, *Résumés de cours. Collège de France 1952–1960*. Paris: Gallimard, 1968.

M. Merleau-Ponty, *La nature. Notes cours du Collège de France*, ed. D. Seglard. Paris: Éditions de Seuil, 1995.

M. Merleau-Ponty, *Nature. Course Notes from the Collège de France*, translated R. Vallier. Evanston: Northwestern University Press, 2003.

M. Merleau-Ponty, *Linguaggio, Storia, Natura. Corsi al Collège de France, 1952–1961*, edited by M. Carbone. Milan: Bompiani, 1995.

M. Merleau-Ponty, "The Eye and the Mind." In *Basic Writings*, edited by T. Baldwin. London: Routledge, 2003.

T. Metzinger, "Out-of-Body Experiences as the Origin of the Concept of a 'Soul.'" *Mind & Matter* 3 (2005): 57–84.

T. Metzinger, *The Ego Tunnel: The Science of the Mind and the Myth of the Self*. New York: Basic Books, 2010.

T. Metzinger, *The No-Self Alternative* in *The Oxford Handbook of the Self*, edited by S. Gallagher. New York: Oxford University Press, 2011.

T. Metzinger, "Minimal Phenomenal Experience: Meditation, Tonic Alertness, and the Phenomenology of 'Pure' Consciousness." *Philosophy and the Mind Sciences* 1, no. 1 (2020): 7.

Milarepa, *The Hundred Thousand Songs of Milarepa,* translated and edited by Qarma C. C. Chang. New York: Shambhala Publications, 1962.

R. N. Mohanty, *Reason and Tradition in Indian Thought. An Essay on the Nature of Indian Philosophical Thinking.* Oxford: Oxford University Press, 1992.

J. Nat Mohanty, *Phenomenology and Indian Philosophy: The Concept of Rationality,* in *Phenomenology and Indian Philosophy,* edited by D.P. Chattopadhyaya, L. Embree, and J. N. Mohanty, 8–19. Albany: State University of New York Press, 1992.

J. Morley, "Inspiration and Expiration: Yoga Practice Through Merleau-Ponty's Phenomenology of the Body." *Philosophy East and West* 51, no. 1 (2001).

J. Morley, "Embodied Consciousness in Tantric Yoga and the Phenomenology of Merleau-Ponty." *Religion and Arts* 12 (2008).

G. Moiraghi, *In cammino verso la cosa. Heidegger dall'estetica all'ontologia.* Milan: Mimesis Milano, 2006 [*On the way to the thing. Heidegger from aesthetics to ontology*]

A. Mookerjee and M. Khanna, *The Tantric Way.* London: Thames and Hudson, 1977.

A. L. Murdoch, *Tapas in the Rigveda.* MA thesis, York University, 1983.

Nāgārjuna, *The Dispeller of Disputes. Nāgārjuna's Vigrahavyāvartanī,* edited and translated by J. Westerhoff. Oxford: Oxford University Press, 2010.

Nāgārjuna, *Fundamental Wisdom of the Middle Way. Nāgārjuna's Mūla-madyamaka-kārikā,* edited and translated by J. L. Garfield. Oxford: Oxford University Press, 1995.

T. Nagel, "What Is It Like to Be a Bat?" *The Philosophical Review* 83, no. 4 (1974): 435–50.

Nāropā, *Iniziazione. Kālacakra,* edited by R. Gnoli. Milan: Adelphi, 1994.

K. Nārāyaṇasvāmaiyar, *Thirty Minor Upanisahds.* Madras: Printed by Annie Besant at the Vasanta Press, 1914.

J. Needleman, "Inner Empiricism as a Way to a Science of Consciousness." *Jacob Needleman Noetic Sciences Review* (Summer 1993).

C. Neri and T. Pontillo, "On the Boundary between Yogakkhema in the Suttapiṭaka and Yogakṣema in the Upaniṣads and Bhagavadgītā." *Cracow Indological Studies* XXI, no. 2 (2019): 139–57.

F. Nietzsche, *The Gay Science,* edited by B. Williams. Cambridge: Cambridge University Press, 2001.

Swami Nikhilananda, ed., *Drgdriśyaviveka. An Inquiry into the Nature of the 'Seer' and the 'Seen,'* translated by Swami Nikhilananda. Mysore: Sri Ramanakrishna Asrama, 1931.

K. O' Brien-Kop, *Rethinking 'Classical Yoga' and Buddhism.* London: Bloomsbury Academic, 2022.

K. O' Brien-Kop, *The Philosophy of the Yogasūtra. An Introduction*, London: Bloomsbury Academic, 2023.

Padmasambhava, *The Tibetan Book of the Dead: The Great Liberation through Hearing in the Bardo*, edited by Guru Rinpoche according to Karma Lingpa, translated by Francesca Fremantle and Chogyam Trungpa. Boston and London: Shambala, 1987.

Padmasambhava, *Il libro tibetano dei morti*, edited by G. Tucci, Milan: Bur, 2019.

A. Padoux, "Tantrism." In *Encyclopedia of Religions*, vol. 14, edited by Mircea Eliade. New York: Macmillan, 1986.

R. Panikkar, *I veda*, ed. M. Carrara Pavan. Milan: Bur, 2012.

Y. Park and G. Kopf, "Philosophy, Nonphilosophy and Comparative Philosophy." In *Merleau-Ponty and Buddhism*, edited by Y. Park and G. Kopf. Lanham, MD: Lexington Books, 2009.

Y. Park and G. Kopf, *Merleau-Ponty and Buddhism*, edited by Y. Park and G. Kopf. Lanham, MD: Lexington Books, 2009.

S. Parker, "Training Attention for Conscious non-REM Sleep: The Yogic Practice of Yoga-Nidrā and its Implications for Neuroscience Research." *Progress in Brain Research* 244 (2019).

Patañjali, *The Yoga Sutras of Patañjali*, edited by E. F. Bryant. New York: North Point Press, 2009.

Patañjali, *Yogasūtra*, edited by Federico Squarcini. Turin: Einaudi, 2019.

Patañjali, *Yoga-Sutras of Patañjali with the Exposition of Vyāsa*, translated by Usharbudh Arya, D. Litt. Honesdale, PA: The Himalayan International Institute of Yoga Science and Philosophy of the U.S.A., 1986.

Patañjali, *Patañjali's Yoga Sutras with the Commentary of Vyāsa and the Gloss of Vāchaspati Miśra*, edited by R. Prasāda. Munshiram: Manoharlal Publishers, 1998.

J. Patočka, "Epoché and Reduktion—einige Bemerkungen." In *Bewusstsein. Gerhard Funke zu eigen*, edited by A. J. Bucher, H. Drüe, and T. M. Seebohm. Bonn, 1975.

J. Patočka, *Le monde naturel come problème philosophique*. La Haye: M. Nijhoff, 1976.

J. Patočka, *Qu'est-ce que la phénoménologie?*, translated by E. Abrams. Grenoble: Millon, 1988.

J. Patočka, "Le subjectivisme de la phénoménologie husserlienne et la possibilitè d'une phénoménologie 'asubjective.' " In *Qu'est-ce que la phénoménologie?*, translated by E. Abrams. Grenoble: Millon, 1988.

J. Patočka, "Weltganzes and Menschenwelt. Bemerkungen zu einem zeitgenössischen kosmologischen Ansatz. Phänomenologische Schriften II." In *Ausgewählte Schriftten*. Stuttgart: Klett-Cotta, 1991.

J. Patočka, "Naturliche Welt und Phänomenologie. Phänomenologische Schriften II." In *Ausgewählte Schriftten*. Stuttgart: Klett-Cotta, 1991.
J. Patočka, *Introduction à la phénoménologie de Husserl*. Grenoble: Millon, 1992.
J. Patočka, *Papiers phénoménologiques,* translated by E. Abrams. Grenoble: Millon, 1995.
J. Patočka, *Essais hérétiques sur la philosophie de l'histoire,* translated by. E. Abrams. Lagrasse: Verdier, 1999.
C. R. Pernet et al., "Mindfulness Related Changes in Grey Matter: A Systematic Review and Meta-Analysis." *Brain Imaging and Behavior* 15, no. 5 (October 2021): 2720–30.
H. W. Petzt, *Auf einen Stern zugehen. Begegnungen mit Martin Heidegger 1929 bis 1976*. Frankfurt am Main: Societäts-Verlag, 1983.
G. Piana, *Elementi di una dottrina dell'esperienza* Milan: Cuem-Libreria Universitaria, 2003.
A. Piarulli et al., "Ultra-Slow Mechanical Stimulation of Olfactory Epithelium Modulates Consciousness by Slowing Cerebral Rhythms in Humans." *Scientific Reports* 8, no. 1 (April 26, 2018).
R. Pine, ed., *The Platform Sutra. The Zen Teaching of Hui-Neng*. Berkeley: Counterpoint, 2006.
Plato, *Complete works,* edited by J. M. Cooper. Indianapolis: Hackett, 1997.
S. Powell, "Etched in Stone: Sixteenth-Century Visual and Material Evidence of Śaiva Ascetics and Yogis in Complex Non-Seated āsanas at Vijayangara." *Journal of Yoga Studies* 1 (2018).
R. Puligandla, "Phenomenological Reduction and Yoga Meditation." *Philosophy East and West* 20, no. 1 (1970).
Puṇyānandanātha, *Kāma-Kalā-Vilāsa* (XIV), translated by A. Avalon. Madras: Ganesh and Co., 1953.
H. Rydenfelt, "Special Issue on Pragmatism and Theories of Emergence." *European Journal of Pragmatism and American Philosophy,* September 11, 2018, online. https://europeanpragmatism.org/cfp-ejpap-special-issue-on-pragmatism-and-theories-of-emergence/.
V. Roebuck, ed., The *Upanishads*. New York: Penguin, 2003, digital edition.
D. M. Rosenthal, "Metacognition and Higher-Order Thoughts." *Consciousness and Cognition,* 9, no. 2 (2000): 231–42.
C. Rovelli, *Helgoland*. Milan: Adelphi, 2020.
A. Sander, "Phenomenological Reduction and Yogic Meditation: Commonalities and Divergencies." *Journal of East-West Thought* 5 (2015).
Śaṅkarā, *Yoga Tarvali,* translated by Swami Narasimhananda, "Yoga-Taravali of Acharya Shankara." *Traditional Wisdom* 124, no. 1 (2019): 1–9.
V. Sarde, "Yoga on Stone': Sculptural Representation of Yoga on Mahuḍī Gate at Dabhoī in Gujarāt." *Journal of Multidisciplinary Studies in Archaeology* 5 (2017).

V. Sarde, "A Medieval Religious Center of Natha and Mahanubhava Sect in Maharashtra." Online resource on *Tattva mag.*, 2021 https://tattvamag.org/a-medieval-religious-center-of-natha-and-mahanubhava-sect-in-maharashtra.

V. Sarde, "Early Images of Nāth Yogis in Maharashtra," online conference, 2020: https://www.youtube.com/watch?v=wsGB3CKb7zg.

Satipaṭṭhāna Sutta, Bhikkhu Anālayo edited by Poggio Nativo. Santa Cittarama Edizioni, 2018.

A. Schopenhauer, *Die Welt als Wille und Forstellung*, Zweiter Tailband. Diogenes, 2017.

K. Schuhmann, *Husserl and Indian Thought*. In *Selected Papers on Phenomenology*, edited by C. Leijenhorst and P. Steenbakker. Dordrecht: Kluwer Academic Publishers, 2004.

R. Schürmann, "Heidegger and Meister Eckhart on Releasement." In *Research in Phenomenology*, vol. 3. Leiden: Brill, 1973.

R. Searle, "Who Is Computing with the Brain?" *Behavioral and Brain Sciences* 13, no. 4 (December 1990): 632–34.

S. Seung, *Connectome: How the Brain's Wiring Makes Us Who We Are*. Boston: Houghton Mifflin Harcourt, 2012.

Sextus Empiricus, *Outlines of Pyrrhonism*, edited by J. Annas and J. Barnes. Cambridge: Cambridge University Press, 2000.

L. Shapiro, *Embodied Cognition*. London: Routledge, 2010.

J. Shear and F. J. Varela, *The View From Within: First-Person Approaches to the Study of Consciousness*, Exeter, UK: Imprint Academic, 1999.

M. Siderits, E. Thompson, and D. Zahavi, *Self, No-Self? Perspectives from Analytical, Phenomenological and Indian Traditions*. New York: Oxford University Press, 2011.

M. Siderits and S. Katsura, ed., *Nāgārjuna's Middle Way*. Somerville, MA: Wisdom Publications, 2013.

R. Sinari, "The Method of Phenomenological Reduction and Yoga." *Philosophy East and West*, 15, 3–4, 1965.

M. Singleton, *Yoga Body. The Origins of Modern Posture Practice*. Oxford: Oxford University Press, 2010.

A. Sironi, ed., *Vijñānabhairava Tantra*. Milan: Adelphi, 1989.

Sri Swami Sivananda, ed., *The Bhagavad Gita*. Rishikesh: The Divine Life Society, 2000.

P. Sloterdijk, *You Must Change your Life. On Anthropotechnics*. Cambridge, UK, and Malden, MA: Polity, 2013.

N. Srinivasan, "Consciousness Without Content: A Look at Evidence and Prospects." *Frontiers in Psychology* (August 2020).

O. Stone and D. Zahavi, "Phenomenology and Mindfulness." *Journal of Consciousness Studies* 28, no. 3–4 (2021): 158–85.

C. C. Streeter et al., "Effects of Yoga versus Walking on Mood, Anxiety, and Brain GABA Levels: A Randomized Controlled MRS Study." *Altern Complement Med* 16, no. 11 (November 2010).

C. C. Streeter, "Treatment of Major Depressive Disorder with Iyengar Yoga and Coherent Breathing: A Randomized Controlled Dosing Study." *The Journal of Integrative and Complementary Medicine* 23, no. 3 (2017).

Svātmārāma, *Haṭhayogapradīpikā. Light on Hatha Yoga,* edited by Swami Muktibodhananda. Munger: Yoga Publications Trust, Bihar School of Yoga, 1985, 1998, online at https://archive.org/details/hatha-yoga-pradipika-swami-muktibodhananda_202206/page/34/mode/2up.

T. Tripiṭaka, ed., *Prajñāpāramitā Hṛdaya Sūtra,* Lapis Lazuli Texts 8, no. 251, apislazulitexts.com/tripitaka/T0253-LL-prajnaparamita-hrdaya/.

E. Thompson, *Waking, Dreaming, Being: New Light on the Self and Consciousness from Neuroscience, Meditation, and Philosophy*. New York: Columbia University Press, 2015.

E. Thompson, "Dreamless Sleep, the Embodied Mind, and Consciousness—The Relevance of a Classical Indian Debate to Cognitive Science." In *Open Mind,* edited by T. Metzinger and J. M. Windt, 37(T). Frankfurt am Main: Open Mind, 2015.

G. Tononi and Gerald M. Edelman, "Consciousness and Complexity." *Science* 282, no. 5395 (December 4, 1998): 1846–51.

G. Tononi, "Consciousness as Integrated Information: A Provisional Manifesto." *The Biological Bulletin* 215, no. 3 (December 2008): 216–42.

G. Tucci, "The Rātnāvali of Nāgārjuna." *The Journal of* the Royal Asiatic Society of Great Britain and Ireland (1934): 307–25.

G. Tucci, "The Rātnāvali of Nāgārjuna." *The Journal of* the Royal Asiatic Society of Great Britain and Ireland (1936): 237–435.

G. Tucci, *Teoria e pratica del mandala*. Rome: Astrolabio, 1949.

Tzongkapha, *The Six Yogas of Naropa: Tsongkhapa's commentary entitled A Book of Three Inspirations,* ed. and trans. G. H. Mullin. New York: Snow Lion Publications, 1996.

Tsongkhapa, *The Great Treatise on the Stages of the Path to Enlightenment,* ed. J. Cutler, G. Newland. New York: Snow Lion Publications, 2002.

Upaniṣad, ed. Raphael. Milan: Bompiani, 2010.

A. Van Lysebeth in *Pranayama: La dynamique du soufflé*. Paris: Flammarion, 1971.

A. Van Lysebeth, *Tantra. El culto de lo femenino*. Barcelona: Urano, 1990.

F. Varela, E. Thompson, E. Rosch, *The Embodied Mind: Cognitive Science and Human Experience*. Cambridge, MA: MIT Press, 1993.

F. J. Varela, "Neurophenomenology. A Methodological Remedy for the Hard Problem." *Journal of Consciousness Studies* 3, no. 4 (1996).

F. J. Varela, *Ethical Know-how*. Stanford: Stanford University Press, 1999.

F. J. Varela, "The Specious Present: A Neurophenomenology of Time Consciousness." In *Naturalizing Phenomenology: Issues in Contemporary Phenomenology and Cognitive Science*, edited by J. Petitot, F. J. Varela, J.-M. Roy, B. Pachoud. Stanford: Stanford University Press, 1997.

Vasgupta, *Śivasūtra* of Vasgupta, edited by R. Torella. Milan: Adelphi, 2013.

C. Villemure et al., "Insular Cortex Mediates Increased Pain Tolerance in Yoga Practitioners." *Cereb Cortex* October 24, no. 10 (2014).

V. A. Wallace, ed., *The Kālacakra Tantra. The Chapter on Sadhana. Together with the Vimalaprabha commentary*, translated by V. A. Wallace. Columbia University's Center for Buddhist Studies, 2010.

A. Wayman, *Analysis of the Śrāvakabhūmi Manuscript*. Berkeley: University of California Press, 1961.

J. Westerhoff, ed., *The Dispeller of Disputes. Nāgārjuna's Vigrahavyāvartanī*, translated by J. Westerhoff. Oxford: Oxford University Press, 2010.

J. Westerhoff, "Nāgārjuna's Catuṣkoṭi." *Journal of Indian Philosophy* (2006) 34, 367–95.

I. Whicher, "Nirodha, Yoga Praxis and the Transformation of the Mind." *Journal of Indian Philosophy* 25 (1997).

K. Wilber, *No Boundary*. Boston: Shambala, 2001.

L. Wittgenstein, *Tractatus Logico-Philosophicus*, translated by D. F. Pears and B. F. McGuinness. London: Routledge, 2001.

W. Woodward, *Gestalt Psychology*, in Vol. 7., *Encyclopedia of Philosophy and the Social Sciences*, ed. B. Kaldis, 383–87. Los Angeles: SAGE, 2013.

Yoga Yājñavalkya, edited by J. Ely, translated by A. G. Mohan. Madras: Ganesh & Co., 2013.

Lama Yeshe, *The Bliss of the Inner Fire. Heart Practice of the Six Yogas of Naropa*. Somerville, MA: Wisdom Publications, 1998.

Lama Yeshe, *La beatitudine del fuoco interiore*. Pomaia: Chiara Luce edizioni, 2003.

Yogabīja, edited by Rām Lāl Śrīvāstav. Gorakhpur: Śrī Gorakhnāth Mandir, 1982.

A. Zaccaro et al., "How Breath-Control Can Change Your Life: A Systematic Review on Psycho-Physiological Correlates of Slow Breathing." *Frontiers in Human Neuroscience* 12 (September 7, 2018): 353.

A. Zaccaro, A. Riehl, A. Piarulli, G. Alfì, B. Neri, D. Menicucci, and A. Gemignani, "The Consciousness State of Traditional Nidrâ Yoga/ Modern Yoga Nidra: Phenomenological Characterization and Preliminary Insights from an EEG Study." *International Journal of Yoga Therapy* 31, no. 1 (January 1, 2021), article 14.

Index

abhyāsa (reiteration), 63, 124, 143, 197n136
Agni, 51–52, 57, 107, 139, 190n46, 190n47, 191n52
appearing (as such), 1, 7, 10, 18, 23, 43–44, 111, 114, 127–128, 140, 158, 165, 187n41, 215n87, 227n126
āsana, 6, 58, 107–108, 111, 117–120, 123–125, 129–132, 134, 137, 193n90, 196n121, 205n96, 214n50, 216n99, 217n106, 217n113, 217n119
Ātman, 3, 18, 49–50, 65–66, 169n3, 221n56
attention, 24, 31, 32, 40, 53, 55, 56, 92, 95, 111, 117–118, 133, 134, 135, 138, 143–145, 151, 152, 154–156, 160, 165
avidyā, 45, 49, 59, 192n75
awareness, 13, 16, 18, 33, 34, 38, 72–73, 126, 131, 136, 152, 153, 158, 166, 167, 170n3, 172n23, 203n72, 248

background, 2, 31–32, 34, 38, 40, 43, 64, 118, 125, 127, 130, 138–139, 145, 149, 153–154, 166, 181n53, 219n11, 222n2
bandha, 45, 108, 138, 213n46
bardo, 75, 203n71, 203n73, 205n105
Being, 5, 16, 18, 19, 29, 35, 37–40, 43–44, 49, 54, 63, 68, 70–72, 74, 111, 125, 127, 136, 143, 153, 161, 162, 164, 177n14, 185n7, 185n14, 186n16, 187n41, 200n36, 208n14, 218n9, 227n126
Bitbol, Michel, 46, 103, 174n40, 196n124, 207n13, 226n100, 227n126
Block, Ned, 13, 170n6
bodhicitta, 79–81, 109, 205n96
bodily dimension, 76, 102, 147, 167
body-as-object, 6, 81, 114, 116, 203n77
Brahman, 3, 47, 49, 50, 53, 65, 76, 169n3, 191n52, 217n117
Buddha, 66, 68, 70, 72–73, 75, 79, 140, 147, 197n132, 199n11, 200n18, 204n87, 206n129
Buddhism: Vajrayāna, 73, 99, 105, 109, 205n96; Mahāyāna, 6, 58, 66, 200n26, 201n42, 201n48

cakra, 107–108, 111, 136, 204n87, 213n49, 221n49
Chalmers, David, 11, 13, 170n5, 171n11, 173n23, 174n41

clear light, 75–76, 81, 82, 202n64, 203n72, 205n105, *See also* clear-light consciousness
cognition, 19, 25, 60, 90, 153
cognitive function, 9, 13, 15, 91, 170n1
cognitive science, 9, 90–92, 210n51
consciousness: a-subjective, 7–10; background, 5, 27, 33, 46, 49, 61, 72, 125, 136, 182n120; clear-light, 6, 79, 81; *continuum* of, 61, 127; embodied, 115, 135; horizon, 5, 2, 21, 27, 31, 33, 34, 35, 37, 38, 72, 125, 127, 129, 136, 166; perceptual, 153; transcendental, 16, 49, 53, 61, 63, 64, 72, 73, 75, 79, 88, 111, 115, 124, 125, 158, 163, 181n71

Dalai Lama, 4, 75, 78, 89, 201n41
David-Néel, Alexandra, 77, 82, 103
dependent arising (*pratītya-samutpāda*), 66–67, 69, 71, 144, 163
Descartes (Cartesian), 16, 29, 39, 90, 96, 126, 128, 182n73
dharma, 56, 58, 66, 68, 73, 100, 201n42, 205n105, 210n3
doing, 7, 43, 53–55, 62, 124–125, 165, 250
dreamless sleep, 13, 14, 47, 172n31

effort, 6, 19, 43, 51, 63–64, 93, 119, 123–125, 132, 141, 155, 163, 218n4, 250
Ego, 24, 59, 79, 81, 129, 164, *See also*, I; cogito, 182n86; pure, 182n75; reduced, 31, 164; transcendental, 93, 128, 219n13
Eliade, Mircea, 4, 57, 61, 190n44, 196n121
embodiment, 5, 12, 18, 19, 73, 89, 116, 153, 167, 249
embodied experience, 2, 74, 88–89, 148, 158, 166
emptiness (*śūnyatā*), 6, 64–66, 69–72, 73, 78–79, 80–81, 83, 85–86, 96, 110, 111, 114, 144, 162, 200n36, 201n42, 204n90, 206n129
enaction, 6, 90, 147
époche, 6, 21, 27–30, 46, 59, 61–63, 125, 130, 131, 138, 147, 179–180n46, 180n47, 181–182n71, 226n100
existence, inherent, 6, 66, 69, 79, 96, 114

flesh (*Chair*), 19, 152, 156, 161–163, 227n113, 227n126
Four Noble Truths, 45, 69, 70, 188n3

Gauḍapāda, 48, 77, 100, 198n3
Gestalt, 5, 25 32, 40, 64, 125, 138, 145, 155, 166, 178n28, 178n29, 183n98, 183n101, 222n16

haṭha yoga, 46, 65, 79, 81, 99–101, 104–105, 110–111, 120, 131, 157, 169n5, 188n4, 206n124, 212n25, 2016n104, 217n112, 225n88
Haṭhayogapradīpikā, 6, 105–106, 108–109, 111, 118, 131, 137, 143, 212n29, 221n52
Heidegger, Martin, 5, 6, 16, 18, 35, 37–43, 46, 53, 68, 70–71, 87–88, 111, 118, 125, 127, 140, 143, 153, 156, 158, 168, 176, 185n7, 200n30, 208n20, 219n11
horizon, vii, 2, 5, 27, 32–34, 39, 40, 43–44, 61, 93, 115, 118, 125–128, 130, 138, 145, 149, 154, 179n39, 208n23, 215n80, 226n24

Husserl, Edmund, 2, 3, 5, 16–17, 21–35, 37–38, 40, 43, 46, 49, 59, 61–64, 67, 72, 77, 81, 88, 92, 93–95, 96, 102, 111, 113–118, 125, 126–128, 133, 135, 143, 145, 147–148, 158, 164, 174n44, 177n5, 177n6, 178n32, 182n73, 182n86, 185n11, 188n42, 203n77, 211n4, 218n11, 221n55, 228n131

I (*See also* Ego): empirical, 30; -ness, 9, 147; psychological, 5, 30, 93, 30; reduced, 93; transcendental, 30
intentionality, 5, 17, 26, 62, 175n44, 227n126
inversion (posture), 119–120, 134, 109

James, William, 10, 94, 95, 170n2

Kālacakra, 6, 75, 79–80, 82–83, 105, 203n75, 204n87, 205n96

letting be (happen), 5, 7, 39–41, 44, 53, 55, 62, 123–125, 131, 156, 165, 219n11, 250
lived-body, 6, 18, 114–116, 128, 133, 135, 148, 161, 203n77, 215n87

Madyamaka, 66, 68–69, 223n23
Marpa, 75, 79, 201n41, 203n74, 205n96
meditation, 2, 14, 22, 58, 60, 64, 81, 82, 152, 166–167, 190n42, 193n92, 196n119, 196n124, 203n72, 203n75, 224n63, 224n643
Merleau-Ponty, Maurice, 7, 16, 18, 19, 86–87, 89–90, 115, 128, 135, 141, 143–164, 183n98, 207n6, 215n79, 219n11, 227n126
Metzinger, Thomas, 12, 129, 26n92, 220n29
Milarepa, 6, 72–75, 79, 201n41, 201n46, 203n74
mindfulness, 152–153, 224n68, 224n69
mudrā, 80–81, 99, 108–109, 111, 205n96, 213n49

nāḍī, 105, 107–108, 212n33, 213n34, 213n46, 221n49
Nāgārjuna, 6, 65–73, 79, 83, 85, 97, 144, 161, 200n18, 201n48
Nāropā, 75, 79–82, 201n41, 203n74, 204n91
nāth, 105, 106, 110, 114, 119, 21n25, 212n26, 217n117, 225n88
natural attitude, 1, 18, 27, 49, 60–62, 68, 80, 93, 95, 99, 113, 125, 130, 137, 138–139, 152, 159
neurophenomenology, 94, 165
nirodha, 15, 59–62, 124, 130, 137, 195n110, 197n135, 197n136, 220n32
nirvāṇa, 72, 73, 192n75

Om, *See* A-U-M, 47–49
out-of-body experience, 115–116

Padmasambhava, 75, 202n68
Patañjali, 15, 46, 56–64, 72–73, 78, 79, 104–105, 110–111, 118, 123–124, 132, 137, 140, 188n3, 188n5, 193n90, 194n103, 195n116, 196n117, 205n96, 216n99, 219n14, 220n32, 221n56
Patočka, Jan, 7, 18, 27, 31, 127–128, 179n42, 182n71

perception, 1, 7, 13, 19, 23–26, 29, 31, 60, 62, 93, 100, 113, 116–117, 133, 135, 140, 145–150, 154, 158–160, 178n21, 179n37, 196n118, 196n119
phenomenology, asubjective, 127, 128, 179n42, 183n91, 220n22
phenomenon, 41, 44, 46, 74, 78, 85, 92, 94, 95, 100, 113, 127, 160, 197n127
Prajāpati, 53, 104, 157, 190n41
prajñā, 14, 47, 48, 49, 64, 72, 83, 189n12, 196n117, 204n95
prāṇa (vital energy), 15, 76, 105–108, 111, 138, 145, 176n59, 213n37, 221n49
prāṇāyāma, 14, 58, 111, 119, 132, 137, 144, 159, 196n121, 204n96, 213n41
prereflective, 1, 10, 11, 114, 126, 143, 146, 150
purification, 1, 5, 6, 21, 50, 56, 58–59, 64, 81, 104–105, 108, 125, 131, 132, 140, 219n11

reduction, 28–29, 33, 37, 43–44, 53, 88, 94, 95, 100, 160, 175n44, 181n53, 182n71, 182n73, 189n10, 226n100
release, 6, 19, 41, 78, 124, 133–134, 136, 187n32, 218n3, 218n9
releasement (*Gelassenheit*), 37, 40, 43, 156, 193n89, 194n98

samādhi (absorption), 17, 58–60, 64, 72–74, 104, 110–111, 123, 125, 174n44, 194n103, 196n117, 196n119, 220n31, 220n32
saṃsāra, 72–73, 80
Śankara, 48, 59, 62, 118, 189n26, 197n132, 216n100
seer, 18, 28, 49, 61–64, 110, 124, 131, 162, 176, 189n26, 192n75, 197n126, 197n130, 197n135
sensation, 116, 117, 133–134, 136, 148, 149, 154–155, 158–159, 190n44, 204n90
senses, 56, 58, 73–76, 77–78, 100–102, 116, 154, 222n19
sensory, 12, 19, 73, 77, 78, 100, 101, 132, 150, 153, 164, 166, 184n 106, 248
siddhi, 110–111, 226n98
Śivaism, 73, 76, 219n13
structural coupling, 16, 89–90, 111
subtle physiology, 105, 111–113, 133, 136, 144

tantra, 58, 73–76, 81, 85, 110, 126, 147–148, 151, 156, 203n75, 205n96, 223n37, 219n13
tapas, 50–53, 55, 57–59, 78, 100, 102–104, 110, 125, 188n4, 190n42, 190n44, 191n52, 193n89, 194n98, 213n43, 213n47, 218n9, 219n11
transcendent, 24–25, 27, 30, 31, 59, 64, 67, 86, 87, 95, 159, 195n111
transcendent object, 24–25, 59, 64, 67, 86–87, 95, 159
transcendental, 5, 26, 29, 30, 31, 35, 43, 49, 63, 64, 75, 93, 96, 115, 116, 128, 143, 146, 148, 153, 160, 175n44, 177n6, 181n71, 182n73, 184n106, n120, 215n87
Thompson, Evan, 2, 16, 172n31, 215n92
touch, 78, 111, 116–118, 148, 150, 154–156, 164, 226n91
Turīya, 48, 111, 140, 162
Tzong Khapa, 6, 80–82, 96, 205n102, 205n117

Upaniṣad, 14–15, 18, 46–47, 49–50, 55–56, 65, 76–77, 100, 106, 138, 162, 172n30, 192n75

Varela, Francisco, 16, 89–96, 111, 130, 136, 143, 146, 153, 165, 175n47, 218n11, 209n37
Veda-s, 46–47, 50–51, 53, 55, 57, 200n26
Vedanta, 49, 65, 76, 105, 175n45, 189n26, 192n75, 193n86, 196n117, 197n32; *advaita*, 48, 49, 62, 66, 114, 197n132
Vijñānabhairava Tantra, 74–76, 151
Vyāsa, 59, 118, 124, 168, 188n3, 216n100

Yoga: *aṣṭāṅga*, 58, 193n87, 205n96; *kriyā*, 57–59, 105; nidrā 48; *rāja*, 57, 105, 111, 131
Yogācāra, 58, 104, 194n94, 194n94, 195n109, 195n116
Yogasūtra, 5, 46, 58–65, 113–114, 118, 124, 173n38, 193n87, 194n93, 198n2, 221n56, 226n98

About the Author

Figure A.1. Giulia Moiraghi. Source: Photo by the author.

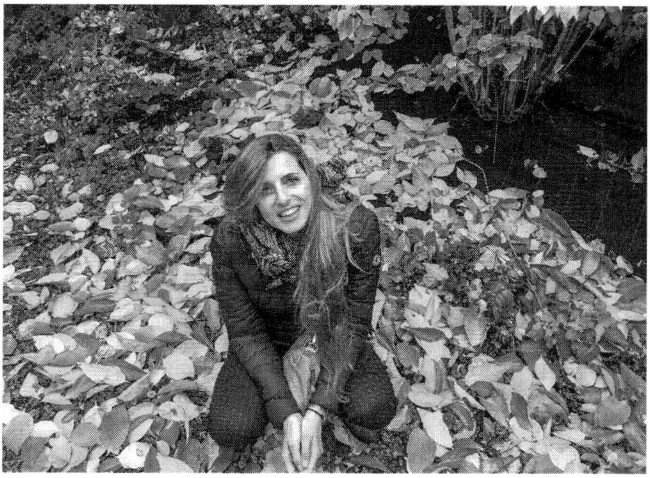

Giulia Moiraghi holds a PhD in philosophy and has been a lifelong dedicated yoga practitioner. After completing her master's degree in contemporary aesthetics at the University of Milan with the highest honors, she pursued her PhD in philosophy at the University of Verona. She authored *In cammino verso la cosa. Heidegger dall'estetica all'ontologia* (*On the Way to the Thing: Heidegger from Aesthetics to Ontology*), and has written several essays on philosophical subjects. On yoga and meditation, she has penned *Cura e Ardore. Il rigore e la passione della pratica yoga* (*Care and Ardor. The rigor and passion*

of yoga practice) and *"La Semplicità"* (The Simplicity)). Giulia is a certified yoga teacher and a member of Y.A.N.I. (National Association of Yoga Teachers), having taught yoga and meditation since 2013. She has developed a phenomenological approach to yoga (Fenomeno Yoga) to bridge Eastern contemplative practices with Western phenomenological research.

She lectures in the Master's Program in Neuroscience, Mindfulness and Contemplative Practices, the International Summer School on Consciousness and Cognition, where she also serves as vice-director, and in the Advanced Course on End-of-Life care: States of Consciousness, Old Traditions and New Therapies at the University of Pisa.

www.fenomenoyoga.it
giuliamoiraghi@yahoo.it

But if you want to know how it really went, here is a longer version:

It all started after years of intense study at university, when I realized that my awareness of the sensory realm was growing weaker and that this dimension needed to be recovered. I felt the urge to reconnect with my body and with lived experience. I began to feel it physically. My health was deteriorating, and after a long period of stomach pain, doctors diagnosed me with celiac disease. That meant saying goodbye to my beloved pastries and many other delicious foods. How was I going to cope with that? As I delved deeper into philosophy, exploring the themes that seemed to matter the most and as I wrote articles and essays, I realized my body did not appreciate this excessive mental pondering and rumination. Even my eyesight was fading, with a rapid loss of diopters. Hours spent sitting hunched over a desk, buried in books, and staring at a computer had also completely disrupted my breathing rhythm, which resulted in blocks when trying to breathe. I couldn't continue like that any longer.

The decision that would directly lead to the life change that awaited me was the humble decision to resume practicing yoga. My fascination with yoga was hardly new; it originated during the long journeys I took to India with my parents as a child. It is thanks to them that I had the opportunity to taste the magic and sacredness of India at such a young age. Among the many experiences I had there, which have not all been a bed of roses, I encountered the practice of yoga. My father was an engaged practitioner for many years, and it was with him, almost playfully, that I began to explore the discipline.

After a somewhat restless childhood, I was relieved to embark on a more stable and disciplined path of life and study, finally in Italy again! Perhaps it was this need for normality that led me, later on, during my university years to choose Western philosophy over Eastern philosophy. I not only needed to rediscover my roots, but I also felt compelled to delve deeply into them.

Although an interest in the Eastern world was still there, my yoga practice at that time became less frequent and sometimes even went dormant for long periods, especially during the "hard study" years. As often happens, I probably needed to take a step back to move forward. The need to embark in research on the body, and its related conscious dimensions surfaced only after having experienced how it felt to go entirely away from it, practically forgetting it.

To start devoting myself to this new path of embodiment, I felt I could no longer settle for the mere declarations of intent typical of many contemporary phenomenologists. Talking about the body was fine; I had written about it too. But merely theorizing or speculating about it was not enough. It was an excellent starting point, but it wasn't transformative. I needed more. I needed to experience it. I had to try, or at least begin to try, to transform my analytical and logocentric mind. I knew that this would be more than just a philosophical interest; it would be a lifelong endeavor.

I decided then to temporarily abandon the realm of theoretical knowledge in order, one might say, to purify, so that I could perhaps catch a glimpse of a broader and more comprehensive dimension. There was a lot at stake, but there was no alternative; that was the only choice for me.

It wasn't just my health that led me in this direction; it was the philosophical research I had pursued that guided me there. Phenomenology was leading me to do this.

That is how I threw myself into the practice with my whole being. I journeyed into a wild and uncharted territory. I didn't miss a single class, and at home, I cherished every available moment to explore and savor the joy of a reawakening body and the unknown conscious dimensions that were surfacing.

Over the years, I found myself enrolled in an official three-year yoga academy. Although I initially had no intention of becoming a yoga teacher and entered the academy more as an interpreter than a student, I emerged after three years and thousands of hours of practice with a certification.

In the ensuing years, the classes I taught grew, and I gradually shifted to full-time teaching, in which together with postures and breathwork and techniques of concentration, I wanted to offer my students some philosophical insights that had ripened through the years of philosophical inquiry and had rooted themselves during the years of practice.

In shifting to a deeper layer of teaching I didn't want to burden the practice with exotic metaphysical concepts, as is often done, especially considering the fact that I was teaching Westerners. I wanted to give them the chance to seriously enter experience without having to categorize it through labels. Rather than adding theory to people's minds, I wanted first of all to allow them to remove all kinds of precomprehensions or expectations in order to meet experience anew. Because of its antidogmatic and anti-ideological connotations, I found phenomenology an incredibly useful tool for conveying some elements that are foundational in yoga, such as the ability to be with what is after having performed the suspensive effort. From this realization, the two-phase method I started to call "doing" and "letting happen" developed.

Later on, I resumed my former philosophical activity of studying, writing, and lecturing, juggling it alongside practice and teaching, both online and in presence. The rest, as they say, is (recent) history: inquiring and experimenting on the mat and the cushion and bringing some of the discoveries I come across into the lectures I deliver, with the hope that yogic practices will eventually find their place in the academic domain and contribute to current research, especially on the theme of consciousness.

Figure A.2. My father and me near Mussoorie in Uttarakhand, India. *Source:* Photo by the author.

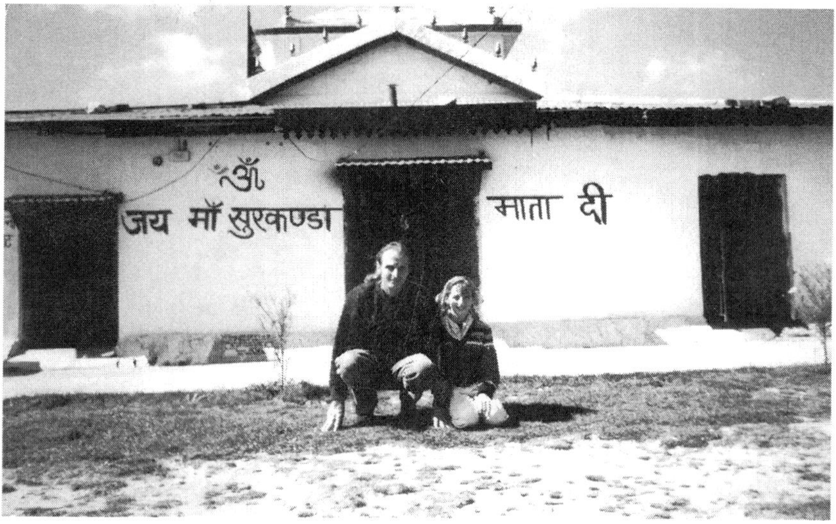

Figure A.3. My father and me practicing in Marina di Grosseto, Italy. *Source:* Photo by the author.

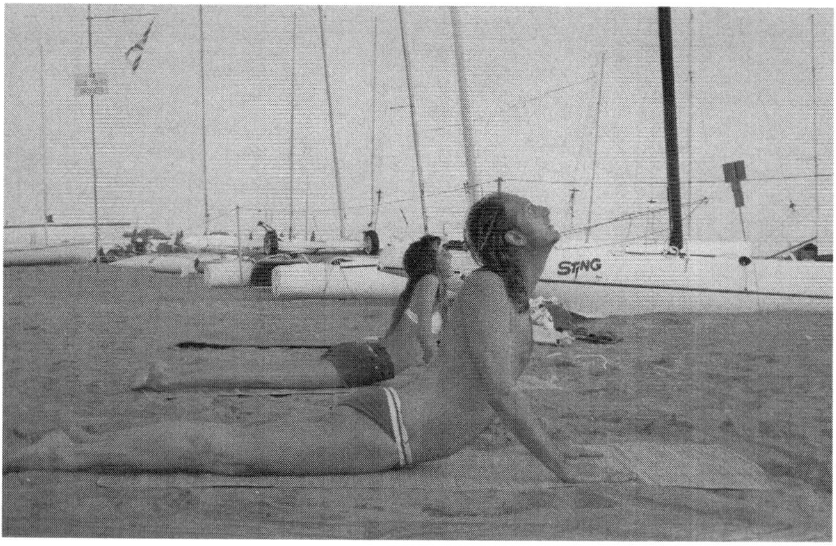